Manual of Childhood Infections

for the British Paediatric Association

Manual of Childhood Infections

E Graham Davies MA FRCP *Consultant and Senior Lecturer in Child Health, St George's Hospital Medical School, London, UK*

David A C Elliman FRCP DCH BA(Open) *Consultant in Community Child Health, St George's Healthcare NHS Trust, London, UK*

C Anthony Hart MB BS PhD FRCPath *Professor and Honorary Consultant in Medical Microbiology, University of Liverpool, Liverpool, UK*

Angus Nicoll MRCP (Paediatrics) *Consultant Epidemiologist, Public Health Laboratory Service, Communicable Disease Surveillance Centre, and Honorary Senior Lecturer, University of London, London, UK*

Peter T Rudd MD FRCP *Consultant Paediatrician, Royal United Hospital Trust, Bath, and Senior Lecturer, University of Bath, Bath, UK*

For the **British Paediatric Association**

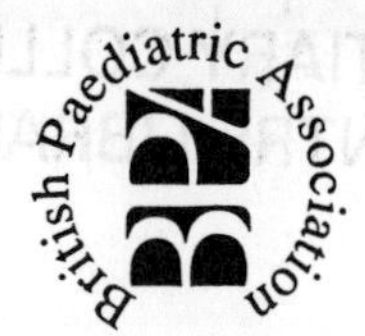

W B SAUNDERS COMPANY LTD
LONDON PHILADELPHIA TORONTO SYDNEY TOKYO

W.B. Saunders Company Limited
24–28 Oval Road
London NW1 7DX, UK

The Curtis Center
Independence Square West
Philadelphia, PA 19106-3399, USA

55 Horner Avenue
Toronto, Ontario M8Z 4X6, Canada

Harcourt Brace & Company
(Australia) Pty Ltd
30–52 Smidmore Street
Marrickville, NSW 2204, Australia

Harcourt Brace Japan
Ichibancho Central Building
22-1 Ichibancho
Chiyoda-ku, Tokyo 102, Japan

A catalogue record for this book is available from the British Library

ISBN 0–7020–1832–5

This book is printed on acid-free paper

Typeset by P & R Typesetters Ltd
Printed and bound in Great Britain by The Bath Press, Avon

CONTENTS

Notice viii

Additional Contributors ix

Acknowledgements xi

Foreword xiii

Introduction xv

Part One – General

1 Congenital Infection 3
2 Neonatal Infection 7
3 The Child with an Upper Respiratory Tract Infection 22
4 The Child with a Lower Respiratory Tract Infection 26
5 The Child with a Bone or Joint Infection 34
6 The Child with Diarrhoea and Vomiting 36
7 Urinary Tract Infections in Children 43
8 Management of Suspected Sexually Transmitted Diseases in Prepubertal Children 47
9 The Child with a Cardiac Infection 51
10 The Child with Bacterial Meningitis 57
11 The Child with Acute Encephalitis 60
12 The Child with Septic Shock 63
13 The Child with Toxic Shock Syndrome 67
14 The Child with a Rash 68
15 The Child with a Pyrexia of Unknown Origin 74
16 The Child with Suspected Immunodeficiency 81
17 Management of the Immunocompromised Child with Infection 89
18 Management of the Child with Systemic Fungal Infection 95
19 The Child with HIV Infection 101
20 Preparation for Travel Abroad 109
21 Management of the Child with an Infection Contracted Abroad 115
22 Refugees and Internationally Adopted Children 122
23 Zoonoses 124
24 Laboratory Diagnosis of Infection 135
25 The Use of Antibiotics 152
26 Infection Control in the Hospital 162
27 Infection Control in the Community 168

Part Two – Specific Infections

28 Amoebiasis 176
29 Arboviruses 177
30 *Ascaris* (Roundworm) 177
31 Aspergillosis 178
32 Botulism (Food-borne and Infant Botulism) 179

33 Brucellosis 182
34 *Campylobacter* Infection 183
35 Candidiasis (Thrush, Moniliasis) 184
36 Cat-Scratch Disease 185
37 Chickenpox and Herpes Zoster (Varicella-Zoster) 185
38 *Chlamydia pneumoniae* Infection 188
39 *Chlamydia psittaci* Infection 189
40 *Chlamydia trachomatis* Infection 190
41 Cholera 191
42 Conjunctivitis 193
43 Cryptosporidiosis 194
44 Cytomegalovirus Infection 195
45 Dermatophytoses: Tinea Capitis, Corporis, Pedis and Unguium 197
46 Diphtheria 199
47 Enterovirus Infection 202
48 *Escherichia coli* Diarrhoea 204
49 Giardiasis 207
50 Gonococcal Infection 209
51 Haemolytic Uraemic Syndrome 210
52 *Haemophilus influenzae* Infection 213
53 Hand, Foot and Mouth Disease 216
54 *Helicobacter pylori* Infection 217
55 Hepatitis A 219
56 Hepatitis B 222
57 Hepatitis C 229
58 Hepatitis E 230
59 Herpes Infections 231
60 Infectious Mononucleosis (Glandular Fever) 234
61 Influenza 235
62 Invasive Helminthiasis causing Multisystem Disease (Cysticercosis, Gnathostomiasis, Hydatid Disease, Schistosomiasis, Strongyloidiasis, Trichinosis) 237
63 Kawasaki Disease 241
64 Legionnaires' Disease 243
65 Leishmaniasis: Visceral (Kala-azar) and Cutaneous Leishmaniasis 244
66 Listeriosis 245
67 Lyme Disease 247
68 Malaria 248
69 Measles 253
70 Meningococcal Disease 257
71 Mumps 266
72 Mycobacterial Infection (Atypical) 268
73 *Mycoplasma* Infections 269
74 Nits and Head Lice 271
75 Parvovirus Infection: Fifth Disease (Erythema Infectiosum or Slapped Cheek Disease) 272
76 Pertussis (Whooping Cough) 273
77 Plague 276

78 *Pneumocytsis carinii* Pneumonia 277
79 Poliomyelitis 279
80 Poxvirus Infection (Including Molluscum Contagiosum) 281
81 Prion Disease (Spongiform Encephalopathies) 283
82 Rabies 284
83 Respiratory Syncytial Virus Infection 287
84 Roseola Infantum, Exanthema Subitum or Sixth Disease (human herpesvirus 6/7 Infection) 288
85 Rotavirus and other Viral Enteropathogens 288
86 Rubella 293
87 Salmonellosis 296
88 Scabies 298
89 Shigellosis 298
90 Staphylococcal Infections 300
91 Streptococcal Infections 302
92 Syphilis (Congenital and Acquired) and Non-venereal Treponematoses 303
93 Tetanus 306
94 Threadworms 307
95 Toxocariasis 308
96 Toxoplasmosis 309
97 Tuberculosis 311
98 Typhoid and Paratyphoid Fevers 319
99 Typhus 320
100 Viral Haemorrhagic Fevers 321
101 Warts and Verrucae 327
102 Yellow Fever 328
103 Yersiniosis 329

Appendices

I Mortality and Morbidity from Infectious Disease in the UK 330
II Neonatal Antibiotic Dosages 340
III Antimicrobials for the Infant and Child (excluding Neonates) 348
IV Notifiable Diseases 1995 362
V Exclusion Periods 364
VI Contraindications to Immunization 374
VII Immunization of the Child with a Potentially Impaired Immune Response 378
VIII Further Reading 383

Index 385

NOTICE

Whilst every effort has been made, both by the authors and the publishers of this work, to ensure that, at press, treatments and drug dosages comply with accepted standards, regional guidelines may vary, drug regimens are continually being revised in the light of new research, and the possibility of human error cannot be eliminated. Therefore, in clinical situations readers are advised to exercise their judgement, and consider information from all sources available. In particular, the manufacturer's recommended does should be checked before prescribing or administering any drug.

BRITISH PAEDIATRIC ASSOCIATION SURVEILLANCE UNIT

Certain conditions should be reported to the BPASU by consultant paediatricians in the UK and Eire. Those currently reportable (1995/6) are highlighted in Part One and are listed below. Normally reports are made through ticking the BPA orange card which is sent to all consultant paediatricians every month. If consultants do not receive these, if they are not certain if a particular case has been reported or they wish further details of the BPASU sceme they should contact the BPASU Scientific Coordinator BPA, 5, St Andrews Place, London NW1 4LB. Tel: 0171-935-1866, Fax: 0171-224-2038. All reporting is voluntary and confidential. The BPASU is part of the British Paediatric Association Research Unit and is the result of a collaboration between the BPA, the Public Health Laboratory Services, the Institute of Child Health, London and other interested bodies. Reference: Lynn R, Hall SM. The British Paediatric Surveillance Unit: activities and developments in 1990 and 1991: CDR 1992; 2: R145–8.

Currently reportable infections (1995/6):
AIDS and HIV in Children, Congenital Rubella, Congenital Syphilis, Invasive Haemophilus Influenzae Infection, Sub-acute sclerosing panencephalitis.

ADDITIONAL CONTRIBUTORS

Dr Barbara Bannister MSc MB BS FRCP
Consultant Physician
Coppetts Wood Hospital, London

Dr Nicola Barrett PhD CBiol MIBIOL
Principal Scientist (Epidemiology)
Communicable Disease Surveillance Centre, Colindale, London

Dr Robert Booy MB BS (Hons) FRACP
Senior Registrar
St Mary's Hospital, London

Dr Gary Brook MD MRCP
Registrar
Coppetts Wood Hospital, London

Dr Andrew James Cant MD FRCP Lond MRCP
Consultant Paediatrician (Immunology and Infectious Diseases)
Newcastle General Hospital
Newcastle upon Tyne

Dr JBS Coulter MD FRCP
Senior Lecturer in Tropical Paediatrics and Honorary Consultant Paediatrician
Liverpool School of Tropical Medicine and Royal Liverpool Children's Hospital, Alder Hey, Liverpool

Dr Rami Dhillon BMED Sci BM BS MRCP
Registrar in Cardiology
Cardiothoracic Unit
Great Ormond Street Hospital for Children, London

Professor Brendan Drumm MD
Professor of Paediatrics & Consultant Paediatric Gastroenterologist
University College, Dublin and The Children's Research Centre, Dublin

Dr Adam Finn PhD BM BCh MRCP
Senior Lecturer in Immunology and Infectious Disease
Children's Hospital NHS Trust, Sheffield

Dr Diana M Gibb MD MRCP
Senior Lecturer in Infectious Diseases and Honorary Consultant Paediatrician
Institute of Child Health, London

Dr Lyda Jadresic MD MRCP
Consultant Paediatrician
Gloucestershire Royal Hospital NHS Trust, Gloucester

Dr James Y Paton MD MRCP
Senior Lecturer in Paediatric Respiratory Disease
Royal Hospital for Sick Children, Glasgow

Professor Tom Rogers MA MRCPath FRCP
Professor in Infectious Disease and Bacteriology
Hammersmith Hospital, London

Dr Michael Sharland MD MRCP
Consultant in Paediatric Infectious Disease
St George's Hospital, London

Dr Alistair Thomson MD D RCOG, DCH, FRCP
Consultant Paediatrician
Mid-Cheshire Hospitals NHS Trust, Crewe

Dr E Jane Tizard MB BS MRCP
Senior Lecturer in Child Health and Honorary Consultant in Paediatrics and Paediatric Pathology
Southmead Hospital, Bristol

Dr JC Tyrrell DM DCH MRCP
Consultant Paediatrician
Royal United Hospital Trust
Bath

Dr Jenny Welch MB BS
Clinical Research Fellow
Sheffield Children's Hospital
NHS Trust, Sheffield

ACKNOWLEDGEMENTS

The Editors also wish to acknowledge the following persons and institutions who made invaluable contributions to the book in various ways:

Miss Susan Ashbrook
Miss Annabel Attridge
Dr Norman Begg
Miss Carol Boutin
Dr Moyra Brett
Dr Sandy Calvert
Professor Alex Campbell
Ms Bernadette Carroll
Mrs Penny Cooper
Mr Ian Costello
Mr Paul Dunn
Miss Lisa Forsyth
Dr Richard Gilbert
Dr Rob George
Dr Tim Healing
Dr Julia Heptonstall
Mrs Carol Joseph
Dr Gil Lea
Dr Marion McEvoy
Dr Jim McLaughlan
Dr Marion Miles
Dr Elizabeth Miller
Dr Elizabeth Mitchell
Dr Philip Mortimer
Miss Lisa Newton
Dr Mary Ramsay
Dr Dan Reid
Mrs Jill Rolfe
Dr David Salisbury
Dr Rosalind Stanwell-Smith
Dr Mark Taylor
Dr Patrick Wall
Dr Jane Watkeys
Mrs Joan Waters
Dr John Watson
Ms Joanne White

Central Public Health Laboratory, London
Department of Health, London
Department of Health & Social Services, Northern Ireland
General Register Office for Scotland
Information and Statistics Division, Common Services Agency, Scotland
Office of Population Censuses and Surveys
Public Health Laboratory Service Communicable Disease Surveillance Centre
Public Health Laboratory Service Malaria Reference Laboratory, London
Scottish Centre for Infection and Environmental Health

FOREWORD

During the past few decades, application of the basic principles of good public health medicine and the widespread acceptance of immunization have led to some outstanding successes in the control of childhood infectious disease. The elimination of poliomyelitis in the UK (except for the rare vaccine-related case), the greatly reduced infection rates from tuberculosis, measles, rubella, pertussis and mumps, and the virtual disappearance from paediatric wards of eppiglottitis and meningitis due to *Haemophilus influenzae* type b are notable examples of the benefits of a comprehensive national programme.

However, any complacency that might exist about infection and its control should have been severely shaken by some recent events—outbreaks of diphtheria in Russia, the resurgence of tuberculosis worldwide, and in the UK the urgent need to carry out a mass immunization programme in schools to forestall a predicted epidemic of measles. There is the still unsolved problem of human immunodeficiency virus (HIV) infection with its growing impact on children. The rapid growth of air travel, relaxed immigration controls and emerging infections appearing worldwide* mean that we must be as aware of the epidemiology of infection in other countries as we are of events in our own 'back yard'.

This authoritative but concise and 'reader friendly' text on infections in childhood is to be warmly welcomed. With the imprimatur of the British Paediatric Association, it has been written by a group who are active in paediatric infectious disease, microbiology, immunization and public health. It is a completely new book and a worthy successor to the *BPA Manual of Infections and Immunisations in Children*. The book is aimed primarily at paediatricians and public health doctors to whom it gives practical and detailed advice on the management of all the important infections of childhood likely to be encountered in the UK and abroad. There is less emphasis on immunization, not because of any lessening of its importance, but because it is so comprehensively covered every 2–3 years in the Department of Health's 'Green Book'†. These two publications should be viewed as complementary or companion volumes, and a considerable effort has been made to make them compatible and consistent in their advice. This manual also reflects the importance of an integrated approach between paediatrics, epidemiology and public health in the control of infectious disease. An emphasis on integration is particularly timely when there is concern that the newly formed independent NHS Hospital Trusts, with their own problems and priorities competing for scarce resources, may pay less attention, *inter alia*, to national or regional initiatives for disease surveillance and the accurate monitoring of adverse events, both essential components of any successful programme of immunization.

A. G. M. Campbell
Emeritus Professor of Child Health, University of Aberdeen
and Chairman, Joint Committee on Vaccination and Immunization, UK

***Centers for Disease Control and Prevention (1994) *Addressing Emerging Infectious Disease Threats*. US Department of Health and Human Services.**

†Department of Health *Immunisation Against Infectious Disease*. HMSO, London (new edition due to be published in 1996).

INTRODUCTION

This handbook is intended for hospital medical staff working with children, paediatricians, specialists in infectious diseases, intensivists, junior doctors and medical students. As a source of information on the treatment and control of infectious diseases, other hospital staff, child-care professionals, doctors working in public health, environmental health officers and health administrators will also find the text useful. The text can be read through in its entirety but as a practical handbook it is designed as a source of information and guidance for the user with a specific problem. Hence there is considerable cross-referencing and some repetition so that the reader does not have to skip around the book excessively. Particular care has been taken to ensure that guidance is compatible with that in the Department of Health's book *Immunisation Against Infectious Disease* (new edition due 1995 or 1996).

Part One gives general guidance on the diagnosis and management of children with specific clinical problems: the child with a rash, the child with a urinary tract infection, the child with a bone or joint infection, etc. When a variety of organisms may be the cause (e.g. otitis media or lower respiratory tract infection), some guidelines on treatment are provided in these pages. There are also special sections on children with congenital infections and zoonoses, and because of the increasing numbers of patients with impaired immunity seen in hospital practice, there are four chapters relating to immunocompromised children including a comprehensive coverage of human immunodeficiency virus (HIV) infection in children. The issue of immunization of the immunocompromised child is discussed in Appendix VII which follows a section on contraindications to immunization. International travel and the numbers of children entering the UK from abroad are increasing, so there are chapters on preparation for travel, management of a child with an infection contracted abroad, and on refugees and adopted children. Finally in Part One there are sections giving guidance on laboratory tests, including the correct methods of specimen collection, the rational use of antibiotics and general principles of infection control in the hospital and community.

Once a specific diagnosis is considered or has been made the reader should consult Part Two, in which individual childhood infections are arranged alphabetically. Each lists the epidemiology (including mode of transmission and incubation periods), clinical features and natural history, diagnosis, management and public health considerations. As this is a practical handbook particular emphasis is placed on methods of diagnosis, management and the action needed to detect and prevent further cases. For some diagnoses antimicrobial treatment is detailed in the relevant chapter, but for most conditions treatment is summarized in two appendices, one being antibiotics for the neonate (Appendix II) and the other antibiotics for the infant and child (Appendix III). There are also appendices giving recent disease statistics for the more important infections, a listing of notifiable diseases and exclusion periods.

The manual details single well-tried approaches to most problems of diagnosis and management of infection. However, there are often acceptable alternatives and we would not wish to imply that these should not be used. If in doubt an expert in paediatric infectious diseases should always be consulted. Similarly, when considering laboratory tests there is no substitute for discussing the case with the relevant medical microbiologist. Because of the public health implications of many infections (these are highlighted for specific infections in Part Two) the local consultant in communicable disease control or director of public health should be informed promptly of such cases. They will often be the persons who have to take action and will also inform the Communicable Disease Surveillance Centre or Scottish Centre for Infection and Environmental Health as appropriate.

We would like to thank all the specialists who contributed particular sections and who are listed on page ix, and the British Paediatric Association who have supported the preparation of the manual. In addition we would like to thank a number of colleagues and institutions (page xi) who commented upon earlier draft sections, provided data and information or assisted in production. Finally, we would like to thank our families and friends who tolerated the long hours which we put in to writing and editing this book.

Graham Davies
David Elliman
Anthony Hart
Angus Nicoll
Peter Rudd

PART 1 – General

1 Congenital Infection

2 Neonatal Infection

3 The Child with an Upper Respiratory Tract Infection

4 The Child with a Lower Respiratory Tract Infection

5 The Child with a Bone or Joint Infection

6 The Child with Diarrhoea and Vomiting

7 Urinary Tract Infections in Children

8 Management of Suspected Sexually Transmitted Diseases in Prepubertal Children

9 The Child with a Cardiac Infection

10 The Child with Bacterial Meningitis

11 The Child with Acute Encephalitis

12 The Child with Septic Shock

13 The Child with Toxic Shock Syndrome

14 The Child with a Rash

15 The Child with A Pyrexia of Unknown Origin

16 The Child with Suspected Immunodeficiency

17 Management of the Immunocompromised Child with Infection

18 Management of the Child with Systemic Fungal Infection

19 The Child with HIV Infection

20 Preparation for Travel Abroad

21 Management of the Child with an Infection Contracted Abroad

22 Refugees and Internationally Adopted Children

23 Zoonoses

24 Laboratory Diagnosis of Infection

25 The Use of Antibiotics

26 Infection Control in the Hospital

27 Infection Control in the Community

CONGENITAL INFECTION

The major congenital infections are summarized in Table 1.1. Most are discussed in more detail in Part Two. The presentation of these infections is varied, from acute illness in the case of herpes simplex or streptococcal infections, to silent disease in most cases of cytomegalovirus (CMV) infection. For many the signs are non-specific and congenital infection should always be considered as a possible diagnosis in the sick neonate. The diagnosis will depend on appropriate use of laboratory tests. One such commonly performed investigation is the 'TORCH' screen (toxoplasmosis, rubella, CMV and herpes serology). This investigation is expensive and has in the past been used rather indiscriminately. It is not indicated for babies who are small for dates but have no other abnormality.

Table 1.1 Congenital infections

Organism/disease	Investigation and management in pregnancy	Investigation and management in the newborn	Refer to Chapter no.
Chlamydia trachomatis	Treat parents/partners with tetracycline or erythromycin after diagnosis of neonatal/infant infection	Rapid. Immunofluorescent test on eye swab or nasopharyngeal aspirate. Oral erythromycin alone for 14 days	40
Cytomegalovirus (CMV)	Rarely diagnosed. Screening inappropriate	Throat swab or urine for culture. CMV specific IgM. Symptomatic treatment. Audiology early	44
Enterovirus	No action if in early pregnancy	Serology. Symptomatic treatment and pooled gammaglobulin. Isolate from other infants	47
Hepatitis B	HBsAg test; if positive, test for HBe antigen/antibody. Test and immunize partner when indicated	Management determined by maternal status. For HBsAg positive, HBe antibody positive—immunize only. For HBe antibody negative—immunize and give hepatitis B immune globulin	56
Hepatitis C	Perinatal transmission can occur	Serology (after maternal antibodies have disappeared)	57
Herpes simplex virus (HSV) infection	Greatest risk in primary genital infection. No indication for serial cervical swabs. Consider caesarean section	Electron microscopy of lesions. Appropriate cultures. Acyclovir for definite or suspected infection	59
Human immunodeficiency virus (HIV) infection	Serology. Consider termination. Give zidovudine during pregnancy and labour. Consider lower segment caesarean section	Isolation unnecessary. Extreme care with body fluids. Mother should not breast-feed. Consider zidovudine for first 6 weeks	19

Human T-cell lymphotrophic virus type I (HTLV-I)	Very rare except in south Japan, South America and Caribbean area. Cause of adult T-cell lymphoma and tropical spastic paresis	Perinatal spread via blood and breast milk known to occur	
Listeria monocytogenes	Blood culture. Cervical swabs. Ampicillin 4–6 g per day in acute infection	Blood culture, lumbar puncture, surface swabs. Ampicillin plus gentamicin	66
Measles	Serology	Very rare. Serology	69
Mumps	Serology. Termination is not indicated	Very rare. Serology	71
Mycobacterium tuberculosis—tuberculosis	Positive tuberculin test (where no previous BCG) needs treatment, even where chest radiography negative	Maternal TB—tuberculin test not indicated. Rarely necessary to isolate infant from mother with active TB until she is non-infectious. Isoniazid (INAH) and BCGfor infant. Infant with TB—INAH and rifampicin	97
Neisseria gonorrhoeae—gonorrhoea	Culture. Ampicillin/benzylpenicillin or Cefotaxime if β-lactamase producer	Culture of conjunctival pus. Topical treatment and benzylpenicillin or cefotaxime IV for 7 days. If mother infected but baby asymptomatic, give single dose of benzylpenicillin	50
Papillomavirus	Detection of HPV DNA by PCR amplification or hybridization	Very unusual for virus to be present at birth. Incubation period several months to 2–3 years	101
Parvovirus	Serology—cordocentesis. May require transfusion for hydrops fetalis	Parovirus IgM. Symptomatic	75

Table 1.1 continued

Organism/disease	Investigation and management in pregnancy	Investigation and management in the newborn	Refer to Chapter no.
Rubella	Serology: IgG and IgM antibodies. Counsel for possible termination following infection before 18 weeks gestation	Symptomatic. Audiology, serology	86
Streptococcus agalactiae (Group B streptococcus)	Cervical swab. Urine culture; ampicillin 2 g 4-hourly where colonized. Consider use when previous morbidity/mortality from group B	Appropriate cultures. Benzylpenicillin/ampicillin/ cefotaxime IV	91
Toxoplasma gondii—toxoplasmosis	Serology on mother. Cordocentesis for fetal serology. Spiramycin until definite fetal infection confirmed. Then pyrimethamine, sulphadiazine and folinic acid, alternating with spiramycin	Serology. Pyrimethamine, sulphadiazine and folinic acid, alternating with spiramycin	96
Treponema pallidum—syphilis	Treponemal serology (TPHA/VDRL tests). FTA test. Benzylpenicillin	Benzylpenicillin	92
Varicella (chickenpox)	Varicella serology. If seronegative and contact, give varicella-zoster immunoglobulin (VZIG). Termination not indicated. Acylovir for acute infection	Varicella-zoster immunoglobulin essential when maternal infection 7 days before to 7 days after delivery; VZIG not indicated at other times or for exposure to infection in neonatal period. Acyclovir for infection acquired in utero	37

Key: AZT, azidothymidine (zidovudine); BCG, bacille Calmette-Guérin; CMV, cylomegalovirus; FTA, fluorescent treponema antibody; HBsAg, hepatitis B surface antigen; Ig, immunoglobulin; INAH, isonicotinic acid hydrazide (isoniazid); TB, tuberculosis; TPHA, *Treponema pallidum* haemagglutination; VDRL, venereal disease reference laboratory; VZIG, varicella-zoster immunoglobulin.

NEONATAL INFECTION

The immaturity of the host defence mechanism in neonates makes them very susceptible to a whole variety of microbial pathogens. This susceptibility is found in term as well as preterm infants. However, it is generally true that the more immature the baby the greater the risk, particularly as immaturity increases the need for invasive intensive care which further compromises the host defences. Severe prematurity also significantly reduces the transfer of maternal immunoglobulin G across the placenta. Babies who are small for gestational age have additional deficiencies in their immune defences and are especially vulnerable to infection.

Neonates not only have a higher incidence of infections but when infected they become more rapidly and more seriously ill. For this reason it is often necessary to treat with antibiotics at the earliest suspicion of infection. Recommendations for antibiotic therapy are summarized in Tables 2.1 and 2.2.

BACTERIAL SEPSIS IN NEONATES

It is useful to divide neonatal bacterial sepsis into two types, according to the time of onset. *Early-onset infection* is that producing symptoms at birth (the infection is established in the baby while in the uterus) or within the first 48 hours of life. The infection often follows a fulminant course, and mortality is high despite antibiotic treatment. The organisms responsible come from the maternal genital tract, and relatively few species are responsible. These are, in order of frequency: group B streptococcus (*Streptococcus agalactiae*), *Escherichia coli*, *Listeria monocytogenes* and rarely, others including streptococci, *Haemophilus* species and anaerobes.

Late-onset infection occurs after 48 hours of age. The responsible organism may have been acquired from the mother's genital tract or may be acquired from the post-natal environment. Infection at this stage may be fulminant but more often has an insidious onset and is more likely to be focal in nature, e.g. meningitis. The list of possible causative organisms includes those responsible for early-onset sepsis plus a large number of possible opportunist pathogens. In recent years the following pathogens have commonly proved troublesome: coagulase-negative staphylococci, *Klebsiella/Enterobacter* species, *Pseudomonas aeruginosa* and *E. coli*. Other causes include: *Staphylococcus aureus*, *Enterococcus faecalis/ faecium* (group D) and *Streptococcus pneumoniae*.

SUSPECTING THE DIAGNOSIS

Early-onset sepsis—risk factors

Maternal

- Unexplained premature rupture of the membranes and/or premature labour (group B streptococcus and *Listeria* infection in particular may promote premature labour).
- Maternal fever.
- Unexplained fetal distress.
- Prolonged rupture (> 24 hours) of the fetal membranes.
- Meconium staining of the liquor in a premature infant (consider *Listeria*).
- Previous baby suffered group B streptococcal sepsis and maternal swabs again positive.

Table 2.1 Common antibiotics and combinations used

	Antibiotic	Used to treat
1.	Penicillin and gentamicin	Early-onset sepsis
2.	Azlocillin and gentamicin	Late-onset sepsis
3.	Vancomycin and ceftazidime	Late-onset sepsis with proven or suspected coagulase-negative staphylococcal infection, plus Gram-negative cover
4.	Vancomycin and ciprofloxacin	As (3) but with resistant Gram-negative isolates
5.	Ceftazidime and gentamicin	Late-onset sepsis with resistant flora
6.	Azlocillin/ceftazidime and amikacin	As (5)
7.	(2) and flucloxacillin	Late-onset sepsis with focal superficial infection
8.	Cefotaxime/ceftazidime and ampicillin (with or without gentamicin)	Empirical treatment of neonatal meningitis
9.	(2), (5) or (6) and metronidazole	Intra-abdominal or post-surgical sepsis, necrotizing enterocolitis
10.	Imipenem†	Broad spectrum; reserve for resistant strains
11.	Trimethoprim	Prophylaxis against urinary tract infections
12.	Erythromycin	Chlamydial, mycoplasmal infections

† **May be superceded by meropenem.**

Baby

- Unexplained birth asphyxia.
- Respiratory distress (note—the radiographic appearance of pneumonia may be indistinguishable from hyaline membrane disease).
- Poor circulatory status (low blood pressure, cold peripheries).
- Unexplained metabolic acidosis.
- Unexplained hypoglycaemia.
- Unexplained neutropenia (neutrophil count<1000/mm^3).
- Rash (consider *Listeria*).

Table 2.2 Best antibiotics for given organisms

Organism	Antibiotic
Group A streptococcus	Penicillin
Group B streptococcus	Penicillin (with gentamicin initially)
Group D streptococcus*	Ampicillin and gentamicin
Streptococcus pneumoniae	Penicillin
Staphylococcus aureus	Flucloxacillin with or without gentamicin (add fucidin for deep infection)
MRSA	Vancomycin
Coagulase-negative staphylococcus	Vancomycin
Listeria monocytogenes	Ampicillin (with gentamicin initially)
*E. coli**	Cefotaxime
Klebsiella, *Enterobacter* spp*	Cefotaxime
*Pseudomonas aeruginosa**	Azlocillin and gentamicin (or ceftazidime)
Bacteroides	Metronidazole
Haemophilus influenzae	Cefotaxime

***Resistance may be a problem. Review antibiotic therapy when culture results available.**
MRSA, methicillin resistant *Staphlococcus aureus.*

- Hepatosplenomegaly.
- Jaundice.

Late-onset sepsis has to be considered as a differential diagnosis for any untoward event that befalls the baby. Such events include:

- Bradycardia and apnoea.
- Poor feeding, increasing gastric aspirates and abdominal distension.
- Irritability.
- Convulsions.
- Increasing jaundice.
- Increasing respiratory distress.
- For ventilated babies: unexplained increased ventilatory requirements; increased volume and 'purulence' of endotracheal secretions; increased shadowing on chest radiograph.
- Unexplained increase or rapid decrease in neutrophil and/or platelet counts.
- Signs or symptoms of necrotizing enterocolitis (see below).
- Signs of focal inflammation such as periumbilical cellulitis, infected drip site, etc.

INVESTIGATIONS

Early-onset sepsis

Blood culture—MOST IMPORTANT. A minimum of 0.5 ml per blood culture bottle should be taken. Take from a peripheral vein by 'clean' venepuncture using the closed system (broken needle technique is not suitable). Peripheral arterial samples are also suitable but are difficult because of the need to use a 'no touch' technique. Samples from a freshly sited umbilical artery catheter (UAC) taken by the person siting the catheter, while still scrubbed up, are acceptable. Note—in symptomatic babies antibiotic treatment should not be delayed. Venous blood cultures should therefore be taken and the first dose of antibiotics given *before* UAC insertion is attempted (other blood tests can wait).

Full blood count including differential white cell count.

Deep ear swab taken by nursing staff using a swab passed through a sterile speculum. The object is to obtain cultures from a site which reflects amniotic fluid infection in utero but has not come into direct contact with the birth canal during delivery. There is no point taking this swab if more than 6 hours has elapsed since birth (by then the external auditory canal will have been colonized).

Maternal cultures Request obstetricians to do a high vaginal swab, blood culture and placental cultures, if possible.

Chest X-ray to look for pneumonia. Appearances of infection may mimic hyaline membrane disease or retained lung fluid.

Lumbar puncture is performed to determine whether meningitis is part of the sepsis. This will have a bearing on the length of treatment and future prognosis. However, it is not essential to do this before giving antibiotics and in an unstable baby this procedure can be delayed. Confirmation of the presence and cause of meningitis can often be made on a post-antibiotic sample using antigen detection tests.

Swabs of any focal site of inflammation—septic spots, etc. (unusual in early-onset infection).

Other tests needed to help in the management of the 'septic' baby include analysis of urea and electrolytes, creatinine, glucose, bilirubin, coagulation screen, group and save serum. Note—'routine' surface swabs are unnecessary in the diagnosis of neonatal sepsis. It is, however, common practice to perform these on babies transferred from other hospitals if part of the hospital's policy for surveillance for methicillin-resistant *Staphylococcus aureus* (MRSA). Urine cultures are unnecessary in early-onset sepsis.

Late-onset sepsis

Routine surveillance cultures of stool and pharyngeal flora performed on infants in neonatal intensive care units (NICUs) have little value in predicting the cause of subsequent sepsis. They may be useful in monitoring trends in predominant colonizing bacterial strains and antibiotic-resistant strains. In ventilated infants there may be some benefit in regular routine culture of endotracheal secretions, though the evidence is not great.

In suspected late-onset sepsis, before starting antibiotic therapy, the following tests should be done.

Blood cultures—as for early-onset sepsis, above.

Full blood count including differential white cell count.

Suprapubic or clean catch urine (see below) but do not delay antibiotics if the child is sick.

Chest X-ray.

Endotracheal tube secretions (in ventilated babies)—usually culture only. Microscopy is rarely helpful.

Lumbar puncture is not always necessary (e.g. in ventilated babies with suspected chest infections). However, a low threshold is needed for doing this test. It can be deferred in a very sick baby in an unstable condition.

Swabs from sites of inflammation, e.g. inflamed umbilicus, infected drip site. Routine surface swabs are not necessary.

TREATMENT

Treat on suspicion—antibiotics can be stopped after 48 hours if cultures are negative.

Suspected early-onset sepsis

Treatment of mother If in utero infection of the baby is suspected, ask obstetricians to take a cervical swab and blood cultures from the mother and start intravenous (IV) ampicillin. Encourage early delivery.

Treatment of the baby Babies should be screened and put on antibiotics. Penicillin and gentamicin is a standard combination to use at this stage, although some units may prefer other regimens including the use of third-generation cephalosporins (but see below). Any symptomatic newborn baby should be admitted to the neonatal unit for treatment and monitoring. Since the symptoms of infection may mimic most neonatal problems, most babies admitted to a neonatal unit are given antibiotics.

If *Listeria* infection is suspected use ampicillin and gentamicin. Suspicion of *Listeria* should be aroused by any of the following:

- Maternal influenza-like febrile illness preceding the onset of labour, especially if there has been spontaneous premature rupture of the membranes.
- Meconium staining of the liquor in a premature baby (unusual in normal circumstances).
- Baby ill with rash (usually a sparse papular eruption) and/or hepatosplenomegaly.
- Gram-positive rods seen in cerebrospinal fluid (CSF).

Penicillin covers 90% of *Listeria* isolates. Ampicillin covers 100% but is not used routinely because *Listeria* is rare, and excessive use of this antibiotic would lead to increased anitbiotic resistance in the Gram-negative flora in the unit—ultimately complicating the treatment of late-onset sepsis. Some units use third-generation cephalosporins (cefotaxime or ceftazidime) in early-onset sepsis. However, such a policy has a number of disadvantages: (a) it provides no cover against *Listeria*, and (b) evidence suggests that excessive use of these agents in neonatal intensive care leads to the emergence of resistant Gram-negative flora in the babies, thus potentially lessening the usefulness of these agents for treating late-onset sepsis. This latter objection is not relevant on ordinary post-natal wards.

Late-onset sepsis

Choice of antibiotics The baby's recent microbiological results should be reviewed, looking particularly for antibiotic-resistant isolates. In ventilated babies, routine endotracheal secretion culture results may be available. Choice of antibiotics for late-onset sepsis should therefore take into account the most recent microbiological data. One cannot assume that the bacteria isolated on screening cultures are the cause of the presumed sepsis, but it is obviously sensible to cover them.

If there is nothing specific to guide antibiotic choice then a combination of azlocillin and gentamicin is a reasonable empirical choice. With the increasing emergence of coagulase-negative staphylococcus as the cause of late-onset sepsis, combinations such as vancomycin and ceftazidime are increasingly used (but note the concerns over cephalosporins listed on p. 11). If intra-abdominal sepsis such as necrotizing enterocolitis or post-surgical sepsis is suspected, add metronidazole. If focal superficial sepsis is present, add flucloxacillin.

If antibiotic-resistant flora are identified, other combinations such as ceftazidime and gentamicin or amikacin with either ceftazidime or azlocillin are used.

If meningitis is suspected, ampicillin and ceftazidime (for babies undergoing neonatal intensive care) or ampicillin and cefotaxime (other babies) are used.

Vancomycin is used if coagulase-negative staphylococci have been isolated. Vancomycin and gentamicin have additive toxicity and the combination should be avoided. If Gram-negative cover is required with vancomycin, use ceftazidime or ciprofloxacin.

Once an isolate and its sensitivities have been obtained, antibiotic treatment should be rationalized.

Treatment of very sick septic neonates In addition to antibiotics, very sick neonates may need the following support.

Ventilation—consider early.

Circulatory—give colloid and inotropic drugs.

Haematological Blood, platelets. Give fresh frozen plasma for coagulation disturbance. White cells are rarely used. If profound neutropenia is found, especially with disseminated intravascular coagulation, consider single-volume exchange transfusion. Recombinant granulocyte colony stimulating factor is a promising new adjuvant therapy for enhancing neutrophil numbers and function in neonatal sepsis which is currently under investigation.

Immunological Fresh frozen plasma provides immunoglobulin and complement factors as well as clotting factors. Intravenous immunoglobulin infusion may also provide benefit in some types of neonatal sepsis.

Renal Sepsis is often associated with renal impairment. Monitor creatinine levels and test urine for blood and protein. *Watch antibiotic levels*.

Gut and nutrition The gut will almost certainly stop working in sepsis, therefore stop enteral feeding. Consider early institution of total parenteral nutrition (TPN), but the precise constitution of TPN needs careful judging as the babies will be catabolic and unable to handle large nitrogen loads.

Hepatic Liver dysfunction, especially conjugated hyperbilirubinaemia, is common in sepsis. Give prophylactic vitamin K.

Monitoring response to therapy It cannot be assumed that the antibiotics will necessarily clear the infection. If the baby remains unwell—and *always* if there are positive blood cultures—further sets of blood cultures should be taken 2–3 days after starting treatment. Persistent positive blood cultures may suggest:

- Inadequate antibiotic levels or regimen.
- Resistant organism.
- Focal infection—abscess, osteomyelitis or endocarditis.

Alteration of therapy and further investigation (e.g. ultrasound, skeletal X-rays and echocardiogram) may be indicated, and the treatment course should be extended in those with a slow microbiological response.

Length of treatment will depend on a number of variables, such as the type of organism and the clinical response. Some guidelines are given below.

- Antibiotics started on possibility of infection but subsequently no clinical evidence of infection and cultures are all negative—48 hours.
- Antibiotics started on suspicion, cultures negative, but patient clinically believed to have been infected and responding to antibiotics—5 days.
- Pneumonia seen on chest X-ray but cultures negative—7 days.
- Positive blood cultures but negative CSF culture—treat for minimum of 10 days from *last* positive blood culture.
- Positive CSF or blood culture—depends on organism (see section on meningitis, p. 14).
- Fungal infections, osteomyelitis, endocarditis and deep abscesses not surgically drained require several weeks of antibiotic treatment; seek advice.

FUNGAL SEPSIS

Invasive fungal sepsis, usually due to *Candida* species, is an occasional problem in neonates. It can occur relatively early on in life (and even be congenital), but more commonly it complicates the management of long-stay patients who have been very sick and have been given large quantities of broad-spectrum antibiotics (with or without dexamethasone).

The diagnosis is suspected on similar grounds to other forms of neonatal sepsis. Absence of a history of previous superficial fungal infection does not rule it out. Tests for fungal sepsis include blood cultures (arterial cultures are considered superior to venous) and suprapubic urine analysis, asking the microbiologists to look specifically for yeasts on microscopy (bag urine specimens are of no use in this situation). Endotracheal secretions should be cultured in ventilated infants and, because there is a high likelihood of associated fungal meningitis, a lumbar puncture should be performed. *Candida* antigen test on serum can be performed, but it is unlikely that the results will be available soon enough to influence the decision to treat; and, in any case, false negative results do occur. Nevertheless, a positive result may be useful in confirming the diagnosis.

Prevention Babies at high risk for fungal infection should receive prophylactic nystatin, ideally given half orally and half by nasogastric tube. All cases of superficial candidiasis should be treated vigorously.

Management Intravenous amphotericin and flucytosine is standard therapy. The latter drug is important because of its ability to penetrate the central nervous system and renal tissues, both being common sites of involvement in neonatal fungal sepsis. Amphotericin is potentially toxic though it is generally well tolerated in neonates. Occasionally acute systemic reactions—pyrexia, tachycardia, hypotension—may occur, and for this reason it is usual to give a test dose of 0.05–0.1 mg before starting therapy in earnest. Then the starting dose is 0.2 mg/kg as a single daily infusion, increasing by 0.2 mg/kg each day to a maximum of 1.0 mg/kg; however, if a good response is achieved it is often possible to stop the escalation short of this maximum dose, thus reducing the incidence of side-effects. Blood levels are not helpful. The drug is given in special pH-tested 5% dextrose and *cannot be mixed with other drugs* (even electrolytes). Fluid volumes may be a problem.

The main toxicity problem is renal. Hypokalaemia (due to renal leak) is very common (try to keep ahead with potassium supplements); if potassium supplements are inadequate, then try amiloride which usually helps. Rising urea and creatinine levels may occur, and should be monitored. It may be necessary to reduce dosage. Avoid other potentially nephrotoxic drugs such as aminoglycosides and vancomycin if possible. Prolonged treatment is usually needed. Once a clinical response has been achieved, amphotericin may be given every other day (at the same dose as daily)—this reduces toxicity. Flucytosine may cause bone marrow suppression–monitor by full blood counts. Blood levels of the drug should be kept below 80 mg/l. Dosage should be reduced if there is renal impairment. Flucytosine is well absorbed and enteral administration can be employed after initial response obtained.

Imidazole drugs (such as miconazole and fluconazole) are relatively untried in this clinical situation. Drug resistance amongst certain species of *Candida* may be a problem.

MENINGITIS

The peak age incidence of meningitis occurs in the neonatal period. It can present as an apparently focal infection (usually in late-onset sepsis) or as part of multisystem sepsis with septicaemia. In this age group the clinical signs are non-specific and there should therefore be a very low threshold for performing a lumbar puncture.

Contraindications to lumbar puncture

- Baby too sick, especially with cardiorespiratory instability: treat with antibiotics anyway and delay lumbar puncture until condition improves.
- Severe coagulopathy or thrombocytopenia: consider deferred lumbar puncture with fresh frozen plasma and platelet cover.
- Known non-communicating hydrocephalus (usually following an earlier intraventricular haemorrhage): perform intraventricular tap. Note—in contrast to other age groups, raised intracranial pressure per se is not a contra-indication to lumbar puncture in neonates.

Treatment

Antibiotic therapy, organism unknown For empirical treatment use ampicillin, and a third-generation cephalosporin (ceftazidime on NICU, otherwise cefotaxime). Gentamicin may also be added to enhance Gram-negative bacillary cover. Try to rationalize treatment when the cause is identified.

Antibiotic therapy, organism known Antibiotics should be given according to the type of micro-organism:

- Group B streptococcus—benzylpenicillin (initially with gentamicin) for 14 days.
- *Listeria*—ampicillin plus gentamicin for 14 days followed by ampicillin alone for a further 7 days.
- Gram-negative bacilli—cephalosporin plus gentamicin for 21 days (minimum), depending on the sensitivity of the organism. Repeated lumbar punctures with CSF bactericidal levels may be needed. Note—intraventricular or intrathecal antibiotics are of no added benefit. Up to 60% of premature neonates with gram negative bacillary meningitis will develop ventriculitis. This may require prolonged treatment with an agent such as ciprofloxacin.

- Coagulase-negative staphylococci—give systemic anti-staphylococcal antibiotics to which the organism (usually present as a complication of ventriculoperitoneal shunt) is sensitive and which penetrate into the CSF. Choice depends on sensitivities—rifampicin and trimethoprim are often used. Additionally, give vancomycin systematically and through the shunt, which may need removal.

Supportive therapy such as ventilation, and inotropic drugs (see section on the treatment of very sick septic neonates, above).

Fluid and electrolyte balance Support cerebral perfusion pressure with colloid, but restrict crystalloid fluids to a minimum to reduce risk of cerebral oedema. Watch out for inappropriate antidiuretic hormone syndrome.

Anticonvulsants Use anticonvulsant drugs if fits occur. Prophylactic usage is not recommended.

PNEUMONIA

Pneumonia should be treated as described for early and late-onset sepsis, above. If the response to antibiotics is poor, consider other causes (viral, chlamydial, etc.).

URINARY TRACT INFECTION

Urinary tract infection is confirmed by obtaining a positive culture, usually with a raised white cell count. Suprapubic or clean catch urine samples are best; bag urine samples are unreliable. Try not to treat on the basis of a single bag urine result. Note—urinary tract infection may be associated with disseminated sepsis, therefore investigate and treat vigorously.

Follow-up There is a high chance of a urinary tract infection in the neonatal period being associated with an underlying abnormality. Therefore, for confirmed infection,

- Examine external genitalia carefully.
- Perform ultrasound examination in all cases.
- Prescribe prophylactic trimethoprim when the treatment course is completed, to be given until the follow-up appointment.
- Arrange follow-up: in paediatric urology clinic if history (e.g. poor urinary stream), physical examination or ultrasonography suggest underlying abnormality, otherwise in appropriate medical clinic.

All babies with a confirmed urinary tract infection in the neonatal period require follow-up, and most require further radiological investigations such as micturating cystourethrography.

GASTROENTERITIS

Gastroenteritis is fortunately unusual in the neonatal period but can lead to serious illness. The usual range of bacterial and viral causes is involved. Any of the recognized infections may precipitate the development of necrotizing enterocolitis (see below). More commonly, severe diarrhoea and vomiting occur, leading to rapid fluid and electrolyte disturbance. Stools should be sent for culture and electron microscopy. Blood cultures (and in sick children a full septic screen) should be performed since *Salmonella* species, in particular, are liable to cause invasive disease at this age. Interestingly, rotavirus infection is often very mild or asymptomatic at this age.

Management is along the usual lines for gastroenteritis in older infants, but there should be a lower threshold for intravenous fluid therapy. Systemic antibiotics are required if invasion is suspected in *Salmonella* infection (use trimethoprim, ampicillin or ciprofloxacin depending on sensitivities). Antibiotics may also be required for *Shigella*, *Campylobacter* and *E. coli* diarrhoeas. Cross-infection is obviously a major risk and the advice of the infection control team should be sought early.

NECROTIZING ENTEROCOLITIS

Necrotizing enterocolitis is a relatively common and potentially devastating disease in which infection of the intestinal wall occurs. The precise pathogenesis remains unclear. The incidence seems to vary dramatically from centre to centre, and within the same unit from time to time. Two forms can be distinguished epidemiologically though not clinically. An 'epidemic' form occurring in clusters suggests that there is an infectious process, and indeed intestinal pathogens can sometimes be isolated (rotavirus, coronavirus and *Salmonella* are amongst those organisms that have been implicated). A 'sporadic' form occurs predominantly in low birth-weight, premature infants, particularly those whose intestines have undergone a period of relative ischaemia prenatally (placental dysfunction and intrauterine growth retardation), at birth (asphyxia) or post-natally (polycythaemia, abdominal surgery).

The hallmark of the disease is the radiological picture of 'pneumatosis intestinalis'—gas in the wall of the bowel itself—though this is not always present in the early stages of the disease and not necessary for the diagnosis. It is thought that damage to the gut wall allows invasion of bacteria including gas producers, which then further compromise the blood supply to the mucosa leading to necrosis, absorption of endotoxin, bacterial invasion to give septicaemia and perforation. Enteral feeding seems to be a cofactor, particularly if formula feeds are used. The diagnosis should be suspected in an infant with any combination of bloody stools, abdominal distension, vomiting—particularly bilious—and non-specific signs of sepsis. Investigate with plain abdominal X-ray (and lateral decubitus view if perforation suspected) and full septic screen, but defer lumbar puncture if the baby is very sick.

Prevention Use of breast milk rather than artificial feeds is protective. In babies known to be at high risk—after abdominal surgery, or babies with growth retardation (especially if fetal Doppler ultrasonography showed reversed diastolic flow), neonatal asphyxia or symptomatic polycythaemia—consider a 10-day period of elective intravenous nutrition with 48 hours of oral vancomycin before feeds are introduced. If possible, avoid umbilical catheters.

Management Infants with necrotizing enterocolitis should be managed in centres with paediatric surgical expertise. Standard treatment, for 10 days minimum, is:

- Nil by mouth and intravenous fluid.
- Intravenous nutrition.
- Antibiotics—azlocillin, gentamicin and metronidazole.
- Surgery may be required for excision of gangrenous bowel, perforation, etc.

OSTEOMYELITIS

Osteomyelitis is rare but it is important not to miss it. The most common causes are *Staphylococcus aureus* and group B streptococci, but Gram-negative bacteria may also be responsible. Presentation is either with a septicaemic illness or, particularly in group B streptococcal cases, the infant may appear relatively well with swelling or immobility of a limb, the latter sometimes mimicking a nerve palsy—for example, upper humeral metaphyseal infection presenting as apparent Erb's palsy. Osteomyelitis should be considered in all cases of *Staphylococcus aureus* bacteraemia or septicaemia, or when sepsis caused by other organisms is slow to respond (especially with persistent positive blood cultures). Clinical signs may or may not be present, e.g. local swelling, tenderness, one limb not moving. In cases with insidious onset, radiographic changes are often present by the time of diagnosis and may show extensive bony destruction which nevertheless will usually heal well after treatment. In contrast to the situation at other ages, isotope bone scanning is not helpful. Treatment involves a prolonged course of antibiotics.

SUPERFICIAL INFECTIONS

Superficial infections should always be taken seriously because of the risk of progression to invasive disease in the immune incompetent child.

Umbilical sepsis A 'sticky' umbilicus is very common. Send a swab for culture (in case infection develops) but do not use antibiotics. Spirit swabbing by nursing staff should suffice.

True periumbilical infection is indicated by a purulent discharge with surrounding erythema. Request swab and blood cultures and prescribe broad-spectrum antibiotics including flucloxacillin.

Paronychia is an infection of the nail fold usually caused by *Staphylococcus aureus* but occasionally by *Candida* species. It is often associated with other superficial staphylococcal infection such as 'septic spots'. Take a swab and blood culture. Treat with oral flucloxacillin if the baby is well; if not, give intravenous flucloxacillin and gentamicin.

Septic spots are sometimes difficult to distinguish from erythema toxicum. If in doubt, puncture a pustule, send a swab and treat as for paronychia.

Candidiasis Treat candidiasis with nystatin or miconazole in neonates. Fluconazole has not been evaluated and is not licensed; however, it should be considered if candidiasis is a persistent or recurrent problem.

Conjunctivitis 'Sticky eyes' are very common and usually do not indicate an infection. Purulent discharge from an eye needs to be taken seriously. Usually these discharges are caused by common bacteria acquired from the environment—*Staphylococcus aureus* and coliform bacteria—and are best treated by neomycin topically. Possible more serious causes should be considered and age of onset may be suggestive:

- If the baby is less than 3 days old it is urgently necessary to exclude gonococcal infection (ophthalmia neonatorum, see Chapter 50).

- In babies over 7 days old, consider *Chlamydia trachomatis* infection (see Chapter 40). Never use topical chloramphenicol without first excluding chlamydial infection. Chloramphenicol partially treats the infection, suppressing symptoms and the true diagnosis. Such babies are at risk of later development of chlamydial pneumonia.

Mothers whose babies are diagnosed as having either gonococcal or chlamydial infection need referral to the department of genitourinary medicine for treatment and contact tracing.

VIRAL INFECTIONS

Respiratory viruses may cause serious respiratory compromise in babies with bronchopulmonary dysplasia. Respiratory syncytial virus (RSV), parainfluenza and influenza viruses, and adenovirus are the biggest culprits. Respiratory syncytial virus is prevalent in the winter months (November to March) each year. It causes common cold symptoms in older children and adults, and can be brought into the unit by them. All these viruses can be rapidly diagnosed by immunofluorescent techniques on nasopharyngeal aspirates. A fine cathether is placed in the posterior nasopharynx and a short, sharp suction applied; the resulting aspirate is flushed through into a trap with sterile saline or viral transport medium. (Note—the test requires epithelial cells stripped off by the suction *not* mucus itself.) Ribavirin treatment should be initiated if compromised babies develop these infections. Cross-infection prevention procedures are very important, particularly hand-washing and cohorting (See Chapter 26).

Herpes simplex virus when contracted in the neonatal period herpes simplex can cause overwhelming infection. It may be acquired from the maternal genital tract or post-natally from contacts excreting the virus.

Prevention If the mother is known to have active cervical disease, deliver the baby by lower segment caesarean section if the membranes have been ruptured for less than 4 hours. Nursing and medical staff with cold sores should wear masks, employ strict hand-washing procedures and use topical acyclovir to shorten the period of viral excretion.

Treatment Exposed babies require close observation and should be *isolated* with the mother. The use of prophylactic antiviral therapy at this stage is controversial. The authors prefer not to use it. First signs of disease may be non-specific (poor feeding, fever, apnoea, jaundice), or specific signs such as vesicular rash (often one or two spots only initially) or keratoconjunctivitis may develop. When infection is suspected, the baby needs a full screen with virological investigation of the CSF, aspiration of fluid from vesicles for electron microscopy and culture, and eye and mouth swabs for viral culture. Treat once the specimens have been collected, with acyclovir for a minimum of 10 days. Note—disease can recur when acyclovir is stopped.

Varicella

Babies born to a mother who develops chickenpox in perinatal period

- Babies born to a mother who develops chickenpox within the period 7 days before delivery to 7 days after birth should be given varicella-zoster immunoglobulin (VZIG); the highest-risk period appears to be 5 days before to 2 days after delivery.

- Mother and baby should be nursed together in their own side-room.
- Breast-feeding should be encouraged.
- The baby should be carefully followed up with continuing care by the community midwife, as chickenpox in the first few weeks of life is life-threatening in 30–50% of unprotected babies. Early antiviral therapy with high-dose intravenous acyclovir 10 mg/kg every 8 hours is indicated if neonatal chickenpox develops.

Management of varicella-zoster virus contacts and cases on the neonatal unit It is important that immediate action is taken in the event of cases or suspected cases as the consequences may be serious for neonates. If a member of staff or a visitor is affected:

- Obtain information on the movements and contacts of the index case and a precise history of when the first lesions were observed.
- Infected staff members should take immediate sick leave and must not return to work until the skin lesions have crusted and further cropping has ceased. A visitor with chickenpox must also not return to the unit until all the crusts are dry.
- Consider the varicella status of all patients, visitors and staff who have had contact with the index case so that specific advice and VZIG prophylaxis can be given if appropriate.
- Inform the infection control team that there has been a chickenpox exposure to the unit.
- The senior nurse in collaboration with the infection control team should create a list of staff and visitors who have had direct contact with the index case and obtain a history of previous exposure to chickenpox and the possibility of pregnancy or immunosuppression.
- Varicella antibody status should be checked in members of staff or visitors without a history of chickenpox.
- A staff member or visitor who has had contact with a case of chickenpox or zoster and who is found to be susceptible to varicella-zoster infection should stay away from the unit from 8–21 days after the initial exposure and should inform the unit should chickenpox lesions develop. Staff members or visitors found to be varicella-zoster virus (VZV) seronegative should not return to normal duties or visits within the neonatal unit for 30 days from the last day of exposure. However, these staff members may be deployed in other low-risk areas, in consultation with the occupational health and infection control teams.
- Staff and visitors with a previous history of chickenpox should be reassured that they are immune to infection. If there is any doubt as to their history of chickenpox recommend a blood test for varicella antibodies, as it is better to be certain than optimistic about protective immunity.

Management of a baby who develops chickenpox on the neonatal unit It may not be possible to move high-dependency babies to an isolation room or ward. Intravenous antiviral therapy with high-dose acyclovir will reduce the period of virus shedding to 72–96 hours but during this period air-borne spread of VZV is inevitable. Measures to reduce transmission include the minimizing of 'hands on' contact and the wearing of single-use disposable aprons and non-sterile latex gloves when attending the patient. Regular cleaning of incubator equipment and accessories with alcoholic chlorhexidine will be helpful. Where practicable, nurse the affected baby with babies who are immune, i.e. have previously transferred maternal VZV antibody. All VZV-susceptible babies (see below) should receive VZIG and the unit should be closed to further VZV-susceptible admissions, depending on the balance of risks individually assessed during the initial 96-hour period.

Management of patients exposed to the index case The following should be given VZIG:

- Babies exposed to varicella-zoster virus within the first month of life (i.e. at risk of developing chickenpox up to 6 weeks after birth) whose mothers have no previous history of chickenpox and are negative for antibody to VZV (see below).
- Babies receiving systemic steroid therapy or who have received systemic steroid therapy within the last 3 months and whose mothers have no previous history of chickenpox and are negative for antibody to VZV (see below).
- Babies who are immunocompromised by disease or its treatment, e.g. bronchopulmonary dysplasia, human immunodeficiency virus (HIV), congenital immune deficiency, malignancy and chemotherapy.
- Babies born before 30 weeks of gestation (regardless of post-natal age) or whose birth-weight was less than 1 kg.

Babies not included in these categories should not be given prophylaxis regardless of their exposure history, as they are not considered to be at high risk of significant morbidity or mortality following chickenpox.

Use of immunoglobulin *In mothers and children who are positive for varicella antibodies the relative increase in systemic antibodies that can be achieved with VZIG is small and no benefit is to be gained from treatment.*

Treatment with VZIG The dose of VZIG in the newborn is 250 mg (1 vial) regardless of weight (the adult dose is 1000 mg). VZIG is given intramuscularly and must not be given by intravenous injection or infusion. In patients with a low platelet count or bleeding tendency, intravenous immunoglobulin at 400–6 00mg/kg can be given instead of VZIG without loss of antiviral potency. Susceptible contacts should be given VZIG when the exposure to varicella-zoster virus has been within the previous 10 days. There is no evidence from the UK data using UK-derived VZIG that administration within 72 hours of contact improves outcome. The administration of VZIG can therefore wait (in most cases) until the results of varicella antibody testing has confirmed the desirability of its use. Patients receiving VZIG may undergo subclinical infection (15%), the infection can be aborted or attenuated or the illness may not be modified (25%). As the incubation period can be delayed after the use of VZIG, a careful watch over contacts for the possible development of chickenpox is required.

Cytomegalovirus

Babies may acquire cytomegalovirus (CMV) transplacentally, from breast milk or from blood products. Premature compromised babies may develop pneumonitis.

Prevention Use CMV-negative blood products and/or white cell filters. If there is accidental exposure to CMV-positive products, consider giving CMV hyperimmune globulin.

Treatment Treat only proven CMV pneumonitis. Ganciclovir (with or without CMV hyperimmune globulin) is probably better than foscarnet.

Enteroviruses

These include coxsackievirus, echovirus and poliovirus. They can cause a wide spectrum of clinical illness. Coxsackieviruses may be particularly dangerous, causing myocarditis, meningoencephalitis and hepatitis. The source of infection is most commonly the mother with a flu-like viral illness in the week preceding delivery. Post-natal transmission leading to outbreaks has also been described. Specimens for viral culture should be sent—CSF, throat swab and stool are the most useful. Note—in seriously immunocompromised neonates, vaccine strain poliovirus may theoretically cause problems. Therefore inactivated polio vaccine (IPV) is used in babies who are going to be staying in the unit.

Enteric viruses See section on gastroenteritis (above) and Chapter 6.

3

THE CHILD WITH AN UPPER RESPIRATORY TRACT INFECTION

The upper respiratory tract consists of the ears, nose, throat, tonsils, pharynx and sinuses. Upper respiratory tract infections (URTI) are common at all ages, and especially in young children. Many of these are minor and self-limiting, but they may also be associated with considerable morbidity, for example the association between URTI and febrile convulsions or wheezy illness. Some of these infections are life-threatening because of upper airway obstruction, for example epiglottitis or diphtheria.

Most children have several URTIs each year in their first decade. Preschool children attending day care are likely to have more frequent infections than those remaining in the home, particularly in the absence of older siblings. When there is a history of very frequent infections, particularly otitis media and sinusitis, immunoglobulin deficiency should be considered. The most likely is an IgA or IgG subclass deficiency (see Chapter 16).

COMMON COLD (ACUTE CORYZA)

Organisms Rhinovirus, adenovirus, coronavirus, respiratory syncytial virus (RSV).

Incubation period Adenovirus 10–14 days; rhinovirus 2–4 days; coronavirus 2–4 days; RSV 2–8 days.

Transmission Direct droplet spread, faeco–oral transmission.

Clinical features Fever, rhinorrhea, sneezing, cough. Poor feeding, especially if nose blocked.

Management is symptomatic; give antipyretics. Some small infants with a troublesome blocked nose will benefit from gentle cleaning of the nose and saline nose drops. Some infants may benefit from a *short* course of decongestant drops.

PHARYNGITIS AND TONSILLITIS

Organisms Adenovirus, enterovirus, group A beta-haemolytic streptococcus, Epstein–Barr virus, *Corynebacterium diphtheriae*.

Clinical features and natural history Fever, sore throat, cervical lymphadenopathy and tonsillar enlargement are seen. It is impossible to distinguish viral infection from bacterial infection clinically—there may be fever and exudative tonsillitis in both. Adenoviral infection is more likely in children less than 3 years old. In some children with already enlarged tonsils, acute infection may cause severe upper airway obstruction. Diphtheria is rare in the more affluent areas of the world because of routine immunization but may still occur. There have been recent outbreaks in what was the USSR (see Chapter 46). Consider this diagnosis in an unimmunized individual who presents with a sore throat and a spreading, grey adherent membrane over the tonsils and pharynx.

Management Children with streptococcal infection should receive antibiotic treatment to relieve symptoms and because of the risk, albeit extremely low, of immune complex disease associated with group A beta-haemolytic streptococcus (glomerulonephritis, rheumatic fever). However most children who develop post-streptococcal glomerulonephritis do not receive medical attention at the time of their initial infection, and the dramatic decline in the incidence of rheumatic fever is not closely related to antibiotic usage. To avoid unnecessary prescriptions of antibiotics the clinician should attempt to decide whether a child has viral or bacterial meningitis with the help of a throat swab if necessary. The antibiotic of choice is penicillin (erythromycin in individuals allergic to penicillin) and must be given for 10 days to minimize the risk of relapse. There is usually a rapid clinical response in children with bacterial infection; those with viral infection continue to have symptoms and fever. Occasionally, severe tonsillar obstruction will require management with a nasopharyngeal airway.

PERITONSILLAR ABSCESS (QUINSY)

Peritonsillar abscess is more common in adolescents and young adults than in young children. It follows severe tonsillitis and causes a very sore throat, severe dysphagia and asymmetrical tonsillar swelling. The treatment is surgical drainage with intravenous antibiotics and subsequent tonsillectomy.

RETROPHARYNGEAL ABSCESS

Retropharyngeal abscess is an unusual condition following bacterial pharyngitis in young infants. There is stridor, fever, drooling, swelling of the neck and lymphadenopathy. This requires surgical drainage and penicillin.

OTITIS MEDIA

Organisms Adenovirus, *Streptococcus pneumoniae*, *Haemophilus influenzae*, group B streptococci, *Moraxella catarrhalis* (previously *Branhamella*), anaerobes such as *Fusobacterium* sp., influenza and parainfluenza viruses.

Clinical features include fever, vomiting, irritability and inconsolable crying. Older children can localize pain to their ears or complain of deafness and dizziness. It is important to examine carefully the ears of all ill children. The eardrum becomes acutely inflamed and may bulge; there is a loss of the normal light reflex. Acute perforation may occur—this often relieves the pain. Recurrent otitis media may lead to 'glue ear' with hearing loss.

Management Relieve pain and fever. Antibiotics are commonly used although many of these infections are viral. (There is considerable controversy about the role of infection in chronic otitis media with effusion.) In older children penicillin may be appropriate because of the incidence of pneumococcal infection, but most paediatricians would use a broad spectrum antibiotic such as amoxycillin, co-amoxiclar or a macrolide, particularly in children less than 3 years old. Myringotomy, with or without grommett insertion, is usually only recommended for children with persistent fluid in the middle ear after a period of close follow-up.

SINUSITIS

The maxillary sinuses increase in size from birth and are usually visible on X-ray between the ages of 2 years and 4 years, by which time the sphenoidal sinuses have also developed. Frontal sinuses are usually not involved in acute infection until school age.

Organisms *Streptococcus pneumoniae*, *Haemophilus influenzae*, *S. pyogenes* (group A streptococci), *Staphylococcus aureus*.

Clinical features Fever, headache, pain and localized tenderness are found. Complications include orbital cellulitis and very rarely intracranial spread (subdural empyema).

Management Give broad-spectrum antibiotics such as co-amoxiclav or a macrolide. Consider the possibility of intracranial spread if severe headaches develop and *always* in the presence of neurological abnormality—computed tomographic (CT) scanning is needed.

ACUTE LARYNGOTRACHEOBRONCHITIS (CROUP)

Croup is a very common condition of young children, most frequently occurring between the ages of 6 months and 4 years.

Organisms Parainfluenza and influenza viruses, respiratory syncytial virus, rhinovirus.

Clinical features In many instances the disease is mild. Following coryzal symptoms a characteristic harsh, barking cough develops, which is typically worse at night or when the child is upset. The symptoms are intermittent and are improved at rest, and the child looks pink, is well perfused and able to drink fluids. In more severe cases there may be increasingly severe respiratory difficulty with chest wall retraction, tachypnoea, tachycardia, agitation and hypoxia.

Management Most children can be managed at home with antipyretics and fluids, but parents should be asked to seek help if the child becomes increasingly distressed and agitated. There is often concern that a child with severe croup may have epiglottitis; it is usually easy to differentiate clinically between the two conditions, but if the croup is very severe the management will be the same—intubation under controlled anaesthetic conditions. The child should be admitted to hospital for careful observation, particularly of the child's colour, respiratory rate, heart rate and chest wall movement. Keep the parent close to the child. Make sure that the nursing staff have clear guidelines as to when to call for medical help. Review the child frequently if there is deterioration. Do not attempt to examine the throat because of the possibility of inducing respiratory obstruction. Pulse oximetry is helpful and non-invasive. Give oxygen as necessary. Although there are anecdotal reports about the value of humidity in this condition, frightening children by placing them in a mist tent is counterproductive. A child who is very agitated and thrashing around is likely to be hypoxic: give oxygen. If the child is deteriorating, becoming hypoxic or extremely agitated, contact an anaesthetist. Each hospital should have guidelines as to which senior medical staff are to be called to a child with an upper airway obstruction. In some hospitals the ear, nose and throat (ENT) surgeon is also called. The child with croup may respond to nebulized adrenaline, 3–5 ml of 1 in 1000 solution, given through oxygen. This effect may last for 20–40 minutes. This should not be used regularly, but is appropriate to 'buy time' while transferring the child to the intensive care unit.

Some studies have shown benefit from the use of steroids in croup and it seems reasonable to use them in severe croup. A suitable dose is 0.6 mg/kg dexamethasone by intramuscular injection as a single dose and then prednisolone 1 mg/kg via nasogastric tube every 12 hours until 24 hours after the child is extubated.

ACUTE EPIGLOTTITIS

Acute epiglottitis is a septicaemic illness caused almost always by *Haemophilus influenzae* type b, producing inflammation and swelling of the epiglottis and subsequent respiratory obstruction. Other organisms occasionally implicated are pneumococcus and *Staphylococcus aureus*.

Clinical features There is acute onset of fever and sore throat. The child may have a muffled voice and drool because of difficulty in swallowing and appear unwell, toxic and lethargic. Stridor is quiet. There may be marked tachycardia but the child may be breathing slowly and carefully. Patients adopt a position that is most comfortable for themselves—often leaning forward. Epiglottitis is a medical emergency as the swollen epiglottis may rapidly produce severe airway obstruction.

Management Keep the child calm with the parents while arranging urgent anaesthetic help and intubation. An experienced anaesthetist and ENT surgeon are essential in case the child requires an emergency tracheostomy because of failed intubation (fortunately rare). Do *not* attempt to examine the throat, take blood or insert a cannula—this should be done once the airway is secured by intubation. There is *no* place for lateral X-ray of neck in the diagnosis of acute upper airway obstruction. Treat with intravenous antibiotic: ceftriaxone or cefotaxime. Recovery is usually rapid and the child may be extubated within 24 hours.

BACTERIAL TRACHEITIS

Organisms *Staphylococcus aureus*, *Haemophilus influenzae* type b.

Clinical features Bacterial tracheitis may complicate laryngotracheobronchitis or may occur as a primary infection. Children with Down's syndrome are especially at risk. The disease presents like severe croup, but with fever and rapidly progressive airway obstruction. Intubation and intravenous antibiotic therapy are required.

FURTHER READING

Kilham HA & McEniery JA (1991) Acute upper airways obstruction. *Current Paediatrics* **1**: 17–25.

Tibballs J, Shann FA & Landau L (1992) Placebo controlled trial of prednisolone in children intubated for croup. *Lancet* **340**: 745–748.

4

THE CHILD WITH A LOWER RESPIRATORY TRACT INFECTION

EPIDEMIOLOGY

The respiratory tract is the most common site of childhood infections, and acute respiratory infections make up 50% of all illnesses in children under 5 years old. Most involve only the upper respiratory tract but about 5% will involve the larynx and lower respiratory tract and may be more serious. Lower respiratory tract illnesses (LRTI) are most common in the first year of life. The incidence of about 20–25 episodes per 1000 children per year over the first 2 years of life decreases with age to around 5 per 1000 children per year in children aged 9–15 years. During the first decade LRTIs occur more commonly in boys but thereafter the rates are similar between the sexes. Hospitalization rates vary considerably, but it has been estimated that 1 in 20 children will be hospitalized because of respiratory infection during the first 4 years of life. Lower respiratory tract infections show marked and unexplained seasonal variations, being most common in the coldest months. This is particularly striking for the annual winter–spring epidemics of bronchiolitis and pneumonia due to respiratory syncytial virus in infants.

PATHOGENESIS

Lower respiratory tract infections develop by two routes. Most agents (respiratory viruses, *Mycoplasma pneumoniae*, *Bordetella pertussis* and *Chlamydia trachomatis*) produce infection by initial involvement of airway epithelium with progression into the parenchyma. In contrast, others—bacteria and viruses such as Epstein–Barr virus (EBV), cytomegalovirus (CMV) and varicella-zoster virus (VZV)—spread from the blood stream into the parenchyma and airways. The development and localization of disease in LRTI then depends on a complex interaction between the organism, host and environmental factors (Table 4.1).

While respiratory viral infections can involve more than one site, inflammation usually predominates at a single site. Certain organisms have affinities for particular parts of the respiratory tract, for example respiratory syncytial virus (RSV) for peripheral airways, for reasons that are not well understood at present. In most circumstances, viruses are only isolated from the respiratory tract during an acute infection. Commonly, one virus tends to predominate in a community at any particular time.

Table 4.1 Risk factors for lower respiratory tract infections in children

Host factors	Environment
Age Sex Low birth-weight Neonatal lung injury Congenital malformation Bottle-feeding Obesity	Passive and active smoking Exposure to infection via siblings Domestic overcrowding Day care Low socioeconomic status Atmospheric pollution

ORGANISMS

The spectrum of organisms that cause LRTIs is wide (Table 4.2) and varies with age. In the newborn, pneumonia is usually due to organisms acquired from the mother's genital tract before or during delivery, e.g. group B streptococci, Gram-negative bacteria, *Listeria monocytogenes*, *Chlamydia trachomatis*, *Mycoplasma hominis*, *Ureaplasma urealyticum*, CMV and herpes simplex virus. After the first month, over 90% of respiratory infections are due to viruses (RSV, parainfluenza and influenza viruses, adenoviruses, rhinoviruses) or *Mycoplasma pneumoniae*. *Mycoplasma* infection rarely occurs before the age of 3 months, and is most common in schoolchildren. Bacterial infections, particularly *Streptococcus pneumoniae* and *Haemophilus influenzae*, causing LRTIs are thought to be uncommon in developed countries. However, the relative importance of these organisms has been difficult to evaluate because of the high carriage rates in the upper respiratory tract found in normal children. Other causes of bacterial pneumonia, e.g. *Staphylococcus aureus*, are uncommon.

Bacterial superinfection during respiratory viral or *Mycoplasma* infections is uncommon in normal children. There are some well-recognized associations between viruses and bacterial infection, e.g. influenza and staphylococcal pneumonia, which are not understood. Double viral infections do occur but seem to be uncommon. If they occur they are often serious, e.g. measles and adenovirus. The importance of host factors such as malnutrition or vitamin A deficiency in superinfection or double infections is not known. Often the specific aetiology of an LRTI cannot be determined, even in retrospect. Developments in microbial diagnostic technology, particularly techniques based on nucleic acid technology such as the polymerase chain reaction, are increasing the proportion of respiratory infections that can be identified definitively.

CLINICAL PRESENTATION AND DIAGNOSIS

The clinical features of LRTIs can include cough with tachypnoea, indrawing, wheeze or stridor. There are well-defined clinical syndromes (Table 4.3) and these clinical patterns are helpful in narrowing the range of likely infectious agents. In infants, clinical features of pneumonia are often non-specific and include fever (> 38.5 °C), refusal to breast-feed and vomiting. At 1–4 years fever (> 38.5 °C) and tachypnoea (respiratory rate >60/min) may occur. Bronchial breathing or reduced breath sounds have been found to be very specific but insensitive indicators of pneumonia.

Definitive diagnosis of pneumonia requires radiological evidence of pulmonary inflammation. Chest radiography is indicated in children with fever and pulmonary findings such as tachypnoea, respiratory distress, decreased breath sounds or bronchial breathing. In the newborn and young infant respiratory signs may be minimal and only non-specific symptoms such as apnoea, anorexia, lethargy or vomiting may be present. In infancy, chest X-rays in the absence of signs are rarely positive. Radiographic changes in pneumonia are not accurate in distinguishing between bacterial and non-bacterial causes. Lobar or segmental consolidation is characteristic of bacterial pneumonia, but bronchopneumonia and interstitial infiltrates can occur in bacterial pneumonia as can alveolar infiltrates in viral pneumonia. An exception is a large pleural effusion where a bacterial origin is likely. In children with immunological deficiency or cardiorespiratory disease, the signs of LRTI may be less obvious and a higher index of suspicion is needed. For

Table 4.2 Relative frequency of organisms causing community-acquired pneumonia in otherwise healthy children

Age group	Frequency		
	Most common	**Occasional causes**	**Rare causes**
NEONATES (< 1 month)	Group B streptococci (typeable) *E. coli* Respiratory viruses Enteroviruses	*Haemophilus influenzae* *Streptococcus pneumoniae* Group A streptococci *Staphylococcus aureus* Varicella-zoster virus CMV Herpes simplex virus	*Mycobacteria* (mostly *M. tuberculosis*) Chlamydia spp. *Listeria monocytogenes*
YOUNG INFANTS (1–3 months) Febrile	Respiratory viruses Enteroviruses	Group B streptococci *Haemophilus influenzae* (type B) *Streptococcus pneumoniae* Group A streptococci *Bordetella pertussis* CMV *Urealyticum* *Pneumocystis carinii*	Varicella CMV Mycobacteria (mostly *M. tuberculosis*) Gram-positive enteric bacilli
Afebrile	*Chlamydia*	CMV *Ureaplasma* *Pneumocystis carinii*	Mycobacteria (mostly *M. tuberculosis*)

INFANTS AND YOUNG CHILDREN (3 months to 5 years)	*Haemophilus influenzae* type b *Streptococcus pneumoniae* Respiratory viruses	*Bordetella pertussis* *Staphylococcus aureus* Group A streptococci *Mycoplasma pneumonia*	Mycobacteria (mostly *M. tuberculosis*)
OLDER CHILDREN (>5 years) AND ADOLESCENTS	*Mycoplasma pneumonia* *Streptococcus pneumoniae* Respiratory viruses	*Staphylococcus aureus* *Chlamydia pneumoniae* Mycobacteria (mostly *M. tuberculosis*)	

Modified from Gilsdorf (1987) *Seminars in Respiratory Infection* 2: 146–151.

Table 4.3 Lower respiratory tract infection syndromes and their clinical features

Syndrome	Presenting symptoms and signs
Croup	Hoarseness, cough, inspiratory stridor with laryngeal obstruction (see Chapter 3)
Tracheobronchitis	Cough and rhonchi; no laryngeal obstruction or wheezing
Bronchiolitis	Expiratory wheezing with or without tachypnoea, air trapping and indrawing
Pneumonia	Crackles or evidence of pulmonary consolidation on physical examination or chest X-ray

organisms entering via the respiratory tract, airway epithelial cells, sampled usually from the nasopharynx, provide excellent material for diagnosis. Viral isolation from the upper respiratory tract usually correlates with lower respiratory tract involvement. Rapid, sensitive and specific immunofluorescence tests are available for many viruses—most notably RSV, parainfluenza and influenza—and are increasingly replacing serology and viral culture. Newer molecular diagnostic tests may offer even greater sensitivity.

Unfortunately, it is often difficult to distinguish between viral and bacterial infections on the basis of clinical, haematological or radiological findings. Definite diagnosis of bacterial infections remains difficult. Some non-specific tests may be useful. There may be a polymorph leucocytosis. Levels of C-reactive protein are more commonly raised in bacterial infections. Cold agglutinins frequently occur in *Mycoplasma pneumoniae* infections, especially with more severe pulmonary involvement. Young children do not usually produce sputum. Culture of pharyngeal swabs is an unreliable substitute because symptomless nasopharyngeal colonization with *Streptococcus pneumoniae* and *Haemophilus influenzae* occurs, particularly in preschool children. Needle aspiration of the lung is regarded as the 'gold standard' for defining bacterial lung infection but is not used frequently in developed countries. Studies using this technique have shown that blood cultures may be positive in as few as 10% of cases. Rapid bacterial antigen detection tests have not proved particularly helpful in clinical practice. In the severely ill or immunocompromised child, more invasive procedures such as bronchoscopy with bronchoalveolar lavage or lung biopsy may be essential to guide therapy. Where positive, culture of blood or aspirated pleural fluid, if present, may confirm bacterial infection.

Special problems The lung is the most common site of serious infection in immunocompromised children. These children are prone to infection particularly when the absolute neutrophil count falls below 500/mm^3. The risk increases with both the severity and duration of neutropenia including those with HIV infection. Neutropenia longer than 2 weeks duration is associated with a high incidence of nosocomial bacterial and/or fungal infections. The array of potential pathogens is wide. Mortality is high. Invasive procedures may be necessary to arrive at a diagnosis.

Children with congenital or acquired immune deficiency including HIV are susceptible to opportunistic pneumonias.

Children with mucous clearance disorders, particularly cystic fibrosis, are also prone to recurrent respiratory infections. In cystic fibrosis, the presence of Gram-negative organisms such as *Pseudomonas aeruginosa* and *Burkholderia cepacia* often make antibiotic treatment more difficult.

MANAGEMENT

Treatment Treatment is most satisfactory when the causative agent is known and a specific and effective medication, if available, can be given.

Respiratory viruses and *M. pneumoniae* cause most cases of tracheobronchitis, bronchiolitis and croup. Symptomatic *M. pneumoniae* infections are uncommon in children under 5 years. Accordingly, antibiotics will not be indicated in most children under 5 especially where confirmation of viral infection can be obtained by rapid diagnostic techniques.

Treatment of RSV infection with nebulized ribavirin has usually been reserved for those at high risk of severe disease or where prolonged illness might worsen an underlying chronic disease (see Chapter 83).

In pneumonia, because of the difficulty of differentiating bacterial from viral infection antibiotics should be prescribed, particularly for the very young or very sick. The initial choice of antibiotic is determined by the child's age and the likely pathogen, guided by knowledge of local microbial sensitivities. Therapy should reviewed later to take account of clinical progress and bacteriological sensitivities.

Supportive care and hospitalization Most children with LRTIs are managed in the community. Supportive care and antibiotics, where indicated, will be all that is required. Only about 10% will be admitted to hospital. In young children especially, this is usually needed because of respiratory distress, severe systemic features or difficulty in feeding. In these more serious cases a number of specific points should be remembered, as follows.

Maintain an adequate airway and ensure oxygenation Hypoxaemia is common. Excessive handling and unnecessary disturbance aggravate this and should be avoided. The development of non-invasive monitors has allowed oxygen saturation to be monitored routinely. Low-flow oxygen administered via nasal cannulae will often be sufficient to maintain the oxygen saturation in the normal range (above 95%). In about 5% of children with severe croup intubation is needed to maintain an adequate airway. About 1–2% of infants with severe bronchiolitis will develop respiratory failure and need mechanical ventilation.

Maintain hydration and nutrition Children with severe LRTIs often have difficulty feeding. Nasogastric or intravenous fluids may be necessary to avoid dehydration and maintain nutrition. Children with pneumonia and bronchiolitis can develop inappropriate antidiuretic hormone secretion and mild fluid restriction is usually advisable.

Clear nasal secretions and encourage sputum clearance Gentle suction clearance of nasal secretions may increase comfort and aid feeding in infants. There is no evidence that physiotherapy is helpful in children with bronchiolitis or pneumonia, but it may have an important role in those children where sputum clearance is impaired.

Drain pleural fluid When pleural fluid is present, it may be useful to aspirate the fluid for diagnostic purposes. Therapeutic aspiration may only be necessary if breathing is compromised or if the clinical response to antibiotic treatment is poor. Predrainage localization of the fluid and selection of the optimal site for drainage using ultrasound or computed tomographic scan can be helpful. Adequate sedation and analgesia will be necessary for safe and painless drainage, especially in infants and young children.

Hospital cross-infection Many respiratory infections are highly contagious. Hospital-acquired respiratory infections are common, spread either by droplets (influenza) or by fomites (RSV). Cross-infection rates of up 25% with RSV infection have been noted in children in hospital for more than 7 days during winter epidemics. Such infections can be associated with significant morbidity and mortality in high-risk infants with immune suppression or cardiorespiratory disease. Effective cross-infection procedures can reduce this rate substantially.

Follow-up For children with pneumonia, careful clinical follow-up to check that the child is better and signs have resolved is all that is necessary in uncomplicated cases. Further chest X-rays do not appear necessary if clinical resolution is occurring. In any child with an unusual, persistent or recurrent pneumonia an underlying disorder such as immune deficiency, cystic fibrosis or a congenital lung disorder should be excluded.

OUTCOME

In developed countries, most LRTIs in children will resolve satisfactorily with appropriate treatment. However, LRTIs remain an important cause of death in childhood. A few LRTIs, particularly with specific karyotypes of adenovirus, can cause lasting structural damage to the lung. The longer-term outcome of LTRI remains controversial. A year after pneumonia, it has been found that children still have residual lung scan defects. Children with past respiratory illnesses show evidence of airways obstruction in later childhood. Young adults with a history of LRTI in the first 2 years of life have an increased incidence of chronic cough. Cohorts with a high infant mortality from respiratory infection continue to show high death rates from chronic bronchitis years later. One study showed a strong association between pneumonia during the first two years of life and reduced lung function in 70 year old men. However, recent prospective studies have found that pre-LRTI lung function is lower in children with wheezing LRTIs. It is not yet clear whether lower lung function predispose to or is a consequence of LRTI.

Prevention Since the immature and rapidly growing lung may be particularly sensitive to permanent injury the prevention and/or improved therapy of LRTIs in early childhood may be vital for pulmonary health in later life. Social and environmental determinants of LRTIs should be minimized. Breast feeding and the high uptake of childhood immunization for pertussis and measles should be encouraged. Influenza vaccination especially for those with chronic respiratory illness should be arranged. Vaccine developments such as highly immunogenic (conjugated) pneumococcal vaccines may further reduce the incidence of LRTIs.

Where vaccination is not available, immuno-prophylaxis may have a role. High titre RSV immune globulin given monthly has been shown to prevent lower respiratory tract infection in high risk infants and children.

While more effective therapies particularly for viral infections need to be developed one simple measure that would have a substantial impact is a reduction in parental smoking.

FURTHER READING

Loughlin GM & Eigen H, eds (1994) *Respiratory Disease in Children: Diagnosis and Management*. Williams & Wilkins, Baltimore.

Chernick V & Kendig EL, eds (1990) *Disorders of the Respiratory Tract in Children* (5th edn). WB Saunders, Philadelphia.

5

THE CHILD WITH A BONE OR JOINT INFECTION

Acute osteomyelitis, an infection of the bone, usually arises by haematogenous spread of bacteria, most commonly in the metaphyseal region of one of the larger bones. It may spread to involve the adjacent joint giving rise to an accompanying pyogenic arthritis. Rarely it may be multifocal. Up to 10% of cases arise by direct extension from an adjacent infected focus or from a penetrating injury. Acute pyogenic arthritis may occur as an extension of osteomyelitis or may arise by haematogenous spread without any overt signs of bony involvement. Most cases are monoarticular (usually hip, knee, ankle or elbow), but in about 10% of cases several joints are affected.

AETIOLOGY

The majority (approximately 80%) of acute bone and joint infections are caused by *Staphylococcus aureus*. The primary focus of staphylococcal infection leading to bacteraemia is usually not evident. In children under 5 years old. *Haemophilus influenzae* type b (Hib) is also an important cause of septic arthritis which has diminished in frequency since the introduction of the Hib vaccination programme. Gram-negative bacilli (particularly *Salmonella* species), *Streptococcus pyogenes* and *Streptococcus pneumoniae* are other important causes. Gram-negative bacilli are more likely to be the cause in compromised individuals such as neonates, those with immune deficiency or sickle-cell diseases. Group B streptococcus is another important neonatal cause (see Chapters 2 and 91). *Neisseria gonorrhoeae* can cause pyogenic arthritis, particularly when perinatally acquired. *N. menigitidis* can cause both infective or reactive arthritis.

CLINICAL FEATURES

In acute cases there is usually a short history (< 24 hours), the child appears ill and is feverish. There is a refusal to move the affected limb or to bear weight on an affected leg. In osteomyelitis there is usually swelling overlying the bone, and tenderness. In pyogenic arthritis the affected joint is hot, swollen and tender. In subacute or chronic osteomyelitis the child appears less ill and may not be febrile, and the local signs are less acute.

DIAGNOSIS

In most acute cases the diagnosis can be made clinically. Orthopaedic surgeons should be involved at an early stage and ideally the child's management should be jointly supervised by the paediatric and orthopaedic teams. In the case of the hip joint, the serious implications of a missed diagnosis make management of suspected arthritis in this joint a matter of urgency. Investigations will show elevations of white cell count, erythrocyte sedimentation rate (ESR) and C-reactive protein (CRP) level (the last two are useful in monitoring response to treatment). Radiographs initially show no bony changes but may show soft tissue swelling and joint effusions (bone changes such as periosteal reaction and areas of rarefaction take at least 10 days to develop). If there is doubt, an isotope bone scan will confirm an inflammatory process in joint or bone. Blood cultures (multiple if possible) should be taken and are positive in approximately 40% of cases of pyogenic arthritis and 60% of cases of acute osteomyelitis. In septic arthritis, microscopy and culture of aspirated joint fluid and (when appropriate) tests for Hib and *Streptococcus pneumoniae* antigens in urine or joint fluid may increase the diagnostic rate. Tests for anti-staphlococcal antibody are generally disappointing in children.

The differential diagnosis of osteomyelitis will include trauma (consider non-accidental injury) and malignancies such as leukaemia, neuroblastoma or osteosarcoma. In acute monoarthritis the differential diagnosis includes reactive arthritis which may follow a viral, bacterial or mycoplasmal infection; non-pyogenic infections such as tuberculosis; haemarthrosis; vasculitis such as Henoch–Schönlein purpura (arthritis may precede onset of the rash); juvenile chronic arthritis or malignancy. A subacute onset or multiple joint involvement may help distinguish these, but if in doubt a diagnostic tap may be required. If the child has an underlying disorder the infecting organism may be unusual; in these cases primary surgical exploration is usually indicated.

MANAGEMENT

The mainstay of treatment is appropriate antibiotic therapy with or without surgical intervention. In pyogenic arthritis drainage of the joint should always be performed and at the same time the joint space is usually washed out. This is both therapeutically and diagnostically useful. Needle aspiration is usually performed, but particularly in the case of the hip joint or if the effusion recurs, open drainage may be needed. In acute osteomyelitis with a short history, no bony changes on radiographs and no underlying diseases, it is reasonable to treat empirically with antibiotics with surgical exploration reserved for cases which fail to respond clinically or develop complications.

Initial antibiotic treatment should be given intravenously in high dosage. Empirical treatment before culture results are available can be given with flucloxacillin and ampicillin in the child over 6 years old, or flucloxacillin and cefotaxime (the latter to cover β-lactamase-producing *Haemophilus influenzae*) in the child under 6 years old. When culture results are available antibiotics can be modified—the combination of flucloxacillin and sodium fusidate (Fucidin) provides good antistaphylococcal treatment, while ampicillin is used for streptococcal and non-β-lactamase-producing *Haemophilus influenzae* infections. Other antibiotics that may be useful are clindamycin or second-generation cephalosporins. In salmonella osteomyelitis ampicillin, co-trimoxazole or ciprofloxacin may be used depending on the sensitivity of the organism. Intravenous antibiotic therapy should be continued for a minimum of 3 days or until the fever has been settled for 48 hours, whichever is the longer. Thereafter oral antibiotic therapy is continued for 3–4 weeks for septic arthritis or 4–6 weeks for osteomyelitis. Measurement of serum bactericidal levels may be useful in ensuring adequate oral therapy, especially when there is an unusual causative organism or there is evidence of persisting inflammation (e.g. persisting high ESR or CRP). In chronic osteomyelitis prolonged antibiotic treatment as well as surgery is required.

6

THE CHILD WITH DIARRHOEA AND VOMITING

Especially in young children, vomiting and (to a lesser extent) diarrhoea may be non-specific indications that a child is unwell rather than indicating a specific problem with the gastrointestinal tract. Vomiting may indicate obstruction (partial or complete, structural or functional) of the bowel, particularly in the neonate. When assessing a child with diarrhoea and vomiting it is essential to be clear how the terms are being used. 'Diarrhoea' usually means the passage of frequent stools or loose stools. It is best assessed on the basis of a change from the previous pattern for that child. Vomiting must be distinguished from possetting and the bringing up of small quantities of feed when a baby breaks wind. The history should include questions about the duration, frequency and magnitude of the problem as well as taking note of the feeding history and any other features of illness that the child may have. General examination including evidence of weight loss should allow exclusion of causes other than gastroenteritis. Some of the more common causes of diarrhoea and vomiting other than gastrointestinal infection are listed below.

- **Diarrhoea**:
  - systemic infection
  - drugs, especially antibiotics and laxatives
  - lactose or cow's-milk protein intolerance (unusual after infancy)
  - toddler diarrhoea—an otherwise well child with often very loose, frequent stools containing undigested food particles
  - malabsorptive syndromes such as cystic fibrosis and coeliac disease
  - Crohn's disease and ulcerative colitis
  - urinary tract infection
  - appendicitis
  - miscellaneous—haemolytic uraemic syndrome (familial cases), Kawasaki disease, malaria, toxic shock syndrome.
- **Vomiting**:
  - same causes as listed above for diarrhoea
  - intestinal obstruction—especially in the newborn or if vomit is bile-stained. Usually accompanied by lack of passage of stools or meconium. Pyloric stenosis will present in the first 2 months of life. In the older child volvulus and intussusception are possible causes. Appendicitis and a Meckel's diverticulum should be kept in mind at any age
  - central nervous system infections such as meningitis and encephalitis
  - metabolic disorders, for example Reye's syndrome, congenital adrenal hyperplasia and some inborn errors of metabolism
  - miscellaneous—drugs, toxins, periodic syndrome, pregnancy, migraine and cerebral tumours.

GASTROENTERITIS

Gastroenteritis can be defined by the onset, usually acutely, of watery or very loose stools, with or without vomiting, due to an infection of the gastrointestinal tract. Infection or other illness outside the gastrointestinal tract must be excluded (see above).

Epidemiology Gastroenteritis (GE) is still one of the most common causes of childhood mortality. The World Health Organization estimates that approximately 5 million children die each year of gastroenteritis worldwide. In England and Wales there has been a dramatic fall in childhood deaths due to GE, from 300–400 per year in the 1970s, to 25 per year in 1986. However, the hospital admission rate for GE is unchanged since the 1970s (about 15 000 per year), and the incidence of the disease seen in general practice is also unchanged, with around 10% of children affected in the first 2 years of life. Although the illness now seen appears to be clinically less severe than previously, it is still an important cause of childhood mortality and morbidity. There is clear evidence for the protective effect of breast-feeding.

Organisms

Endemic The cause of endemic GE varies around the world. In the UK no pathogen can be isolated from the stools in around 50% of children admitted with gastroenteritis.The main pathogens are shown in Table 6.1.

Food/water-borne Nearly 50 000 cases of food poisoning were notified in England and Wales in 1993. The causative organism can usually be predicted by the incubation period and symptoms (Table 6.2). No cause is found in around half of all cases. Early referral of outbreaks to the consultant in communicable disease control is important.

Foreign travel Malaria must be considered in a child recently returned from abroad with a fever and either vomiting or diarrhoea. Other diagnoses to consider include travellers' diarrhoea (enterotoxigenic *E. coli*), amoebiasis, cholera and helminth infection (if an eosinophilia is present).

Table 6.1 Infective agents causing gastroenteritis in the UK

	Infective agent	No. of cases	Percentage
Viral (73%)	Rotavirus	600	42.3
	Adenovirus	182	12.8
	Astrovirus	155	10.9
	Calicivirus	74	5.2
	SRSV (includes Norwalk virus)	23	1.6
	Corona/Breda virus	3	0.2
Bacterial (19.3%)	*Campylobacter* spp.	94	6.6
	Salmonella spp.	83	5.9
	Shigella spp.	49	3.5
	E. coli	45	3.2
	Plesiomonas spp.	1	0.07
Protozoal (7.7%)	*Giardia lamblia*	18	1.3
	Cryptosporidium parvum	91	6.4

Data for children attending Alder Hey Children's Hospital, Liverpool, UK (1984–87). Other causes include *Yersinia enterocolitica* and *Entamoeba histolytica* (and *Isospora belli* and *Microsporidia* in the immunocompromised).

Table 6.2 Food poisoning: causes and features

Incubation period	Fever	Vomiting	Cause	Clinical features, isolation of cause
< 3 hours	–	+	Chemical	Neurotoxic or histamine-like reaction
1–7 hours	–	++	*Staphylococcus aureus* or *Bacillus cereus* enterotoxin	Isolate toxin in food, vomit or stool
8–14 hours	–	+/–	*Clostridium perfringens* enterotoxin	Isolate toxin in food, vomit or stool
16–36 hours	+	+/–	*Shigella* sp. *Salmonella* sp. *Vibrio parahaemolyticus* Enteroinvasive *E. coli* *Yersinia enterocolitica*	Isolate toxin in food, vomit or stool
12–36 hours	–	–	*Clostridium botulinum*	Botulinism Descending flaccid paralysis
1–7 days	–	+	*Vibrio cholerae* Enterotoxigenic *E. coli* Norwalk virus *Campylobacter* sp.	

Adapted from *Management of Outbreaks of Foodborne Illness*, Department of Health, 1994.
Other infections may be food-borne but do not typically cause gastroenteritis: examples are brucellosis, toxoplasmosis and some other parasitic infestations.

Immunocompromised host Pathogens include cytomegalovirus, *Cryptosporidium parvum*, *Isospora belli*, Microsporidia and atypical mycobacteria. A more interventional approach to diagnosis and treatment may be required, with early referral to a specialist unit.

Pseudomembranous colitis (antibiotic-associated diarrhoea) Various antibiotics (especially ampicillin, erythromycin, clindamycin and co-trimoxazole) can produce colonic overgrowth of toxin-producing *Clostridium difficile*. This cytotoxin produces multiple plaque-like lesions on the mucosal surface. Bloody diarrhoea ensues. The spectrum of severity ranges from mild colitis to toxic megacolon. The diagnosis can be confirmed on finding *C. difficile* toxin in the stool. Treatment consists of replacing the causative antibiotic with oral vancomycin (or metronidazole) for 1 week.

Virulence A number of different mechanisms are involved in the pathogenesis of gastrointestinal infection. Examples include adherence to mucosal surface by fimbrial adhesins, enterotoxin production (for example heat-labile cholera toxin), cytotoxin production (for example the Shiga toxin of *Shigella dysenteriae* type 1) and invasion by *Salmonella* sp.

Clinical features

History Particular note should be made of the presence of bilious vomiting, blood or mucus in diarrhoea, reduced urine output, altered level of consciousness, other affected family members, foreign travel, previous gastrointestinal problems, and medication already received. Viral infections are relatively short-lived (48–72 hours) and are often accompanied by both diarrhoea and vomiting. Respiratory tract symptoms are common, especially in rotavirus infection. In contrast, bacterial infections are mainly associated with diarrhoea and there may be significant systemic upset. Infection with *Campylobacter jejuni* causes an illness of variable severity. Apart from diarrhoea and vomiting, there is often abdominal pain, fever and general malaise. Bloody diarrhoea is common in infections with *Shigella* sp., and young children may have relatively long-lasting febrile convulsions. *Yersinia enterocolitica* may be associated with an abdominal mesenteric adenitis that can be confused with appendicitis.

Examination—plot on growth chart. The most important points are to assess the state of dehydration of the child, and to identify whether there is any other pathology mimicking gastroenteritis. *Dehydration* is a clinical diagnosis (Table 6.3). A recent clinic weight (from the parent-held record) can be useful in assessing fluid loss. Hypernatraemic dehydration can be difficult to assess. The child will usually be drowsy, and other signs of dehydration may be masked.

Management

Children with gastroenteritis die of dehydration. The priority of management is therefore to rehydrate the patient when necessary. Gastrointestinal infections increase the amount of fluid being secreted into the bowel, either through the action of a toxin, or by direct invasion of the mucosa. Rehydration aims to correct those losses. Children who are not clinically dehydrated should continue on their normal diet, and be reassessed if symptoms persist.

Oral rehydration therapy If the child is breast-fed, then the mother should be advised to continue to breast-feed throughout the illness, increasing the length and frequency of breast-feeding. Extra fluids such as oral rehydration solutions

Table 6.3 Clinical assessment of dehydration

Sign	Degree of dehydration		
	< 5%	5–10%	> 10%
Skin	Normal	Loss of turgor	Mottled, cold, with poor capillary return
Fontanelle (if open)	Normal	Depressed	Deeply depressed
Eyes	Normal	Sunken, with reduced intraocular pressure	Sunken, with reduced intraocular pressure
Lips	Moist	Dry	Dry
Peripheral pulses	Normal	Normal	Poor volume and tachycardia
Blood pressure	Normal	Normal	Low
Behaviour	Normal	Lethargic	Prostration, coma
Urine output	Normal	Long periods between micturition	Anuric

Table 6.4 Basic fluid requirements in children

Age	Daily fluid (ml/kg) requirement
Up to 6 months	150
6–12 months	100
1–2 years	80
3–4 years	70
5–8 years	60

(ORS) can be offered if necessary. Any supplemental formula feeds should be stopped. If the child is formula fed, then this should be stopped. Oral rehydration therapy should be given alone for a period of 12–24 hours, the aim being to rehydrate the child in this time. The parents should be warned that although the vomiting and diarrhoea will decrease, they will probably not stop completely. If vomiting is a persistent problem, then very small, frequent feeds (e.g. 20 ml every 20 minutes) is best. A number of commercial ORS are now available (Dioralyte, Rehidrat), and the parents should be instructed how to make them up (the powder is added to a bottle, followed by a measured amount of boiled water and left to cool). The amount given depends on the child. At least the child's maintenance fluid requirements should be given, and the fluid deficit made up. The child should then be given further volumes of ORS with each loose stool. In practice most parents allow their child to drink as much as they want, and this is safe as long as the ORS has been made up correctly.

Intravenous rehydration therapy Children who are shocked (over 10% dehydration) or those vomiting or not taking sufficient oral fluids will need intravenous rehydration therapy (IVRT). The principles of fluid management are:

- Resuscitate.
- Replace deficit.
- Provide daily maintenance.
- Replace ongoing losses.

Resuscitation should be with 20–40 ml/kg of plasma or normal saline. In a shocked child this can be given over 30–60 minutes. More may be needed: assess on the basis of pulse, blood pressure and peripheral perfusion. Replacing deficit requires an estimate of the deficit from a clinical assessment of the child's percentage dehydration:

$$\text{Deficit (ml)} = \text{dehydration(\%)} \times \text{body weight (kg)} \times 10$$

The deficit should usually be replaced over the first 24 hours. Briefly, if the child has a normal serum sodium concentration, use 4% dextrose/0.18% saline. If the serum sodium level is low, then use 0.45% saline. In hypernatraemic dehydration, rehydrate more slowly over 48 hours, using 0.45% or 0.9% saline initially. Potassium chloride should be added in standard amounts, once the child has passed urine. Providing daily maintenance requires a knowledge of basic fluid requirements, which vary with age (Table 6.4). Ongoing deficits should be based on the clinical or measured assessment of continuing fluid loss. In severe secretory diarrhoea (e.g. cholera) this can be massive.

Return to normal diet A gradual return to normal feeds is no longer considered necessary. After 24 hours of oral rehydration therapy the child should go back to normal full-strength milk and solids.

Admission, investigation and treatment

- Admit children:
  - needing IVRT
  - with oliguria (consider haemolytic uraemic syndrome).
  - with a history of severe illness
  - with adverse social circumstances
  - with a doubtful diagnosis.
- Investigations (not warranted in most episodes of mild GE) include:
  - stool microscopy—trophozoites, cysts, spores
  - stool culture/agglutination—*E. coli*, *Salmonella*, *Shigella*, *Campylobacter*
  - stool virology—electron microscopy/ELISA/culture
  - blood culture if child febrile
  - full blood count and electrolytes if child is pale, oliguric or needing IVRT.
- Treatment—There is no place for antiemetics, antidiarrhoeal agents, changing to a different cow's milk preparation or starvation. Antibiotics are needed very rarely. They should be used under the following circumstances:
  - invasive salmonellosis (in children under 6 months old or where the infective organism is *Salmonella typhi* or *S. paratyphi*)
  - shigellosis if the child is toxic and febrile
  - amoebiasis
  - cholera
  - giardiasis
  - severe *Campylobacter* infection
  - gastroenteritis due to *Clostridium difficile* toxin
  - gastroenteritis due to enterotoxigenic *E. coli* (travellers' diarrhoea).

Chronic persistent diarrhoea With rapid introduction of normal feeds, there does not appear to be an increase in temporary food intolerance, which normally occurs in up to 20% of children after GE. All children with GE should be advised to seek further medical advice if the diarrhoea recurs, or persists over 10 days. The stools should then be sent for culture, and tested for the presence of reducing sugars (Clinitest, significant if 1% or greater).

Diagnoses to consider include:

- Lactose intolerance—strongly positive Clinitest (> 2%). Return to ORS, then slowly reintroduce normal formula feed. If lactose intolerance persists, then change to alternative milk (see below).
- Reinfection or persisting infection may indicate immunodeficiency. Consider investigating further (see Chapter 16).
- Cow's-milk protein intolerance is a diagnosis of exclusion without a jejunal biopsy. It gives a clinical picture of continuing diarrhoea and poor weight gain after GE, without either of the above. Treat by changing to an alternative milk (casein/whey hydrolysate) for 3 months.

URINARY TRACT INFECTIONS IN CHILDREN

Urinary tract infections (UTIs) in children are common. There is a paucity of comprehensive and prospective population-based studies on the annual incidence and prevalence. One exception is a Swedish study, which found that the prevalence of UTIs before the age of 11 years was 3% in girls and 1% in boys. This study also showed that the first UTI occurs most commonly during the first year of life. During the first 3 months, the female to male ratio is 0.4. After this there is an increasing female preponderance.

DEFINITION

The definition of a UTI is the presence in an uncontaminated urine sample of more than 10^8 organisms per litre in a symptomatic child. This definition is confounded by a number of problems. The first is that urinary infections may occur with lesser number of organisms. Secondly, based on large population studies it is known that between 1% and 2% of school-age girls and approximately 0.03% of school-age boys have asymptomatic bacteriuria. While asymptomatic bacteriuria can be detected during the first year of life in approximately 0.7% of girls and 2.7% of boys. Thirdly, it is difficult to obtain uncontaminated urine samples from children who are not toilet trained, and significant culture results may be obtained which in fact may represent single organism contamination. Pyuria, although more commonly found in older children with UTIs, may not occur (particularly in the infant), and its absence does not exclude a UTI. In addition, white cell lysis may occur if there is a long delay before the sample is examined microscopically, particularly if it is left at room temperature or if the urine pH is very high.

Obtaining a urine sample A midstream urine specimen or a clean catch specimen is ideal. In sick infants in whom there should be no delay in initiating treatment a suprapubic bladder aspirate should be performed. This is a safe procedure which is easily learned and should be a service provided by paediatric departments. If the suprapubic aspirate fails and the infant is ill enough to warrant antibiotic therapy then a catheter specimen of urine should be obtained immediately after the first dose of antibiotic.

Hollister urine collection bags are widely used; they are applied after the perineum has been washed, the child is held upright and the bag is taken off as soon as a sample is produced. However, contamination rates are high and although a negative culture result is reliable, a positive culture result obtained by this method may not necessarily indicate infection. Repeat urine samples are often needed and results may be confounded if antibiotics have already been started. The use of urine collection bags is best discouraged, certainly within a hospital setting.

Immediate microscopy of a freshly obtained unspun specimen is the 'gold standard' and this can be achieved with basic training. This forms standard practice in some hospital units and general practices. The advantage is that an immediate diagnosis can be made and only those samples where abnormalities are found on microscopy need be sent to the laboratory. The use of a combined dipstick that contains nitrite to detect bacteriuria and leucocyte esterase for the detection of pyuria in freshly collected urine specimens has been found in recent studies to have very low false negative rates and high predictive values. However, there are limitations, as the rare infections caused by *Pseudomonas* or group B streptococci will not be identified, and urine must stay in the bladder for at least an hour for the bacterial conversion of nitrate into nitrite to occur. As yet, this method is not recommended.

There is wide variation in the use of dipslides for urine culture and transport. With this method urine is dropped onto the slide, which is coated in culture medium. The advantage of this method is that urine culture can start when the urine is still fresh, thereby minimizing the proliferation of contaminants. The disadvantage is that urine microscopy is not possible.

If there is going to be a delay in the specimen reaching the laboratory it can be refrigerated for up to 24 hours at 0–4 °C to prevent the proliferation of contaminants.

ORGANISMS

Bacteria giving rise to UTI originate from the bowel flora. In boys there is circumstantial evidence that preputial organisms may be important. There are a number of reports that quote a significantly lower risk of UTI in circumcised boys. This point, however, has not been analysed prospectively. *Escherichia coli* is by far the most common infecting organism, causing between 65% and 85% of infections. Other organisms such as *Proteus* sp., *Klebsiella* sp., other coliforms and enterococcus cause between 1% and 10% of infections. The possibility of urinary calculi should be considered in all children with *Proteus* urinary infection.

CLINICAL PRESENTATION

The modes of presentation of a UTI, especially in younger children and infants, are numerous and very often non-specific. There may be systemic symptoms such as fever, found to be present in an average of 60% of children over 1 year old and in over 80% of children under 1 year old. Other symptoms are vomiting, irritability, jaundice, failure to thrive, screaming, abdominal pain, dysuria and frequency. In children presenting with dysuria and frequency it is important to think of other possible diagnoses such as vulvovaginitis (which may be accompanied by vaginal secretions not seen in a true UTI), threadworms, diabetes and hypercalciuria.

MANAGEMENT

Most children with a UTI are only mildly unwell. For these, treatment with 5–7 days of oral antibiotics is sufficient, although the optimum length of treatment is not known. Most community-acquired infections will respond to trimethoprim. Other suitable antibiotics are nitrofurantoin and nalidixic acid, but these are not suitable for systemically unwell children as significant tissue concentrations are not achieved. In addition, nitrofurantoin is often poorly tolerated, particularly if given in liquid form, as it causes nausea and vomiting. For sensitive organisms amoxycillin can be used for a therapeutic course but bacterial resistance is common, as it is with oral cephalosporins such as cephalexin. The antibacterial therapy should be modified according to the infecting organism sensitivity pattern once this is known. Lack of clinical improvement within 48 hours can be due to inappropriate antibiotic therapy or to underlying urinary obstruction. Single dose therapy with either amoxycillin or trimethoprim has been recommended for girls more than 5 years old with normal urinary tracts.

In acutely sick children and infants, intravenous therapy should be used for at least 48 hours or until improvement occurs. Parenteral cephalosporins such as cefuroxime or cefotaxime are good first-line therapy. Aminoglycosides may be used with careful drug level monitoring but are rarely necessary unless the organism sensitivity pattern dictates. Azlocillin, ceftazidime and ciprofloxacin should be reserved for *Pseudomonas* infections. Some children—particularly infants and neonates—may be severely unwell, with dehydration presenting with signs of shock which may be associated with electrolyte imbalances and renal failure; early detection and correction are crucial. A transient decrease in the kidneys' urine concentrating ability is common in episodes of pyelonephritis, and an increased water intake during the episode is needed.

Urinary tract abnormalities, vesicoureteric reflux and renal scarring Abnormalities of the urinary tract may be detected on renal imaging of children presenting with UTI. The incidence of these abnormalities varies according to the nature of the studies. Most abnormalities are already present at the time of the first investigation. Obstructive uropathies and neuropathic bladder are specific problems which must be looked for, as there is no doubt that surgical intervention and intermittent catheterization in the latter case can avert deterioration in renal function.

Vesicoureteric reflex (VUR) is found in 20–50% and renal scarring in around 10% of all children with a UTI. The natural history of VUR is one of progressive resolution with age, particularly in cases of mild reflux. Renal scarring is associated with problems during pregnancy such as pre-eclampsia, and if extensive may lead to hypertension and renal failure.

Recommendations from a Royal College of Physicians working party (see Further Reading below) advise renal tract investigation of all children after their first documented UTI regardless of gender or age at the first episode (see Further Reading). The purpose is to exclude obstruction, to identify VUR early and to institute urinary prophylaxis in the hope that renal scarring will be prevented. The working party formulated guidelines for renal tract imaging. Children under 1 year old should have an abdominal radiograph, renal ultrasound scan, micturating cystogram and dimethyl succinic acid (DMSA) scan, the last to be performed 2–3 months after the acute episode. In sick infants an ultrasound scan should be done during the acute illness to look for obstructive uropathies such as posterior urethral valves in boys or pelviureteric junction obstruction in either sex. There was more discrepancy within the working party as to the extent of renal imaging needed in children aged 1–7 years. The consensus view is shown in Table 7.1.

Antibiotic prophylaxis is recommended in young children with VUR, in infants under the age of 6 months and in children with normal urinary tracts but repeated infections. There is no consensus about how long prophylaxis should be given for. It is thought that the risk of renal damage diminishes appreciably after the age of 5 years and prophylaxis is often stopped at this point. However, some clinicians would stop earlier in cases of mild VUR with no renal scarring. In the presence of scarring and persistent VUR some clinicians would continue prophylaxis until puberty. There is considerable variation on this practice point.

Children, usually girls, who suffer with recurrent UTIs associated with bladder instability but otherwise have a normal urinary tract may benefit from antibiotic prophylaxis to prevent symptomatically troublesome infections.

The most commonly used prophylactic antibiotic is trimethoprim and it is well

Table 7.1 Renal imaging after first confirmed urinary tract infection

Age 0–1 year	Age 1–7 years	Older than 7 years
Ultrasound scan Abdominal X-ray* Micturating cystogram (when urine sterile) DMSA scan (3 months post-infection)	Ultrasound scan Abdominal X-ray* DMSA scan Intravenous urogram *If above abnormal* or *acute pyelonephritis* or *family history of VUR* or *reflux nephropathy*: ↓ Micturating cystogram†	Ultrasound scan Abdominal X-ray* *If above abnormal* or *recurrent UTIs*: ↓ DMSA scan or Intravenous urogram†

***This investigation may not add significant information.**
†Considered appropriate by most members of the working group but this was not a consensus view.
Guidelines from a working group of the Royal College of Physicians (see Further Reading).

tolerated. Nitrofurantoin is also used, but the liquid form suitable for infants is poorly tolerated, giving rise to gastrointestinal symptoms, particularly nausea. Amoxycillin, cephalosporins and nalidixic acid are not suitable as bacterial resistance develops and rapidly spreads. In spite of their wide use, the role of antibiotics in preventing renal scarring has not been established in a prospective controlled study. New scar formation or progression of existing scars has been seen regardless of the presence or absence of recurrent infection, although there are many uncontrolled retrospective studies that support an association between infection and scar progression.

Urethral catheterization carries a significant risk of infection. There are a number of reports on the occurrence of a UTI after either micturating cystography or cystoscopy. For this reason it is strongly recommended that antibiotic prophylaxis should be given for 48 hours in full therapeutic dosage at the time these procedures are carried out.

FURTHER READING

Royal College of Physicians (1991) Guidelines for the management of acute urinary tract infection in childhood. Report of a Working Group of the Research Unit, Royal College of Physicians. *Journal of the Royal College of Physicians* **25**: 36–42.

Winberg J, Anderson HJ, Bergstrom T, Jacobsson B, Larson H & Lincoln K (1974) Epidemiology of symptomatic urinary tract infection in childhood. *Acta Paediatrica Scandinavica* (suppl. 252) **63**: 1–20.

Verrier Jones K (1990) Antimicrobial treatment for urinary tract infections. *Archives of Diseases in Childhood* **65**: 327–330.

MANAGEMENT OF SUSPECTED SEXUALLY TRANSMITTED DISEASES IN PREPUBERTAL CHILDREN

There are a number of aspects to be considered when sexually transmitted disease is suspected in a prepubertal child. When should such a disease be suspected? When a potentially sexually transmitted disease (STD) is found in a child, what is the likelihood of this actually being due to sexual activity? If a child is suspected to have been sexually abused, what infections should be sought in the absence of any specific clinical indications? There are no simple answers to any of these questions. For management of individual infections, refer to the appropriate chapters.

WHEN TO SUSPECT A SEXUALLY TRANSMITTED DISEASE

Many young girls have a clear or slightly milky, vaginal discharge without any symptoms. This is usually of no significance and requires no treatment. However if the discharge is purulent, has an offensive odour or is causing symptoms and/or signs in the genital area investigations ought to be carried out to exclude infection. Chlamydial, trichomonal, and gonorrhoeal infection need to be specifically looked for and excluded. Although the presence of a foreign body should always be borne in mind, it is uncommon and an examination under anaesthesia need only be carried out to exclude it if all other diagnoses have been ruled out.

SEXUALLY TRANSMITTED DISEASE AND SEXUAL ABUSE

It has become increasingly apparent that sexual contact is the most common explanation for these diseases when they have not been acquired perinatally. In some, no other explanation should be entertained, whereas in others alternative modes of transmission occasionally occur. Perinatally acquired anogenital warts and chlamydia may not present in the perinatal period. Some authorities suggest that anogenital warts can first appear up to 2 years after birth. Table 8.1 is compiled from a number of sources and is offered as a guide to the significance of some infections which may be sexually transmitted. Wherever sexual abuse is considered possible on the basis of one of these infections, others should be sought. The local social services department must be involved at an early stage.

The overwhelming majority of children (as high as 97% in young children) who have been sexually abused do not develop an STD. However, it is appropriate to look for *Chlamydia*, *Neisseria gonorrhoeae* and *Trichomonas* in all those where genital-to-genital contact is suspected as infection may be asymptomatic. Oral and/or anal gonococcal infection must also be considered where the alleged behaviour puts the child at risk. Remember that screening for STDs should ideally take place 10–21 days following the last incident. Accompanying symptoms or signs may suggest further investigations. When a child has been repeatedly abused by strangers, consideration should be given to testing for other STDs including human immunodeficiency virus (HIV) and hepatitis B. If this is to be done, antibody levels should be measured at presentation and again at 3 months and 6 months after exposure. Testing should not be done without counselling the parents and child.

It is useful to have a standard kit to test for the main STDs (gonorrhoea,

Table 8.1 Infections that may be sexually transmitted

Infection	Incubation period of acquired disease	Modes of transmission	Definitive diagnosis	Probability of abuse
Chlamydia	7–14 days	Intrapartum Sexual contact	ELISA/IFAT Culture*	++ (+ + + if child > 3 years)
Gonorrhoea	3–4 days	Intrapartum Sexual contact	Culture	++ (+ + + if child > 2 years)
Hepatitis B	Up to 3 months	In utero Intrapartum Sexual contact Blood-borne	Serology	+ + +[a]
Herpes simplex	2–14 days	Intrapartum Sexual contact Autoinoculation Direct contact	Culture and EM	++
HIV	Up to 6 months	In utero Intrapartum Sexual contact Blood-borne	Serology	+ + +[a]

Anogenital warts	Up to 2 years	In utero Intrapartum Sexual contact Autoinoculation Direct contact	Clinical	(++ > 2 years)
Syphilis	Up to 3 months	In utero Intrapartum Sexual contact	Serology	+ + +[a]
Trichomonas	1–4 weeks	Intrapartum Sexual contact	Culture and microscopy	+ + +

***Culture is essential in medicolegal cases as there are too many false positives with ELISA.**
ELISA, enzyme-linked immunosorbent assay; EM, electron microscopy; IFAT, immunofluorescent antibody test.
++, abuse likely; + + +, abuse almost certain.
[a]If in utero, intrapartum and blood borne infection can be ruled out by testing the mother and excluding the possibility of blood borne transmission post natally.

chlamydial infection and trichomoniasis) available wherever a child suspected of being abused is likely to be examined. The exact contents of this kit will need to be decided in conjunction with the local microbiology service. A swab and slide for *gonococcus*, a swab in *Trichomonas* medium and the preferred local option for *Chlamydia* would comprise a reasonable basic kit. The specimens should be conveyed to the laboratory as soon as possible after they have been taken. If they are to be used in evidence in court, it is important that the 'chain of evidence' is maintained.

FURTHER READING

Royal College of Physicians (1991) *Physical Signs of Sexual Abuse in Children*. RCP, London.

Hobbs CJ, Hanks HGI & Wynne J (1993) *Child Abuse and Neglect, a Clinicians Handbook*. Churchill Livingstone, Edinburgh.

THE CHILD WITH A CARDIAC INFECTION

Infection of the heart results in endocarditis, myocarditis or pericarditis, but there is overlap between these conditions. Connective tissue diseases can cause cardiac inflammation and mimic infection. Acute rheumatic fever (post-infective) and Kawasaki disease (not a proven infection) have important cardiac sequelae. Cardiac involvement in the acquired immune deficiency syndrome can cause ventricular dysfunction or pericardial effusion. These conditions form part of the differential diagnosis but are not further considered here.

ENDOCARDITIS

Epidemiology and causes Infective endocarditis (IE) is an infection of the endocardium or heart valves. Most affected children have congenital heart disease (CHD). The pathogenesis of endothelial injury and formation of vegetations is related to turbulent and high-velocity blood flow (e.g. aortic stenosis, ventricular septal defect). For this reason IE is very rare in isolated secundum atrial septal defect. The incidence of IE in neonates without CHD is increasing in association with advances in life support and the use of central venous lines. The presence of prosthetic material within the cardiovascular system predisposes to IE.

Gram-positive cocci are commonly responsible (90% where an organism is isolated). Viridans streptococci form the largest group and usually produce a subacute illness. They form part of the normal oral flora; bacteraemia follows mucosal disruption such as dental extraction. Other responsible streptococci are enterococci, pneumococci and beta-haemolytic streptococci. The latter two are associated with a high mortality; pneumococcal IE follows an acute course. Staphylococci (usually *Staphylococcus aureus*) are responsible for 20–30% of cases of IE. *Staphylococcus aureus* is the most likely cause of acute disease in those with previously normal hearts and in injecting drug abusers. The course is often fulminant. There is a rising incidence of *Staphylococcus epidermidis* IE following cardiac surgery; this is the main agent responsible for prosthetic valve endocarditis.

Gram-negative bacteria, Gram-positive bacilli and fungi are uncommon causes of IE and are associated with a high mortality. Rarely, IE is due to anaerobes or *Coxiella burnetii* (Q fever).

Clinical presentation Fever, typically low-grade, is usual. It may be absent in 10% of cases. Non-specific features are common: malaise, anorexia, weight loss and fatigue. Arthralgia or arthritis occurs in a quarter of patients. Chest pain is unusual but may be related to pulmonary embolism. Murmurs are present in 90% of affected children. However, as most children have pre-existing structural heart disease, a new or changing murmur is found in only 25%. Heart failure occurs in a third and is related to valvular regurgitation. Splenomegaly is found in over 50% of patients. It is usually non-tender; but pain and tenderness may indicate splenic infarction or abscess formation. Petechiae of the extremities or mouth are common; splinter haemorrhages, Osler's nodes, Janeway lesions and Roth's spots are not. A variety of embolic neurological defects may present in 20% of patients. In infants, IE is acute and presents as overwhelming sepsis with bacteraemia, cardiac failure and a murmur. Amongst injecting drug abusers with

IE, two-thirds have previously normal hearts, two-thirds have extracardiac sites of infection and in one-third the affected tricuspid valve is regurgitant. Pulmonary complications include infarction, abscess formation and effusions.

Diagnosis Blood cultures are mandatory; ideally four sets in the first 24 hours, followed by a further two sets during the next 24 hours. In 90% of cases, the first two sets will be positive. In fungal endocarditis, blood cultures may be positive only intermittently and the organism is slow to grow. Blood culture-negative IE occurs in 10%, due to: prior antibiotic administration; rickettsial, chlamydial or viral infection; slow-growing or nutritionally variant organisms; anaerobes; non-bacterial thrombotic vegetations; mural endocarditis; right-sided endocarditis or fungal endocarditis (especially *Aspergillus* sp). Measurement of antibodies against *Staphylococcus aureus* may be of value.

Elevation of the erythrocyte sedimentation rate is usual and recovers with successful therapy. Anaemia is present in 40% and, less commonly, haematuria. Echocardiography will detect vegetations in two-thirds of patients; but a 'negative echo' does not exclude vegetations. The transoesophageal modality is more sensitive than the transthoracic. Valvular regurgitation can be detected by echocardiology before it is clinically apparent.

Management Intravenous bactericidal antibiotics are required for 4–6 weeks, except in the case of fully penicillin-sensitive streptococci, when oral amoxycillin may be substituted for benzylpenicillin and gentamicin after 2 weeks. Synergy between agents may produce a rapid bactericidal effect and allow lower doses of each agent. The microbiologist should be closely involved. Therapy can usually be withheld until initial Gram stain or positive blood culture results are available. In seriously ill patients, antibiotics should be started immediately after initial blood cultures have been taken. Benzylpenicillin and an aminoglycoside are recommended. If *Staphylococcus aureus* is suspected, flucloxacillin replaces benzylpenicillin. If the disease follows recent cardiac surgery, vancomycin can be used as hospital-acquired *Staphylococcus epidermidis* or *S. aureus* infection is likely.

There should be clinical improvement within a few days. Daily physical examination should concentrate on the detection of embolic phenomena and valvular regurgitation, implying progression of local disease. The success of treatment can be monitored by measurement of C-reactive protein. Initially, daily electrocardiography will allow detection of arrhythmias and conduction defects. Echocardiography should be performed at least weekly. Surgical intervention is indicated for acute valvular destruction, removal of infected prosthetic material, large, mobile left-sided vegetations and persistent or recurrent infection.

Prevention of further cases Good dental hygiene is essential to reduce the risk of IE. Antibacterial prophylaxis is required for any procedure that induces a bacteraemia in patients with a structurally abnormal heart, whether congenital or acquired, native or operated. Patients who have had successful surgical ligation or transcatheter occlusion of patent ductus arteriosus and those who have undergone direct suture repair of secundum atrial septal defect no longer require prophylaxis after 6 months have elapsed. Recommendations for prevention of IE in children with heart disorders are given in Table 9.1.

MYOCARDITIS

Epidemiology and causes Most cases of myocarditis are related to viral infection, most commonly coxsackie B viruses. They are usually sporadic, although epidemics may occur. Spread is by the faeco–oral route or by droplet infection; intrauterine infection may occur in late pregnancy. Less common causes include coxsackie A, ECHO, rubella, herpes simplex and varicella-zoster viruses.

Clinical presentation is variable but can be fulminant in infants. There may be a history suggestive of recent viral illness. There are signs of reduced cardiac output with cool periphery and pallor. Cardiac failure is common with tachypnoea, tachycardia, a third heart sound and hepatomegaly; less common is an apical pansystolic murmur of mitral regurgitation.

Diagnosis Viruses are infrequently isolated but should be sought in stools, urine, sputum and throat swab. Paired viral sera will diagnose active infection if there is a fourfold increase in antibody titres. Blood cultures are indicated as it may be difficult to distinguish myocarditis from other cardiac infections. Levels of C-reactive protein are usually elevated. Electrocardiographic abnormalities are common and include sinus tachycardia, conduction disturbances (notably complete heart block) and classically, low-voltage QRS with flattened or inverted lateral T waves. Pathological Q waves may indicate severe damage. Echocardiography invariably shows ventricular dilatation with impaired function affecting one or more chambers, and no structural abnormality. Secondary mitral regurgitation may be present. In infants, anomalous origin of the left coronary artery must be positively excluded. Endomyocardial biopsy is not recommended routinely.

Management Cardiac output must be maintained and heart failure treated. Cautious administration of digoxin and diuretics is usual, with captopril a useful adjunct. Inotropic agents are often required and dobutamine with or without dopamine is suitable. Arrhythmias demand effective control; patients with complete heart block should be paced. Hypoxaemia and anaemia need correction. The case for using steroids or other immunosuppressive agents is inconclusive. The prognosis for the newborn is poor but better in older children. Cardiac transplantation may be appropriate for those with persistent, severe ventricular dysfunction.

PERICARDITIS

Epidemiology and causes Causes of pericardial effusion in childhood include Still's disease, Kawasaki disease and viral infection. This section concentrates on the more serious purulent pericarditis which comprises about 90% of cases of acute pericarditis in children under 2 years old. Infection spreads either directly or haematogenously, most commonly from the lungs. The usual organisms are *Staphylococcus aureus*, *Haemophilus influenzae* and pneumococci, but streptococci, meningococci and anaerobes also occur. Tuberculous, fungal and hydatid pericarditis are rare in the UK.

Clinical presentation This diagnosis should be suspected in any septicaemic child who develops cardiomegaly. Patients present with pyrexia, tachycardia and tachypnoea. There may be evidence of pericardial effusion or a friction rub (they may occur together). Older patients may complain of chest pain. Cardiac

Table 9.1 Prevention of endocarditis in children with heart disorders*

Regimen	Dose
Dental procedures* under local or no anaesthesia	
• No penicillin in previous month—oral amoxycillin 1 hour before procedure:	
< 5 years old	750 mg
5–10 years old	1500 mg
> 10 years old	3 g
• If penicillin given in previous month or penicillin-allergic—oral clindamycin 1 hour before procedure:	
< 5 years old	150 mg
5–10 years old	300 mg
> 10 years old	600 mg
If previous endocarditis, add gentamicin to the above	
Dental procedures* under general anaesthesia	
• No penicillin in previous month, no history of endocarditis—amoxycillin:	
< 5 years old	250 mg IV at induction; then 125 mg orally at 6 hours
5–10 years old	500 mg IV at induction; then 250 mg orally at 6 hours
> 10 years old	1 g IV at induction; then 500 mg orally at 6 hours

Special risk group Prosthetic valve or history of endocarditis

- No penicillin in previous month

< 5 years old	amoxycillin 250 mg IV + gentamicin 2 mg/kg IV at induction; then amoxycillin 125 mg orally at 6 hours
5–10 years old	amoxycillin 500 mg IV + gentamicin 2 mg/kg IV at induction; then amoxycillin 250 orally at 6 hours
> 10 years old	amoxycillin 100 mgIV + gentamicin 2 mg/kg IV at induction; then amoxycillin 500 mg orally at 6 hours

- Child is allergic to penicillin, or penicillin given in previous month:

Vancomycin	
All ages	20 mg/kg IV over 100 min; then gentamicin IV 2 mg/kg at induction
OR	
Teicoplanin	
All ages	6 mg/kg IV + gentamicin IV 2 mg/kg at induction
OR	
Clindamycin	
< 5 years old	75 mg IV at induction. Repeated oral/IV 37.5 mg at 6 hours
5–10 years old	150 mg IV at induction. Repeated oral/IV 75 mg at 6 hours
> 10 years	300 mg IV at induction. Repeated oral/IV 150 mg at 6 hours

***Dental procedures that require antibiotic prophylaxis are extractions, scaling and surgery involving gingival tissues. Prophylaxis is indicated for tonsillectomy, adenoidectomy and procedures on the middle ear; it should also be given for genitourinary procedures including bladder catheterization.**

tamponade can develop with even a moderate-sized effusion if accumulation is rapid.

Diagnosis Pericardial effusion is suggested radiologically by a rapidly increasing cardiothoracic ratio without increased pulmonary vascular markings. In over 90% of cases, there is ST segment elevation on the electrocardiogram. Other typical (although non-specific) changes include low-voltage QRS with flattened or inverted T waves (see myocarditis). Echocardiography is a sensitive tool for the detection of pericardial effusion. Blood cultures are positive in most cases. Cerebrospinal fluid culture may be indicated. If pericardiocentesis is performed, microbiological examination of the fluid must include Gram stain, microscopy and culture for bacteria (including *Mycobacterium*), viruses and fungi.

Management Children with purulent pericarditis require urgent drainage, about half for tamponade. Should pericardiocentesis fail, immediate surgical drainage is indicated. Free drainage should be maintained as fluid is likely to reaccumulate. Antibiotic therapy should be tailored to the causative organism. If this is unknown, intravenous flucloxacillin and ampicillin in combination are suitable. If *Haemophilus influenzae* is suspected, cefotaxime should replace ampicillin. In some cases, an aminoglycoside may be added. Intravenous therapy should be continued for 3–4 weeks. As with all of the conditions discussed in this chapter, general supportive measures are very important in sick children; these include oxygen, appropriate volume expansion and inotropic support. If necessary, these should be provided on an intensive care unit. Follow-up for at least a year will be needed to detect constrictive pericarditis, which can develop rapidly.

FURTHER READING

Garson A, Bricker JT & McNamara DG, eds (1990) *The Science and Practice of Pediatric Cardiology*. Lea & Febiger, London.

Longman LP & Martin MV (1993) The prevention of infective endocarditis—paedodontic considerations. British Society for Antimicrobial Chemotherapy. *International Journal of Paediatric Dentistry* **3**: 63–70.

THE CHILD WITH BACTERIAL MENINGITIS

Despite advances in treatment for bacterial meningitis, this condition remains the most important bacterial cause of mortality and morbidity in children in this country.

EPIDEMIOLOGY

The peak ages of incidence are infancy and early childhood. The incidence has fallen in the UK following the introduction of the conjugated vaccine against *Haemophilus influenzae* in 1992. The most common causative organisms at various ages are shown in Table 10.1.

Table 10.1 Common causative organisms of bacterial meningitis

Age of child	Common cause	Empirical antibiotic treatment
0–1 month	Group B streptococcus *Escherichia coli* (usually K1 serotype) *Listeria monocytogenes*	Cefotaxime and ampicillin +/−gentamicin
1–3 months	*Neisseria meningitidis* *Haemophilus influenzae* type b (Hib) *Streptococcus pneumoniae* Group B streptococcus *Escherichia coli* *Listeria monocytogenes*	Cefotaxime and ampicillin
3 month–5 years	*Neisseria meningitidis* *Haemophilus influenzae* type b (Hib)—rare in the UK since 1992 *Streptococcus pneumoniae*	Ceftriaxone or cefotaxime
6 years or more	*Neisseria meningitidis* *Streptococcus pneumoniae*	Ceftriaxone or cefotaxime

NATURAL HISTORY AND CLINICAL FEATURES

The onset of symptoms may be relatively insidious or there may be rapid progression with coma and prostration. Meningitis may present with fever, vomiting, lethargy and (in the younger child) convulsions. In the older child headache, photophobia, vomiting and anorexia are common presenting symptoms. However, with slower onset illness, the symptoms and signs are often non-specific, especially in very young children. Doctors dealing with young children with acute febrile illnesses should have a high index of suspicion and a low threshold for performing a lumbar puncture. Whereas in the older child neck stiffness is the characteristic sign, this may not be present in the child under 18 months. The classical purpuric rash of meningococcal sepsis occurs in about half to two-thirds of cases of meningitis caused by this organism. However, occasionally such a rash may be caused by the other meningitic pathogens. A non-specific maculopapular rash may also occur in meningococcal disease. Arthritis may complicate *Haemophilus influenzae* and meningococcal meningitis and in the latter is often multifocal.

Outside the neonatal period, the causative organisms are spread by respiratory secretions and droplet transmission. Usually the bacteria first colonize the nasopharynx and from there invade via the blood to the meninges. Asymptomatic nasopharyngeal carriers of these organisms are not uncommon in the population. Pneumococcal meningitis may be associated with chronic middle ear sepsis, may follow skull fractures or may complicate congenital defects in the coverings of the central nervous system.

Diagnosis Lumbar puncture with cerebrospinal fluid (CSF) examination provides the basis for diagnosis. A Gram stain and cell count should be performed. In cases of bacterial meningitis, a white blood cell count of more than 50×10^6/l is usual, although more than 20×10^6/l is abnormal. Polymorphonuclear leucocytes should predominate: mononuclear cells are seen in tuberculous and viral meningitis, and in partially treated cases of bacterial infection. Tuberculous and viral cases can usually be differentiated by history and clinical signs. In tuberculous infection, as with bacterial meningitis, CSF glucose concentration is low, and protein levels are elevated.

The causative organism can usually be cultured from the blood and occasionally from synovial fluid. In meningococcal sepsis, a throat swab will often grow the organism even after the first dose of antibiotics. Gram stain and culture of material obtained from skin lesions may also be used to confirm the diagnosis. Antigen detection tests such as latex agglutination may detect bacterial capsular polysaccharide in CSF, blood or urine, and enable identification of the causative organism to be made when cultures are negative. These are useful if prior antibiotic therapy has been given or if lumbar puncture is contraindicated because of raised intracranial pressure.

Isolates of *Streptococcus pneumoniae* should be sent to the Streptococcus and Diphtheria Reference Unit, Central Public Health Laboratory (Tel: 0181 200 4400) for serological classification and epidemiological typing. This provides information on circulating strains which is important for the selection of appropriate pneumococcal vaccines.

MANAGEMENT (see also Chapter 70)

Children with suspected meningococcal sepsis should be given parenteral benzylpenicillin or ampicillin prior to transfer to hospital. In hospital, blood cultures should be performed and a lumbar puncture considered. Intravenous antibiotic therapy should not be delayed; it is acceptable to start this before lumbar puncture particularly when there are clinical signs of meningococcal infection. The fundi should be examined for evidence of papilloedema before a lumbar puncture is performed. In the unconscious child, intracranial pressure may be high, even in the absence of papilloedema, and a lumbar puncture may increase the risk of coning. In these cases lumbar puncture should be avoided. Nevertheless, treatment of presumed meningitis without a bacteriological diagnosis is unsatisfactory, and because other serious illness may have similar signs, management of this condition without a lumbar puncture should be the exception rather than the rule. In children older than 3 months, ceftriaxone or cefotaxime is the recommended empirical treatment of choice (see Table 10.1 and Appendix III). These agents achieve more than adequate CSF bactericidal levels against the major bacterial pathogens and, so far, resistance has not been a problem. In infants less than 3 months old, ampicillin is added empirically to cover *Listeria monocytogenes*. Dexamethasone has been shown to reduce the incidence of neurological sequelae in non-neonatal meningitis caused by pneumococcus and *Haemophilus influenzae*, though this has not been proved in meningococcal meningitis. Dexamethasone 0.6 mg/kg per day in four divided doses should be commenced in all cases of non-neonatal meningitis without a purpuric rash, ideally with or before the first dose of antibiotics.

Complications of meningitis include inappropriate antidiuretic hormone secretion and cerebral oedema. Once any accompanying dehydration has been corrected, crystalloid fluids should be restricted though colloid infusions may be necessary to support the circulation and maintain cerebral perfusion pressure. Rifampicin is given to close contacts and the index case to eliminate nasopharyngeal carriage following infections with *H. influenzae* type b and meningococcus (see Chapters 52 and 70). Long-term complications of meningitis include sensorineural deafness (in up to 10% of cases) as well as motor and intellectual impairment. Children should be followed up, and hearing tests performed.

Multiply resistant pneumococcal infection may prove to be a problem as it already is in certain parts of the USA.

11 THE CHILD WITH ACUTE ENCEPHALITIS

Acute encephalitis is a rare but potentially very serious condition in children. It is characterized by acute brain dysfunction (encephalopathy) and is most commonly due to inflammation of brain tissue induced directly or indirectly by microbial infection. Acute encephalopathy can also be caused by a variety of non-infective processes including toxin exposure, metabolic disturbance, tumour, trauma, vascular mishaps, hypoxia, uncontrolled hydrocephalus and status epilepticus.

ORGANISMS

A large number of microbial agents can cause encephalitis either by direct invasion of the brain or by an immunologically mediated process leading to inflammation and demyelination in which the organism cannot be demonstrated in nervous tissue (post-infectious encephalomyelitis). Table 11.1 lists the important causes.

Table 11.1 Infective causes of acute encephalitis

Viral causes	Non-viral causes
Arboviruses	*Mycoplasma pneumoniae**
Rabies	*Mycoplasma hominis*
Herpes simplex (I and II)	Leptospira species
Enteroviruses	*Borrelia burgdorferi* (Lyme disease)
Mumps	Tuberculosis
Respiratory syncytial virus	Listeriosis
Influenza	Typhus fever
Measles*	Rocky Mountain spotted fever
Lymphocytic choriomeningitis	Falciparum malaria
Rubella*	Toxoplasmosis
Varicella-zoster virus*	Trypanosomiasis
Epstein–Barr virus	Acute bacterial meningitis
Cytomegalovirus	

***These organisms usually produce the post-infectious form of disease.**

EPIDEMIOLOGY

The incidence of encephalitis induced by any particular organism varies with the prevalence of that organism in the community. For instance, clusters of cases of mycoplasmal or influenza-associated encephalitis are likely to be seen during epidemic years for those particular organisms. Worldwide, the incidence varies considerably in different geographical areas, and sometimes seasonally, depending on the prevalence of arboviruses, rickettsial infections and rabies. The incidence is relatively low in the UK but good epidemiological data are not available. In Finland an incidence of 8.8 per 100 000 children under 16 years of age has been reported.

Transmission Arboviruses are insect-borne; rickettsiae, *Borrelia burgdorferi* and typhus are tick-borne. Other causative agents may be spread by droplets (respiratory pathogens) or by the faeco-oral route (enteroviruses).

NATURAL HISTORY AND CLINICAL FEATURES

In the directly invasive forms of the illness, encephalitic symptoms are normally present from the start (monophasic process), while in the post-infectious forms they usually develop as a second phase after the initial systemic illness (biphasic process). These two forms are not always clinically distinguishable and indeed some agents can induce encephalitis by either or both mechanisms. The early symptoms are usually non-specific, commonly with fever and vomiting. Symptoms and signs of systemic infection (for example rash, lymphadenopathy or pneumonia) may be present. Many agents causing encephalitis, particularly those involving direct invasion, also produce a meningitic process in which case there is a combined clinical picture of meningism (headache, vomiting, nuchal rigidity and photophobia) and encephalitis. The symptoms and signs of the latter include drowsiness (which may proceed to coma), altered behaviour, convulsions, focal or generalized paresis, cranial nerve palsies, ataxia and the signs and symptoms of raised intracranial pressure. Many organisms seem to be capable of producing a clinical picture anywhere along the spectrum from pure aseptic meningitis to pure encephalitis.

More specific clinical pictures are produced by some agents. The post-infectious encephalitis associated with chickenpox usually produces predominantly signs of cerebellar dysfunction. Focal convulsions and deficits are characteristic of herpes simplex virus encephalitis.

Diagnosis

Not all acute encephalopathy will be infective in nature and non-infective causes should be considered and excluded. The majority of cases are, however, associated with infection, and the diagnosis may be evident from the characteristic clinical picture of the infection—for instance a common childhood exanthematous illness. A careful history covering recent illness or medication, possible exposure to rabid animals and foreign travel is important. In a considerable number of cases the precise microbial diagnosis will not be evident. It is important to initiate specific therapy for treatable causes while pursuing investigations into the aetiology. It should be remembered that acute bacterial or tuberculous meningitis may sometimes produce predominantly encephalitic symptoms.

Investigations should include radiology—computerized tomography, or preferably magnetic resonance, scanning of the brain and usually a chest radiograph. It is important to initiate early a comprehensive battery of investigations to try to establish a microbial diagnosis. This will include appropriate viral and bacterial cultures, Mantoux test, viral (and other) serology and analysis of samples by polymerase chain reaction to look for microbial nucleic acid. Cerebrospinal fluid is usually the most useful sample for analysis but care should be taken to assess the risks of lumbar puncture if there is a possibility of raised intracranial pressure. In some cases with a history of foreign travel, specialist advice from tropical medicine experts may be useful both for clinical management and for help in directing samples to specialist reference laboratories.

MANAGEMENT

Treatment may be divided into supportive and specific therapies.

Supportive care It is essential for recovery that careful attention is paid to keeping the brain in optimal condition. The child should ideally be managed in a centre with paediatric intensive care facilities. Correction of biochemical disturbances and maintenance of fluid balance are vital. Haematological, haemodynamic and respiratory support may be required. Convulsions will need to be controlled and electroencephalographic monitoring may be helpful in this respect. Raised intracranial pressure may need monitoring using invasive techniques in selected cases.

Specific therapies Empirical antibiotic therapy (see Table 10.1 in Chapter 10) should usually be initiated to cover the possibility of acute bacterial meningitis and should be continued until this diagnosis has been excluded. It may sometimes be necessary to commence empirical antituberculous therapy.

Of all the viral encephalitides only that due to herpes simplex virus (HSV) has been shown to respond favourably to specific antiviral therapy. Although the later findings in this condition are fairly characteristic, the early features may be non-specific. Acyclovir (500 mg/m^2 three times daily) should therefore be commenced in all cases of encephalitis where the aetiology is unclear and will need to be continued until either a firm alternative diagnosis is made or, in the absence of the typical features of HSV encephalitis emerging, there is a negative polymerase chain reaction for HSV on cerebrospinal fluid. There is no evidence to support the use of other antiviral agents in encephalitis. A few of the bacterial causes (for example Lyme disease or rickettsial disease) are also amenable to specific therapy.

In some of the post-infectious encephalitides where there are multifocal areas of demyelination, corticosteroid therapy may be of benefit.

PREVENTION OF FURTHER CASES

Acute encephalitis in children in the UK is often caused by common organisms and preventative strategies are dealt with in Part Two. For Japanese B and tick borne encephalitides there are vaccines available which should be given to travellers to endemic areas (see Chapter 20). Vaccines are not generally available for the other arbovirus encephalitides—travellers to endemic areas should be given advice on minimizing exposure to vector insects.

FURTHER READING

Davies EG & De Souza C (1993) How to investigate and manage the child with suspected acute encephalitis. *Current Paediatrics* **3**: 106–113.

Levin M (1991) Infections of the nervous system In *Paediatric Neurology*, 2nd edn (ed. Brett EM) pp. 603–665. Churchill Livingstone, Edinburgh.

THE CHILD WITH SEPTIC SHOCK

EPIDEMIOLOGY AND CAUSES

Organisms responsible for septic shock in infants and children include *Neisseria meningitidis* (most common), *Escherichia coli*, *Haemophilus influenzae* type b, *Klebsiella* spp., *Salmonella* spp. and other Gram-negative bacteria; *Staphylococcus aureus* and *Streptococcus pneumoniae* are the most frequent Gram-positive pathogens. Group B *Streptococcus agalactiae* and *Escherichia coli* are more common causes of septic shock in infants less than 3 months old. Surgical patients usually develop septicaemia due to enteric organisms. Immunosuppressed patients may develop septicaemia due to unusual and opportunistic organisms, though Gram-negative bacteria cause the major mortality.

TERMINOLOGY AND PATHOPHYSIOLOGY OF SEPSIS

Septicaemia is defined as the presence of organisms in the blood stream accompanied by clinical features of sepsis (tachypnoea, tachycardia, pyrexia or hypothermia, and neutrophilia or neutropenia).

Sepsis is the clinical expression of the host's response to bacteria, specifically to constituents of the cell wall of Gram-negative bacteria—endotoxins—as well as exotoxins produced by Gram-negative organisms. Bacterial infection results in activation of macrophages which produce the lymphokines interferon γ, granulocyte macrophage colony stimulating factor, tumour necrosis factor (TNF-α) and Interleukin 1 (IL-1). These substances are beneficial to the hosts in mediating the protective inflammatory response, but in severe infection, high levels of TNF-α and IL-1 cause serious damage. Acting with the inflammatory mediators prostaglandin E_2 (PGE_2), released by neutrophils, and platelet activating factor, a state of shock can develop with damage to the endothelial cells of blood vessels resulting in leakage of plasma from the circulation with consequent vascular collapse, as well as breakdown of the normal coagulation mechanisms. The devastating effects of fulminant septicaemia result from the host's response to the bacteria, and future strategies for the prevention of septic shock will not come from the development of new antibiotics but from agents antagonistic to endotoxins, the cytokines or inflammatory mediators (see below).

CLINICAL PRESENTATION

Full clinical assessment must include observations of temperature, pulse rate, blood pressure, respiration rate, mental status, conscious level and urine output. Early features of sepsis typically include fever and tachycardia. Respiration rate may be normal or mildly raised with an irregular breathing pattern. Urine output may be mildly reduced, reflecting mild dehydration, but mental status and conscious level are unaffected. Later features may include hypothermia, a marked tachycardia, sustained tachypnoea and respiratory irregularity, depressed conscious level and a clinically appreciable reduction in urine output. Hypotension may also be present but its presence is not essential to the diagnosis of septic shock. Blood pressure may be maintained until a late stage by vasoregulatory mechanisms, especially in a young child. These mechanisms preserve central blood pressure at the expense of impaired perfusion to limbs and organs. Impaired perfusion may be recognized by cold peripheries, poor capillary refill, tachycardia, tachypnoea or oliguria. Skin–core temperature gradient should be measured with thermistor probes on a toe and in the rectum: a large skin–core temperature difference (over 3 °C) is a sensitive marker for severe shock. A capillary refill time prolonged beyond 2 seconds in a room-warm limb is a reliable marker for reduced skin perfusion. Hypoxaemia or poor cerebral perfusion may result in restlessness or irritability in a child. Measurement of hypoxaemia with a saturation monitor is a valuable adjunct to clinical examination.

INVESTIGATION

Haemoglobin levels may fall rapidly. The white blood count (showing neutrophilia or, more seriously, neutropenia) and blood lactate concentration (elevated) are helpful measures of response to shock. Blood glucose concentration is often low, and potassium and calcium levels may be low and need correcting. Evidence of multiorgan failure should be sought with clinical and laboratory evidence of disseminated intravascular coagulation (DIC), adult-type respiratory distress syndrome, acute renal failure, hepatobiliary dysfunction and central nervous system (CNS) dysfunction.

DIAGNOSIS

The underlying cause can often be inferred from careful history and examination of the patient. Blood cultures should be taken before antibiotics are given: the causative organism usually can be isolated within 24 hours. Bacterial antigen detection in urine or plasma may establish the diagnosis in children who have previously received antibiotics.

MANAGEMENT

See also Chapters 13 and 70.

Immediate treatment is with urgent antibiotic therapy to cover the likely causative organisms, parenteral fluids, vasoactive agents and oxygen. Early drainage of purulent foci should be performed. The first choice of antibiotic for paediatric medical patients is cefotaxime (initial dose 200 mg/kg per day IV in 4 divided doses). This may need variation or supplementation if surgical or immunocompromised patients are being treated. Children should be stabilized and nursed in an area designated for high-dependency care within the paediatric ward. Patients with evidence of impaired peripheral perfusion (see above) should initially be resuscitated with 4.5% albumen 20–40 ml/kg over 10–30 minutes, followed by a further 20-40 ml/kg albumen over the next hour.

Admission to a paediatric intensive care unit Patients who do not respond to immediate treatment are likely to require ventilatory support and should be admitted to a paediatric intensive care unit (PICU). The criteria for admission to a PICU should not be based solely upon the need for ventilatory support. Resuscitation should be continued (with albumen, fluid and inotropic drugs) and stability maintained while arrangements are made for admission and throughout the period of transfer. The airway should be stabilized—often with endotracheal intubation—and intravenous access secured. Facilities for intermittent positive pressure ventilation and cardiopulmonary resuscitation should be available. If an ambulance journey is required the child should be accompanied by experienced paediatric, anaesthetic and nursing staff.

Management Invasive monitoring of blood pressure, pulse and urine output and differential core–peripheral temperature monitoring should be established. Central venous pressure (CVP) monitoring may allow colloid to be given with confidence until the CVP is approximately 12–15 cmH_2O. This should be followed by a reduction in the core–peripheral temperature difference. Children with Gram-negative septic shock may require several times the calculated circulating volume of colloid owing to capillary leak, which is a major feature of the condition. It is important not to be misled by the fluid volumes required into slowing infusion rates or discontinuing volume expansion too early. Once adequate volume replacement has been completed as shown by CVP and blood pressure, persistent of signs of impaired peripheral perfusion suggests that either myocardial failure due to endotoxinaemia or peripheral vasoconstriction may be present. Myocardial function can be assessed by echocardiography to measure end-diastolic volume.

The child with established septic shock should be electively intubated and ventilated. This is an urgent requirement if the airway is compromised or there are abnormalities of breathing rate or pattern. Ventilation reduces the work of breathing and myocardial workload. Intermittent positive pressure ventilation can avert the severe deterioration which may occur during a period of unexpected decompensation and reduces the risk of pulmonary oedema. Midazolam 100 μg/kg per hour is given for sedative effect during ventilation; it is also an anticonvulsant. Intravenous opiate infusions such as morphine 20–40 μg/kg per hour or alfentanil 30–60 μg/kg per hour can be used for sedative and analgesic effect.

Cardiovascular support Dopamine 2.5–5 μg/kg per minute, an inotrope with vasodilator action, should be commenced as first-line supportive treatment when there are signs of impaired perfusion which have not responded to the initial measures. Dobutamine 2.5 μg/kg per minute may be added for further inotropic effect and increased to a dose of 20–40 μg/kg per minute while maintaining renal perfusion using dopamine at a maximum of 5 μg/kg per minute. If hypotension persists despite adequate CVP the introduction of a third inotrope such as adrenaline 0.1–1.0 μg/kg per minute or isoprenaline 0.1–2.0 μg/kg per minute may be considered while keeping dopamine at the renal dose of 5 μg/kg per minute. Noradrenaline may be used a fourth inotrope. Vasodilators which reduce afterload on the heart and improve perfusion, include glyceryl trinitrate patch 5 mg per day, and nitroglycerine 1 μg/kg per minute. Nitroprusside has also been used. Prostacyclin 5–20 ng/kg per minute acts as a potent vasodilator and an inhibitor of platelet aggregation, which may reduce the risk of DIC. The place of prostacycline, nitroprusside and glyceryl trinitrate vasodilators in the management of septic shock has not been established in double-blind trials in children.

Fluid and electrolyte balance In septic shock it is important to address fluid balance under the headings of restoration of intravascular volume, maintenance fluid and replacement of ongoing losses. In view of the large amounts of colloid used for the first category, (volumes may exceed 100 ml/kg), it is advisable to restrict maintenance crystalloid to half the recommended amount. Ongoing fluid losses (e.g. nasogastric aspirates) should be measured over a time period and replaced with the same volume of 0.9% saline IV over a subsequent similar time period. Regular electrolyte and blood glucose measurements should be performed. If blood glucose concentration is low, dextrose 10% infusion at 0.5 ml/kg per hour should be commenced. Higher dextrose concentrations may be needed if there is a poor response.

Disseminated intravascular coagulation Many patients in septic shock show evidence of DIC with deranged clotting studies, thrombocytopenia and raised fibrin degradation products. The management of DIC is supportive during correction of the underlying cause. Patients with severely deranged clotting studies should be given fresh frozen plasma or cryoprecipitate. Platelet infusions may be required for patients with severe thrombocytopenia and active bleeding (e.g. from puncture sites), but their effect only lasts 6–8 hours. Low-dose heparin (10 units/kg per hour) should be considered for individual patients with impending peripheral gangrene and severe coagulation derangement, though this area is controversial. Results of trials of various specific treatments targeted at the disorders of haemostasis that contribute to DIC are awaited.

Areas of controversy Administration of corticosteroids is often contemplated as a supplementary treatment in septic shock. Although early corticosteroid treatment appears beneficial in animals and adult humans, evidence also suggests that in established septic shock steroid therapy may be detrimental. Little data are available from children, and therefore corticosteroids are not currently recommended.

Plasmapheresis and blood exchange have been used to reduce the concentrations of circulating endotoxin and cytokines. There is no convincing evidence of their success.

Modulators of the inflammatory response in sepsis are being extensively studied. These include monoclonal antibodies against endotoxins and cytokines, nitric oxide synthase inhibitors (such as *N*-monomethyl-L-arginine, L-NMMA) and other agents such as polymyxin B and taurolin (anti-endotoxins) and pentoxiphylline (a cytokine antagonist). No trial data yet exist on their overall efficacy or safety.

FURTHER READING

Jafari HS & McCracken GH (1992) Sepsis and septic shock: a review for clinicians. *Paediatric Infectious Disease Journal* **11**: 739–749.

THE CHILD WITH TOXIC SHOCK SYNDROME

See also Chapters 90 and 91.

Toxic shock syndrome was first defined in 1978 in a series of children with *Staphylococcus aureus* infection. Since then a similar illness following streptococcal infection has been described. Although it is unusual to isolate *Staphylococcus aureus* from blood culture in this syndrome, the bacterium is usually isolated from other (often superficial) sites. Several exotoxins are known to mediate the disease, including a staphylococcal enterotoxin, also known as toxic shock syndrome toxin 1 (TSST-1), a protein of molecular weight 22 049 with a known nucleotide sequence. The streptococci identified in toxic shock have been exotoxin-producing M1 and M3 strains.

EPIDEMIOLOGY

Toxic shock syndrome is rare in children. Although thought initially to be predominantly associated with menstruation and tampon use, this is true in only about half the cases. It has been described following apparently mild staphylococcal skin infection, osteomyelitis and empyema, but most consistently in association with bacterial tracheitis. The cases associated with streptococcal infection have been from two main groups—children with varicella infection and children with relatively innocuous streptococcal upper respiratory tract infections.

CLINICAL FEATURES

There is usually a rapid onset of illness with a high fever, vomiting, diarrhoea, headache, pharyngitis, myalgia and hypotension. Multisystem organ failure results from hypotension with poor tissue perfusion and polyclonal activation of T cells with release of cytokines and other inflammatory mediators. Fatal complications include irreversible shock, disseminated intravascular coagulation (DIC) and arrhythmias. There are very specific dermatological features. These include a diffuse scarlatiniform rash on the trunk and arms, which tends to be more marked on the flexor surfaces. The palms and soles may become oedematous and the eyes become red. Desquamation may occur in the recovery phase.

Diagnosis The differential diagnosis includes Kawasaki disease and staphylococcal scalded skin syndrome. Most cases of staphylococcal toxic shock have been associated with sterile blood culture, but cultures may be positive in streptococcal infection. Although the portal of entry may not be apparent, investigations should include throat swab with skin wound and vaginal swabs where appropriate. The haematological findings include leucopenia with a high band count, thrombocytopenia and features of DIC with a prolonged coagulation time and raised fibrin degradation products. Other laboratory abnormalities may reflect multi-organ failure if this is present.

MANAGEMENT

This section should be read in conjunction with Chapters 12, 90 and 91.

With the rapid onset of the disease, treatment must be prompt and aggressive. A prognostic scoring system may be useful (see Table 70.2). Intensive monitoring is important to assess the degree of intravascular depletion. Large volumes of fluid may be required, supported by inotropic drugs. In patients mechanical ventilation is required. Appropriate antibiotics should be given. Treatment of DIC with fresh frozen plasma may be necessary. Metabolic abnormalities may occur as a result of renal failure and require appropriate treatment.

14

THE CHILD WITH A RASH

Just as a fever may not always be caused by an infectious disorder, a rash may not be the result of an infection. The aim of this chapter is to help the clinician decide the likely cause of a rash. Definitive diagnosis and subsequent management are described later in the book. Rashes in the neonate are not covered in this section.

DIAGNOSIS

Diagnosis is based on the history, general examination, features of the rash itself and, in some cases, specific laboratory investigations. In many cases it may not be possible to make an exact diagnosis (in young children, over half the cases diagnosed as measles are in fact due to something else). This may not matter, as long as important diagnoses have been excluded. However, there are some conditions where the possible consequences are such that an accurate diagnosis is essential. An obvious example is suspected rubella in a pregnant woman or one of her close contacts. Bearing in mind these caveats the following framework is suggested.

History

- Features of rash:
  - duration
  - site
  - evolution (changes in site, appearance and possible cropping)
  - presence of pruritus.
- Accompanying symptoms:
  - presence of prodromal illness
  - current symptoms—fever, malaise, headache, etc.
- Past history:
  - immunizations
  - possible contacts
  - foreign travel
  - known or suspected allergies
  - previous similar episodes.
- Miscellaneous:
  - current or recent medication
  - pets
  - similar illness in locality of residence, at school or playgroup, etc.

Examination A complete general examination is necessary. Points to which particular attention should be paid include:

- General appearance, i.e. does the child look well or unwell?
- Fever.
- Lymphadenopathy.
- Splenomegaly.
- Mucous membranes (conjunctivae and mouth).

The rash

- General appearance:
  vesicular
  maculopapular
  punctate
  haemorrhagic.
- Distribution of rash—look particularly at the soles of the feet, palms of hands, behind the ears and at the mucous membranes.
- Are all areas and elements at the same stage of evolution or is there evidence of cropping? Has there been scratching?

Investigations These investigations will depend on the possible differential diagnoses, but may include:

- Full blood count.
- A 'saved sample' for serology.
- An appropriate specimen for viral culture.
- Blood cultures.

Table 14.1 should help in deciding the aetiology of most rashes. Reactions to drugs and other allergic reactions commonly give rise to a maculopapular or punctiform rash and rarely to a vesicular eruption.

Scabies often produces a mixed papular and vesicular rash around the fingers, wrists and elbows. Scratching may obscure the characteristic linear burrows.

Table 14.1 Types of rash

	Prodrome	Fever	General malaise	Distribution of rash	Pruritus	Special features
Vesicular rashes						
Chickenpox	None or short coryzal	Mild to moderate	Mild	Mostly truncal	Yes	Contact with sufferers is common; crops
Dermatitis herpetiformis	Nil	Nil	Nil	Trunk	Yes	Sporadic cases eventually leave depigmentation
Eczema herpeticum	Nil	Moderate to high	Moderate	In areas of eczema	Yes	May be seriously ill
Hand, foot and mouth disease	Nil	Minimal	Minimal	Palms, soles and inside mouth	No	Often occurs as minor epidemics
Herpes simplex gingivostomatitis	Nil	Moderate to high	Moderate (may be dehydrated)	Mouth and lips	Yes (at onset)	Frequent history of contact with cold sores
Impetigo	Nil	Nil	Nil	Face and hands	Yes	Vesicles often replaced by yellow crusting
Insect bites	Nil	Nil	Rare	Variable	Yes	Usually isolated lesions

Molluscum contagiosum	Nil	Nil	Nil	Variable	No	Characteristic pearly vesicles with central dimples
Maculopapular and punctate rashes						
Enteroviral infections	Short	Mild	Mild	General	No	Rash often pleomorphic
Fifth disease	Uncommon; mild fever and respiratory symptoms	Mild, if any	Minimal	Face ('slapped cheeks') trunk and limbs	No	Rash may come and go. Heat brings it out. Can have a reticular pattern
Glandular fever	Malaise, mild fever and sore throat	Moderate	Common	General	No	Exudate in throat especially marked Swollen glands and spleen
Kawasaki disease	Mild fever, malaise and sore thorat	Moderate to high and persistent	Mild to moderate	General	No	Palms and soles, lips and conjunctivae affected
Measles	Rising fever, cough and conjunctivitis	Moderate to high	Substantial	Around ears, then face, then trunk. Confluent	No	Koplik's spots in mouth before rash on 4th day of illness

Table 14.1 continued

	Prodrome	Fever	General malaise	Distribution of rash	Pruritus	Special features
Meningococcal disease	None or short with coryza or fever	Variable	Profound	Variable	No	Petechial rash may be preceded by maculopapular rash
Pityriasis rosea	Nil	Nil	Nil	Trunk	Initially	Usually in older children; herald patch at onset
Roseola infantum	High fever and irritability	Moderate	Moderate	Trunk then face	No	Dramatic improvement in child when rash appears on 4th or 5th day
Rubella	Short, mild fever and malaise	Mild	Mild or absent	Face then trunk and limbs	No	Posterior occipital lymphadenopathy
Scarlet fever	Fever and sore throat	Moderate to high	Moderate	Face, then rapidly generalized	No	Rash blanches on pressure; strawberry tongue and periora pallor

Haemorrhagic rashes						
Acute lymphoblastic leukaemia	Mild, non-specific	Absent or mild/moderate	Moderate	Anywhere, including mucous membranes	Nil	Pallor, lymphadenopathy and hepato-splenomegaly may be present
Henoch–Schönlein purpura	Mild, sometimes symptoms of upper respiratory tract infection	Mild or moderate	Moderate	Mainly limbs, especially legs and buttocks	No	Rash is urticarial initially. Arthralgia, joint swelling and abdominal pain often present
Idiopathic thrombocyto-penic purpura	Nil to mild	Nil	Nil	Anywhere, including mucous membranes	Nil	Child is usually well, apart from effects of bleeding
Inherited bleeding disorder	Nil	Nil	Nil	Anywhere, including mucous membranes	Nil	Spontaneous bruises. Family history may be present
Meningococcal disease	None or short with coryza or fever	Variable	Severe	Variable	No	Petechial rash may be preceded by maculopapular rash

15

THE CHILD WITH A PYREXIA OF UNKNOWN ORIGIN

The definition of pyrexia of unknown origin (PUO), also called fever of unknown origin (FUO), varies between different authors. Petersdorf suggested a minimum temperature of 38.3 °C for 3 weeks and at least 1 week of intensive hospital investigation, whereas some standard paediatric textbooks set a shorter minimum period of 1 week of fever (see Further Reading).

IMPORTANCE

True PUO is not a common disorder in hospital paediatric practice. Often the patient recovers before a definitive diagnosis has been made or a viral infection is assumed, but the syndrome is important for a number of reasons. The underlying disorder may have serious implications for the individual, e.g. malaria or neoplasia. A delay in diagnosis may put other individuals at risk from an infectious disease, e.g. tuberculosis. In order to make a diagnosis, a patient may be detained in hospital and extensive investigations carried out. These consume valuable resources in terms of expense and professional time, and may also be hazardous, causing morbidity and rarely death. Therefore it is important that there is some structure to the investigations rather than a 'scatter-gun' approach.

POSSIBLE DIAGNOSES

The list of conditions that may present as a PUO is almost endless, including infectious diseases, autoimmune disorders and neoplasia. The disorders listed in Table 15.1 are those most likely to be encountered in a western European country.

MANAGEMENT

Age is not very helpful in guiding the diagnosis (Table 15.2).

All children with a PUO should have:

- A full blood count and film.
- A thick blood film for malaria parasites if there is any possibility of this diagnosis.
- Repeated blood cultures.
- Epstein–Barr virus serology.
- Serum saved for other possible serology.
- Urine microscopy (this is important to determine the presence of red and white cells) and culture.
- Tuberculin test.
- Chest X-ray.

Further investigations should be based on the possible diagnoses suggested by a full history and examination (Table 15.3). 'Blind' imaging is rarely helpful (the exception is abdominal ultrasonography which is non-invasive), nor is bone marrow biopsy. The value of white cell scans in children has not been proved.

When a diagnosis cannot be made, consideration must be given to the possibility of factitious fever (Munchausen syndrome by proxy). Admission and close observation to ensure that the child is not being given anything to raise the temperature artificially is essential. This can sometimes be difficult to detect.

Table 15.1 Likely causes of PUO

Category	Disease
Specific bacterial infection	Brucellosis *Campylobacter* infection Cat-scratch disease Legionellosis Rheumatic fever *Salmonella typhi* infection Tuberculosis
Localized infection	Abscess: abdominal, dental, hepatic, pelvic, perinephric, rectal, subphrenic Cholangitis Endocarditis Mastoiditis Meningitis Osteomyelitis Pneumonia Pyelonephritis Sinusitis
Spirochaete infection	Leptospirosis Lyme disease Syphilis
Viral disease	Cytomegalovirus infection Epstein Barr virus (Infectious mononucleosis) Hepatitis HIV infection
Chlamydial disease	Psittacosis
Rickettsial disease	Q fever
Fungal disease	Histoplasmosis
Parasitic disease	Giardiasis Malaria Toxocariasis Toxoplasmosis Trypanosomiasis
Autoimmune disorders	Juvenile chronic arthritis Polyarteritis nodosa Systemic lupus erythematosus Undefined vasculitis

Table 15.1 continued

Category	Disease
Neoplasms	Atrial myxoma Hodgkin's disease Leukaemia Lymphoma Neuroblastoma Wilms' tumour
Miscellaneous	Anhidrotic ectodermal dysplasia Chronic active hepatitis Diabetes insipidus Drug fever Fabry's disease Factitious fever Familial dysautonomia Familial Mediterranean fever Hypothalamic central fever Ichthyosis Inflammatory bowel disease Kawasaki disease Pancreatitis Periodic fever Pulmonary embolism Serum sickness Thyrotoxicosis

Table 15.2 Distribution of types of causes of PUO by age

	Age		
Disorder	**0–11 months** ($n = 21$)	**12–59 months** ($n = 40$)	**60 months or over** ($n = 52$)
Infection	9 (43%)	11 (28%)	21 (40%)
Autoimmune disorders	1 (5%)	5 (13%)	9 (17%)
Neoplasia		6 (15%)	5 (10%)
Miscellaneous	7 (33%)	9 (22%)	4 (8%)
Factitious fever			4 (8%)
Undiagnosed	4 (19%)	9 (22%)	9 (17%)

Adapted from Chantada *et al.* (1994) Fever of unknown origin in Argentinian children. *Paed. Inf. Dis.* 13: 260–263.

Table 15.3 Pointers to likely diagnoses and helpful investigations

History/examination	Likely diagnoses	Investigations to be considered
Pica	Toxocariasis Toxoplasmosis	Specific serological tests
Exposure to wild or domestic animals	Toxoplasmosis Leptospirosis	Specific serological tests
Possible tick bite	Lyme disease and arbovirus infection	Specific serological tests
Travel abroad	See Chapter 21	
Palpebral conjunctivitis	Measles Coxsackievirus infection Tuberculosis Infectious mononucleosis Cat-scratch disease	Specific serology except tuberculin test for TB and histology for cat-scratch disease
Bulbar conjunctivitis	Kawasaki disease Leptospirosis	None specific Isolation of organism from urine or serology
Uveitis	Sarcoidosis Juvenile chronic arthritis Systemic lupus erythematosus Behçet's syndrome Kawasaki disease	Chest X-ray and Kveim test
Chorioretinitis	Cytomegalovirus infection Toxoplasmosis Syphilis	Specific serological tests

Table 15.3 continued

History/examination	Likely diagnoses	Investigations to be considered
Blisters	Infection with pneumococci, other streptococci, meningococci Malaria *Rickettsial* infection	Blood cultures Blood films Serology
Localized bone tenderness	Osteomyelitis	X-ray and bone scan
Hectic fever with rigors	Septicaemia with renal, liver or biliary disease Malaria Brucellosis Localized pus	Blood cultures and ultrasound scan Blood film Serology, blood and bone marrow culture Ultrasound scan
Red throat	Infectious mononucleosis Cytomegalovirus infection Toxoplasmosis Typhoid (*Salmonella typhi*) Kawasaki disease Leptospirosis	Serology Serology Serology Isolation of organism (blood culture) Clinical diagnosis *Leptospira* in urine
Abdominal pain and tenderness	Inflammatory bowel disease Collection of pus	Barium meal/enema Abdominal ultrasound scan
Rash	See Chapter 14	
Lymphadenopathy	Reactive hyperplasia Cat-scratch disease Cytomegalovirus infection	Serology, tuberculin testing. If nodes remain enlarged without explanation biopsy may be needed as well as bone marrow

	Infectious mononucleosis Mycobacterial infection Toxocariasis Toxoplasmosis Hodgkin's disease Other malignancy	examination
Jaundice	Brucellosis Cholecystitis Hepatitis A Hepatitis B Infectious mononucleosis Leptospirosis Pancreatitis	Specific serology for most cases of jaundice. Seek *Leptospira* in urine. Cholecystitis is a clinical diagnosis. Pancreatitis is accompanied by a raised serum amylase level
Absence of sweating	Anhidrotic ectodermal dysplasia Family dysautonomia Atropine poisoning	Careful examination of skin, nails, hair and teeth Tests of autonomic function Toxicology
Erythrocyte sedimentation rate above 100 mm/h	Kawasaki disease Tuberculosis Malignancy Autoimmune disease	Tuberculin test
Pyuria	Urinary tract infection including tuberculosis	Renal imaging Early morning urine collections (for TB culture)

FURTHER READING

Behrman RE, Kliegman RM, Nelson WE & Vaughan VC, eds (1992) *Nelson Textbook of Pediatrics*, p. 652. WB Saunders, Philadelphia.

Lorin MI & Feigin RD (1992) Fever without localising signs and fever of unknown origin. In *Textbook of Pediatric Infectious Disease* (eds Feigin RD & Cherry JD) pp. 1012–1022. WB Saunders, Philadelphia.

Petersdorf R (1992) Fever of unknown origin: an old friend revisited. *Archives of Internal Medicine* **152**: 21–22.

THE CHILD WITH SUSPECTED IMMUNODEFICIENCY

Although many of the rare major primary immunodeficiencies are now very well defined, more minor degrees of susceptibility to infection in childhood are both common and poorly understood. Indeed, the combination of immunological naïvety and immaturity is universal in the first years of life with consequences familiar to any parent and any children's doctor. It is often very difficult to decide, on clinical grounds, whether a child has had more than an average number or severity of infections by chance or because of an underlying problem. A formal strategy for investigation is hard to formulate. However, some guiding principles can be set out.

For practical purposes, recognized immunodeficiencies can be divided into defects of specific immunity, namely, lymphocyte function including the production of antibodies—and defects of non-specific immunity including neutrophils, complement components and other problems such as breakdown of the protective barriers of the skin and mucosa.There are clear deficiences in these barriers around the time of birth and also significant defects in other aspects of non-specific immunity. The main universal deficiency in early childhood is, however, in specific immunity. Most babies encounter no pathogens prior to entering the birth canal, and from then onwards face an onslaught involving one new potential pathogen after another until, after some years, they achieve a broad repertoire of immunity. Distinguishing between the immunodeficiency of immaturity and that due to a primary (and permanent) immunodeficiency disorder may not always be easy.

NATURAL HISTORY AND CLINICAL FEATURES

Apart from the common presentation of frequent or unrelenting infection, brought forward by a parent or another physician, or the unusual but obvious case of a family history of a specific disorder, several other features should signal the possibility of an immunodeficiency. Erythematous rashes in small infants may signal graft-versus-host disease due to maternal lymphocytes in the baby's blood in severe combined immunodeficiency. Delayed separation of the umbilical cord is seen in leucocyte adhesion defects and sometimes in other congenital neutrophil disorders. Unexplained poor growth and persistent diarrhoea are also common features. Recurrent opportunist infection with severe diarrhoea during infancy may result from severe combined immunodeficiency. There are several rare syndromal associations producing immunodeficiency including aortic arch defects, partial albinism and short-limbed dwarfism. Children presenting with ataxia may have ataxia-telangiectasia, a chromosomal breakage disorder with immunodeficiency.

Immunodeficiency may present later in childhood. Surprisingly, severe congenital immunodeficiency disorders may not come to light for several years. Persistent ear infections and lower respiratory tract problems, sometimes presenting as asthma can turn out to be due to antibody production defects. Rashes and poor growth remain prominent features. Recurrent skin sepsis does not usually turn out to be due to underlying problems but rather is due to colonization with a virulent strain of *Staphylococcus aureus* which may also affect other members of the family. However, particularly when there is persistent infection, rashes, lymphadenitis, more deep-seated infection or unusual bacterial isolates, an underlying immunodeficiency should be sought. It is worth trying to establish whether there is a predictable temporal pattern to recurrent infection, as neutropenia may be cyclical. The spectrum of immunodeficiencies currently recognized are not usually seen in association with recurrent urinary tract infection. The association of recurrent infection with severe allergy or unusual autoimmune disorder should also merit investigation of immune function.

Human immunodeficiency virus (HIV) infection will need to be considered in the differential diagnosis of children with recurrent infections, particularly those from high-risk backgrounds. Tactfully, it is necessary to introduce the subject of testing to the family and if they agree, counselling before and after the test by a trained counsellor is required.

Understanding of the subtleties of immune function is still in its infancy. A considerable proportion of children with a pattern of recurrent infection suggestive of immunodeficiency cannot be given a specific diagnosis. Presumably they have an as yet unrecognized problem. An example is the child with frequent and severe attacks of herpes labialis.

The important primary immunodeficiency disorders are listed in Table 16.1.

EXAMINATION

This should focus on growth parameters, the skin and the presence of any rash, the respiratory tract including the tympanic membranes (and when appropriate hearing assessment), the presence or absence of lymphoid tissue, tonsillar tissue, palpable lymph nodes and the presence of an enlarged liver and spleen.

INVESTIGATIONS

Tests for immunodeficiency will often be carried out alongside those for other disorders with overlapping presentation such as cystic fibrosis and recurrent aspiration. In general, the following situations should prompt investigation for immunodeficiency:

- Single infections with unusual organisms.
- Recurrent infections with common organisms—especially bacterial.
- Infections associated with failure to thrive.
- Infections associated with severe allergy or unusual autoimmune disorder.
- Family history of immunodeficiency.

Blood count The simplest test is the blood count with differential white cell count. Patients will sometimes have had several done previously and an important abnormality such as lymphopenia may have gone unnoticed—children with severe combined immunodeficiency (SCID) are often persistently lymphopenic ($< 2.8 \times 10^9$/l). Persistent neutropenia is occasionally seen but the degree of associated infectious problems correlates poorly with the neutrophil count. In cyclical neutropenia the neutrophil count falls to abnormally low levels in a regular 3–4-weekly cycle, diagnosable only by twice-weekly blood counts over a period. Eosinophilia may be a feature of some T-cell disorders and also certain bone marrow disorders. Abnormalities in platelet number and size are seen in Wiskott–Aldrich syndrome which may present with infections, bleeding or both. A careful examination of the blood film may reveal abnormal leucocyte granular morphology in Chédiak Higashi syndrome.

Lymphocyte tests Lymphocyte immunophenotyping ('subsets') is now widely available, providing a more sophisticated count of the different functional types of lymphocytes. Age-related normal values for the main types (CD3, all T cells; CD4, helper subset; CD8, suppressor/cytotoxic subset; CD16, natural killer cells;

Table16.1 Important primary immunodeficiency disorders

Disorder	Inheritance (predominant mode)	Common presenting features	Important tests
Humoral deficiencies			
Selective IgA deficiency	?	Respiratory/gastrointestinal infections	Serum/salivary IgA
IgG subclass deficiency	?	Respiratory infections	Serum Ig and subclasses
Deficient anti-carbohydrate responses	?	Respiratory and other invasive bacterial infections	Response to pneumococcal vaccine
Agammaglobulinaemia (Bruton)	XL	Bacterial infections	Serum Ig B cell numbers
Common variable immunodeficiency	?	Bacterial infections Opportunistic infections	Serum Ig and subclasses Lymphocyte numbers and function
Hyper-IgM syndrome	XL	Bacterial and opportunistic infections	Serum Ig and subclasses Lymphocyte function
Complement defects	Most AR	Bacterial infections, esp. meningococcal Autoimmune disorders	Total haemolytic complement

Table16.1 continued

Disorder	Inheritance (predominant mode)	Common presenting features	Important tests
Combined immunodeficiencies (SCID)			
Reticular dysgenesis	AR	Bacterial/fungal infections Opportunistic infections Chronic diarrhoea Failure to thrive	Serum Ig and subclasses Lymphocyte numbers and function
Adenosine deaminase deficiency	AR	As above	As above, and specific metabolite assays
Purine nucleoside phosphorylase deficiency	AR	As above	As above, and specific metabolic assays
X-linked SCID	XL	As above	As above
Autosomal SCID	AR	As above	As above
Syndromal deficiencies			
Ataxia-telangiectasia	AR	Ataxia Bacterial and viral infections Malignancy	Alpha-fetoprotein DNA radiosensitivity
Wiskott–Aldriche syndrome	XL	Bleeding Bacterial infections Malignancy	Platelet morphology Serum Ig and subclasses Lymphocyte numbers and function

Di George syndrome	?	Cardiac defect Hypocalcaemia Abnormal facies Bacterial/opportunistic infections	Chest X-ray Lymphocyte numbers and function DNA studies (deletion on chromosome 22)
Neutrophil deficiencies			
Congenital neutropenia	AR	Bacterial and fungal infections	FBC and bone marrow examination
Cyclical neutropenia	AD	Intermittent infections especially gingivostomatitis	Repeated FBCs
Chronic granulomatous disease	XL and AR	Pneumonias Deep abscesses	NBT test
Leucocyte adhesion molecule deficiency	AR	Delayed cord separation Bacterial, fungal and viral infections	Specific leucocyte monoclonal antibody studies
Hyper-IgE syndrome	AR	Skin infections Cold abscesses Pneumonias	Serum IgE
Neutrophil chemotactic defects	?	Bacterial infection Delayed wound healing	Neutrophil chemotaxis

Key: ?, often familial but no distinct mendelian pattern; AD, autosomal dominant; AR, autosomal recessive; FBC, full blood count; Ig, immunoglobulin; NBT, nitroblue tetrazolium; SCID, severe combined immunodeficiency; XL, X-linked.

CD19/20, B cells) are now available, although specialist help with interpretation is often useful. More sophisticated markers of abnormalities which may be associated with certain specific immunodeficiencies can also be determined. Functional tests of the ability of lymphocytes to proliferate and produce cytokines (such as interleukin 2) in response to different stimuli (mitogens such as phytohaemagglutinin or antigen such as *Candida* or tetanus) in vitro are rapidly becoming more widely used.

Antibody tests Assays for immunoglobulin (Ig) levels are the most widely known and used tests of immune function. Measurement of total serum IgG, IgA, IgM and IgE is available in most hospitals and IgG and IgA subclasses can also be measured. Particular caution is needed in the interpretation of these tests in early childhood. Normal newborns have undetectable levels of IgA, IgM and IgE. Maternal IgG is present and blood levels wane until the second half of the first year. Many laboratories do not quote well-defined paediatric normal ranges for their own assays which may be unreliable at the low levels detectable in small children. Furthermore, low values particularly of one or more IgG subclasses can be a transient finding of no great significance. It is therefore advisable to investigate any child with suspected humoral immunodeficiency in conjunction with a centre experienced in handling and interpreting paediatric material. Repeat investigations and assays of 'functional' antibody production should be undertaken before gammaglobulin therapy is considered.

Evidence is accumulating that tests of specific antibody responsiveness are a more sensitive index of humoral immune function than are measurements of total immunoglobulin levels. The presence of naturally occurring IgM isohaemagglutinins can be detected in routine cross-matching laboratories. These antibodies are, however, not found in those of blood group AB or, reliably, in infants under 9 months of age. Serology to a number of common pathogens and vaccine antigens is available in most centres. However, many of these assays are really set up to detect seroconversion as a basis for retrospective diagnosis of infection and may be inadequately sensitive for immunological investigation. Serum can often be sent to reference laboratories for more sensitive analysis by special arrangement, and this is particularly useful for measuring antibodies against previously given vaccine antigens—such as diphtheria, tetanus, polio, *Haemophilus influenzae* type b (Hib) and measles, mumps and rubella (MMR)—or additional vaccines given during the course of investigation. Hib, pneumococcal, influenza and injectable typhoid (Vi) vaccines can all be used in this way, with the added benefit of providing some potentially useful protection. Pneumococcal polysaccharide vaccine is particularly useful in this respect, since being a pure polysaccharide it is the least immunogenic and therefore potentially the most discriminating test when investigating partial humoral immunodeficiencies. It should, however, be noted that normal children do not reliably respond to this vaccine before 2 years of age.

Neutrophil tests The pathophysiology of neutropenia is often classified for conceptual purposes into either a failure of maturation and release of neutrophils from the marrow or an increased peripheral destruction (often antibody-mediated). Bone marrow examination will often, but not invariably, help distinguish between these two mechanisms. Demonstration of anti-neutrophil antibodies may also be helpful.

There are two well-defined groups of functional neutrophil disorders. Chronic granulomatous disease, which is a failure of neutrophil production of microbicidal oxidative products, is diagnosed by a simple slide test called the nitroblue tetrazolium (NBT) test. More sophisticated tests can then be performed to confirm the diagnosis. Bactericidal tests can be used to identify other less well-characterized neutrophil killing defects. Deficiency of leucocyte adhesion molecules such as leucocyte function antigen 1 (LFA-1) is due to an absence of the cell surface receptors important for the migration of leucocytes out of the circulation. All leucocytes are affected and there are consequences for specific immunity, but the main manifestations relate to failure of normal neutrophil function. These patients have high leucocyte counts and severe cutaneous and deep seated infections without pus. Diagnosis is by detailed leucocyte immunophenotyping. Defective neutrophil chemotaxis and adherence can also be demonstrated in the laboratory. Individuals with recurrent cutaneous and pulmonary infection, rashes and very high circulating IgE levels (> 5000 iu/l)—hyper-IgE syndrome or Job syndrome—also appear to have a defect in neutrophil chemotaxis, although the reason for this is not clearly understood. Other less well-defined neutrophil function disorders are associated with defective chemotaxis but they are difficult to diagnose and characterize, because measurement of chemotaxis is fraught with difficulties and results can vary considerably from time to time in any one individual.

Complement tests Deficiencies of many of the individual components of the complement cascade have been described. These are rare. Affected individuals tend to suffer from autoimmune disorders as well as infections. Recurrent sepsis occurs in those with C3 deficiency, alternative pathway deficiencies and to a lesser extent in early classical pathway component deficiencies. Recurrent meningococcal infection complicates deficiencies anywhere in the cascade, particularly the later (lytic) components. However, very few individuals with single episodes of invasive meningococcal disease have underlying complement disorders. Recurrent meningococcal disease or a family history should prompt investigation. Screening can be performed using a total haemolytic complement (CH_{50}) test in which antibody-sensitized red cells are lysed in the presence of test serum indicating the integrity of the whole cascade.

MANAGEMENT

General principles It is important to minimize exposure to potentially serious pathogens. Chickenpox and measles are particularly dangerous in children with cell-mediated immunodeficiencies. Prophylaxis should be given after exposure (see Chapter 37). Children with SCID should ideally be kept in strict isolation until arrangements for transfer to a bone marrow transplant centre can be made. In SCID and some other severe deficiency states blood products should be irradiated because of the risk of graft-versus-host disease.

Antimicrobials In most cases of minor immunodeficiency, the mainstay of management is the use of antibiotics given either in response to infection or on a long-term prophylactic basis. In the latter case most immunologists use co-trimoxazole at a quarter of the daily therapeutic dose. There is large anecdotal experience of the regimen both in immunodeficient children and in the prevention of urinary tract infection (before it became customary to use trimethoprim alone in that setting). Since immunodeficient children are being treated to prevent respiratory and cutaneous infection and, in some severe cases, opportunistic infection with *Pneumocystis carinii*, the combination drug is preferred. Opportunistic fungal infections can be difficult to treat and studies are currently in progress to assess the prophylactic use of antifungal drugs in conditions such as chronic granulomatous disease.

Gammaglobulin Intravenous immunoglobulin (IVIG) therapy is now widely used in cases of severe antibody deficiency. This treatment should not be embarked upon lightly as it is very costly and administration involves considerable disruption to the patient's life, even when arrangements can be made for administration at home. Most children with minor immunoglobulin deficiencies such as IgA or IgG subclass deficiency do not require IVIG and can be managed on prophylactic antibiotics unless breakthrough bacterial infections occur and put the child at risk of chronic lung damage. Intravenous immunoglobulin is potentially dangerous in those with IgA deficiency who may develop an anaphylactic reaction to the trace amounts of IgA present in the infusion. Although all commercially available products are made from carefully screened donors, IVIG is not totally without risk of transmission of viral infection, particularly hepatitis. In severe cases, IVIG therapy can transform the patient's life from one of chronic invalidity to near normal health. Management involves careful monitoring of the clinical course as well as adjusting dosages to maintain appropriate serum immunoglobulin levels. It is recommended that this is done in conjunction with a specialist centre wherever possible.

Cytokines and growth factors The cytokine interferon gamma has been shown to reduce the frequency of infections in patients with chronic granulomatous disease under certain conditions. It is curently used in the UK in selected patients. Granulocyte and granulocyte macrophage colony stimulating factors (GCSF and GMCSF) can increase neutrophil counts in neutropenic patients. Experience with these agents in children with primary immunodeficiency remains limited and requires expert supervision.

Bone marrow transplantation remains, for the moment, the only curative treatment for immunodeficiency. It is performed only in children with major defects such as SCID. Results are best when there is a matched sibling donor and when the diagnosis can be made during the first months of life. Success in SCID transplants particularly depends on early diagnosis and transplantation. For those without a matched sibling donor, parent to child haploidentical (mismatched) transplantation can be attempted using fractionation of the donor marrow to remove mature lymphocytes capable of causing graft-versus-host disease.

Genetic counselling Since most of the primary immunodeficiencies are inherited, counselling is important and (where appropriate) antenatal diagnosis should be considered. In an increasing number of disorders the gene has been identified, allowing first-trimester diagnosis. In other conditions such as some SCID cases this is not yet possible but second-trimester diagnosis can be performed on fetal blood. Female carrier detection can be performed for some X-linked conditions such as X-linked SCID and chronic granulomatous disease.

FURTHER READING

Watson JG & Bird AG (1990) *Handbook of Immunological Investigations in Children*. Wright, London

MANAGEMENT OF THE IMMUNOCOMPROMISED CHILD WITH INFECTION

Those working in paediatric medicine increasingly have to deal with children whose immunity to infection is compromised. This may be by virtue of immaturity of immune responses (very low birth-weight infants, particularly those who are sick); primary defect of immune function (congenital immunodeficiency); or more commonly through acquired defects of immunity secondary to human immunodeficiency virus (HIV) infection, chemotherapy or other immunosuppressive treatment (including corticosteroids). Other immunocompromised children include those who have been splenectomized, and those with sickle cell anaemia, cystic fibrosis and primary ciliary dyskinesia syndrome.

Infections in immunocompromised children are liable to be more frequent and more severe. They may show atypical features and may be caused by atypical (opportunistic) organisms. Since immunocompromised children are susceptible to a wide variety of organisms it is not always easy to predict the class of organism causing infection, let alone the species. However, there are some general rules depending on whether the predominant defect lies within phagocytic cells (usually the neutrophils), antibodies or the cell-mediated immune system.

NEUTROPHIL DISORDERS

Neutropenia The most commmon of these problems is neutropenia. This may be congenital or autoimmune in origin but most commonly it will be secondary to myelosuppressive chemotherapy or radiotherapy. Affected children tend to suffer infection with bacteria—particularly staphylococci and Gram-negative bacilli, including *Pseudomonas aeruginosa*. They may also develop fungal infections with *Candida* and *Aspergillus* species, and this is most likely to occur if the neutropenia is profound ($< 0.1 \times 10^9$/l) and prolonged (> 1 week), and if broad-spectrum antibiotics have been used extensively.

A significant fever (> 38 °C) in a significantly neutropenic child ($< 0.5 \times 10^9$/l) should be treated very seriously. A careful examination is required, looking for focal signs of infection—skin, mouth, chest, abdomen and perineum being particularly important. Blood cultures from any indwelling central line and by direct venepuncture should be collected, swabs taken from any focal infective lesions and a chest radiograph performed. Empirical broad-spectrum antibiotic therapy should be commenced immediately. Suitable therapy includes an antipseudomonal β-lactam (such as piperacillin or ceftazidime) and an aminoglycoside. Some centres use single broad-spectrum agents such as ceftazidime alone or imipenem, but most still use combination therapy. The most common organism isolated from blood cultures in this situation is the coagulase-negative staphylococcus and this is usually associated with an indwelling central venous catheter. Gram-negative bacillary sepsis is less common but is more feared because of the possibility of a fulminant illness with endotoxic shock. *Staphylococcus aureus* and streptococcal species are also found. If blood cultures are positive, antibiotic therapy can be tailored appropriately. However, quite commonly they are negative and if the fever does not settle this presents a problem—empirical changes in antibiotics become necessary and must be made by the third day of unremitting fever. The choice at this stage is either a new combination of antibacterials such as a glycopeptide (vancomycin or teicoplanin) and an anti-Gram-negative agent (ceftazidime, ciprofloxacin) or the addition of intravenous amphotericin to cover fungal infection. The latter should be introduced for patients at high risk of fungal infection (prolonged and profound neutropenia). The process of empirical change is repeated again after 48 hours if the fever persists without localizing signs and with negative cultures. By this stage it should be obligatory to add amphotericin.

When focal signs develop during episodes of febrile neutropenia new problems are faced. Soft tissue infections can occur anywhere but are found particularly around the head and neck and the perineal region. These often produce relatively mild signs of inflammation (until neutrophils return) but usually do cause some local swelling and with disproportionately severe pain. White cell infusions may have a role in containing these local infections. 'Embolic' skin lesions may occur from circulatory dissemination of infection. Necrotic skin lesions are characteristic of pseudomonal sepsis (ecthyma gangrenosum).

Intra-abdominal focal sepsis is relatively common in neutropenic patients particularly after chemotherapy which induces a mucositis. Characteristic features of typhlitis (necrotizing colitis) are diarrhoea with or without bleeding, abdominal pain, distension and, later, an ileus. Management should be conservative with fluid therapy, nasogastric drainage and antibiotics—metronidazole should be added to the regimen though good evidence to support its usefulness is scarce.

Pneumonia in neutropenic children will present with the usual symptoms, though chest pain is more common in this group than in immunocompetent children. Chest signs are notoriously unreliable and radiography while confirming the presence of a likely infective process rarely gives specific clues as to the microbial diagnosis. It is reasonable to start empirical treatment with a standard neutropenic broad-spectrum antibiotic combination; but if there is failure of response after 24–48 hours then bronchoalveolar lavage (BAL) should be undertaken to try to obtain a microbial diagnosis. It should be borne in mind that children who are neutropenic because of chemotherapy will also have depressed cell-mediated immunity and therefore be susceptible to the whole gamut of opportunistic pneumonias. Specimens obtained at BAL should therefore be tested accordingly.

Neutrophil function disorders Children suffering from neutrophil function disorders are liable to the same spectrum of infections as neutropenic children, though generally infection is less fulminant and more focal in nature. Unless the patients have indwelling venous lines, staphylococcal infections are usually of the coagulase-positive (*S. aureus*) variety. Skin and lymph node sepsis and pneumonia are common, while more deep-seated focal infection in liver, brain or bone may also occur. Depending on the defect there may be a tendency to less intense inflammation than might be expected. Fungal infection, particularly with *Candida* and *Aspergillus* species, also occurs. Treatment is with antibiotics and judicious surgical intervention. Adjuvant treatments with recombinant cytokines such as granulocyte colony stimulating factor (GCSF) or interferon gamma have been shown to be useful in some situations.

ANTIBODY DEFICIENCY

As well as occurring in primary immunodeficiencies, antibody disorders are found amongst children with HIV infection, on prolonged immunosuppressive treatment, after bone marrow transplantation and in protein-losing states such as enteropathies and nephrotic syndrome. Splenectomized and sickle-cell patients produce poor antibody responses to capsulated organisms and this is part of the explanation for their similar disease susceptibility. Bacterial infections are the hallmark of antibody deficiency states whether partial, as in IgA or IgG subclass deficiencies, or profound, as in X-linked agammaglobulinaemia. The predominant bacterial types are different from those causing problems in neutrophil disorders. Capsulated organisms such as *Streptococcus pneumoniae* and *Haemophilus influenzae* are the most common pathogens found, though Gram-negative and staphylococcal infections also occur. Infections are most common in and around the respiratory tract (otitis, sinusitis, pneumonia) but more disseminated infections may occur—bacteraemia, cellulitis, meningitis, septic arthritis. Febrile episodes with or without focal signs should be treated early with a broad-spectrum antibiotic such as co-amoxiclav or ceftriaxone. Care should be taken if immunoglobulin infusions are to be given during a febrile episode since reactions are more common at this stage. If there is failure of response to first-line antibiotics, other infective organisms to consider include *Mycoplasma* and *Ureaplasma* species which can cause arthritis as well as respiratory and genital infections in these patients. While 'pure' antibody deficiencies rarely result in opportunistic infections, some syndromes such as common variable hypogammaglobulinaemia may include subtle defects of cell-mediated immunity. Therefore, opportunistic infection (see below) may need to be considered when treating these patients.

Non-bacterial infections can occur in pure humoral deficiency states. *Giardia lamblia* can cause acute or chronic diarrhoea and may require repeated courses of treatment. Some viruses, particularly enteroviruses, are poorly handled in profoundly hypogammaglobulinaemic patients. Thus vaccine strain poliomyelitis may occur, and echoviruses may produce a chronic infection of the nervous system or muscle tissue. These viral infections are rare in those already on immunoglobulin replacement therapy. When they occur they are very difficult to treat though they may respond to initiation of very high-dosage intravenous immunoglobulin or intraventricular immunoglobulin for established central nervous system infection.

CELL-MEDIATED IMMUNE DEFICIT

Children with primary congenital disorders of the T lymphocytes, those undergoing chemotherapy, immunosuppressive therapy (including steroids) or bone marrow transplantation and those suffering from moderately advanced HIV disease will all be vulnerable to a wide variety of different pathogens, including opportunistic infections. Since disordered cell-mediated immunity usually results in defective antibody production these disorders therefore produce a combined immunodeficiency, and the spectrum of microbial susceptibility includes bacterial pathogens. The wide range of potential pathogens in these children is shown in Table 17.1. A history of antimicrobial prophylaxis is helpful since its usage will alter the balance of possibilities. For instance, *Pneumocystis carinii* pneumonia (PCP) is much less likely to occur if the child has been given prophylactic co-trimoxazole. If the child is also neutropenic this also alters the spectrum of possibilities.

Initial management of febrile episodes without localizing signs should be treated with broad-spectrum antibiotics (as for the neutropenic child if neutropenic, otherwise as for the antibody-deficient child—see above). Many

Table 17.1 Pathogens in immunocompromised children

Neutrophil disorders	
Bacteria	Staphylococci, enteric Gram-negative bacilli
Fungi	*Candida* spp, *Aspergillus* spp.
Antibody disorders	
Bacteria	Encapsulated organisms —*Streptococcus pneumoniae*, *Haemophilus influenzae* Gram-negative staphylococci
Viruses	Enteroviruses
Protozoa	*Giardia lamblia*
Cell-mediated immune disorders	
Bacteria	Intracellular pathogens—*Salmonella* spp., *Listeria monocytogenes*, *Mycobacteria, Legionella* spp.
Viral	Herpes group (herpes simplex virus, varicella-zoster virus, cytomegalovirus, Epstein–Barr virus) Respiratory (adenovirus, influenza virus, respiratory syncytial virus, measles) Enteric (rotavirus, adenovirus) Papovavirus
Fungal	*Candida* spp., *Aspergillus* spp., *Cryptococcus neoformans*, *Pneumocystis*, *Nocardia*
Protozoa	*Toxoplasma gondi*, *Cryptosporidium parvum*
Helminths	*Strongyloides stercoralis*

episodes will settle on this regimen, but if not a wide diagnostic trawl needs to be initiated. Pneumonitis has the widest spectrum of causes and early intervention is needed with bronchoalveolar lavage to look for bacteria, fungi (including *P. carinii*), mycobacteria and viruses (a panel of respiratory pathogens should be included in the screening as well as cytomegalovirus, other herpesviruses and measles). If BAL fails to provide a diagnosis and the patient fails to improve, more aggressive diagnostic intervention such as lung biopsy may prove necessary.

Gastrointestinal infections may occur with common or opportunistic pathogens. Acute episodes of diarrhoea may fail to resolve completely and the resulting chronic symptoms may lead to nutritional problems and failure to thrive. Stools need to be examined for the usual bacterial and viral pathogens and particular care taken to look for *Giardia lamblia*, *Cryptosporidium*, *microsporum* sp. and *Isospora belli*. These are notorious for causing chronic diarrhoea in patients with human immunodeficiency virus infection and disease.

Central nervous system infection may present as acute meningitis. In addition to the usual pathogens, *Cryptococcus neoformans*, *Salmonella* species and *Listeria monocytogenes* all need to be considered. Encephalitic illness may be generalized and acute or subacute due to a wide variety of pathogens, especially cytomegalovirus, Epstein–Barr virus and enteroviruses. Focal encephalitis presenting as focal neurological deficit or focal convulsions may occur due to reactivated *Toxoplasma* infection (usually in older childen who have had previous exposure to *Toxoplasma*), herpes simplex or focal fungal infections in disseminated *Aspergillus*, *Candida* or *Nocardia* infections. Computerized tomography or magnetic resonance imaging will help define some of these infections.

Skin and lymph node infections can be due to bacteria including *Salmonellae, Mycobacteria* (mainly atypical) and fungal infection.

PREVENTION OF INFECTION IN THE IMMUNOCOMPROMISED CHILD

Prevention should start with education of the family and their health professionals about the risks of infection and the need to seek prompt medical advice after infectious contacts such as with chickenpox or measles. In children beginning chemotherapy, antibody status against measles and herpesviruses (varicella-zoster virus, herpes simplex virus and cytomegalovirus) should be measured on samples taken before blood products (and thus passive antibody) are given. This will help determine subsequent susceptibilities. During periods of neutropenia precautions against nosocomial infection are required. Avoidance of high-risk foods such as salad or fruit without skin is sensible, but completely sterile food is unnecessary unless gut decontamination is being attempted. Broad-spectrum, non-absorbable antibiotic combinations are rarely used in children as they are poorly tolerated and of doubtful usefulness. Non-absorbable antifungals should, however, be used prophylactically in all neutropenic patients. The role of the new absorbed azole drugs is still under evaluation (see Chapter 18). Prophylactic absorbable antibiotics are used in some centres; quinolones such as ciprofloxacin

Table 17.2 Antibiotic prophylaxis in the immunocompromised

Penicillin	Sickle-cell anaemia, nephrotic syndrome, and some complement disorders
Flucloxacillin	Some neutrophil disorders
Co-trimoxazole (daily)	Immunoglobulin, some neutrophil disorders
Co-trimoxazole (3 times a week)	Cell-mediated disorders including HIV infection
Nystatin/fluconazole	Neutrophil and cell-mediated disorders
Itraconazole	When high risk of *Aspergillus* infection (under evaluation)
Acyclovir	Cell-mediated disorders (special circumstances)

have replaced co-trimoxazole in this situation. There are, however. concerns about using these powerful therapeutic tools on a prophylactic basis particularly when they are not yet licensed in children. In other situations such as the partial immunoglobulin deficiencies prophylactic antibiotics have an important role (Table 17.2).

In some circumstances judicious use of vaccination and immunoglobulin may be helpful (see Appendix VII).

MANAGEMENT OF THE CHILD WITH SYSTEMIC FUNGAL INFECTION

The great majority of systemic fungal infections that are seen in paediatric practice in this country are opportunistic, in that they afflict children who are susceptible by virtue of some severe debilitating disease, such as acute leukaemia, or as a consequence of the treatment of that disease. The principal fungal groups are *Candida* spp., *Aspergillus* spp. and *Cryptococcus neoformans*. Surveys in the USA have highlighted *Candida* as a leading cause of hospital-acquired bloodstream infections in patients suffering from a broad range of medical and surgical conditions that might increasingly be seen in paediatric intensive care units (PICUs). *Candida albicans* is the principal pathogenic species, although the proportion of systemic candidal infections due to non-*albicans* species has also noticeably increased. Cryptococcosis is the leading systemic mycosis in acquired immune deficiency syndrome (AIDS) patients, although it can also occur in lymphoma and in the chronically immunosuppressed, classically presenting in these groups as meningitis. There are also fungi that hitherto have been rare human pathogens but are believed to be generally increasing in incidence in the immunocompromised. These include *Fusarium* sp., *Pseudoallescheria boydii*, and phaeohyphomycetes such as *Phialophora*. Histoplasmosis, blastomycosis and coccidioidomycosis rarely arise in the UK, typically following acquisition of the causative agent (a dimorphic fungus) from endemic areas in other countries.

ANTIFUNGAL DRUGS

The antifungal armamentarium is still limited in terms of the number of drugs that have proven efficacy and are relatively safe for treating systemic mycoses (Table 18.1). The polyene amphotericin B is still widely regarded as the 'gold standard' therapeutic agent, even though efficacy data from controlled trials are scant, despite its use over three decades.

The advantages of amphotericin B are its broad antifungal spectrum of activity and the fact that fungal resistance to the drug has rarely been documented. The disadvantages are that the normal mode of administration, by slow intravenous infusion, is often accompanied by unpleasant febrile reactions, and nephrotoxicity is an almost invariable complication of prolonged treatment. A liposomal preparation of amphotericin (Ambisome) is now licensed for use in the UK for the same indications as 'conventional' amphotericin. Its principal advantage is that the incidence of nephrotoxicity is greatly reduced even when much higher daily doses are given. Whether at the same time this is associated with greater efficacy is unclear, especially in paediatrics where experience with the drug is as yet limited. More recently, another formulation comprising amphotericin complexed with cholesteryl sulphate (Amphocil) has been licensed. Again, data in children are very limited, but (as for Ambisome) kidney sparing would be an expected property such that it also could replace conventional amphotericin in the event of nephrotoxicity. A third lipid formulation of the drug (ABLC) is currently under evaluation. The place of these new formulations and how precisely they should be used is yet to be established, especially bearing in mind that they are considerably more expensive than conventional amphotericin. In view of the lack of clear evidence of greater efficacy, the present recommendation is to consider their use in place of amphotericin when renal function is already impaired or is rapidly deteriorating. There have been a few reports of use of amphotericin with intralipid, also with the aim of preventing nephrotoxicity; however, this preparation has yet to be properly evaluated and so its use cannot be recommended.

Flucytosine has a narrower spectrum of activity, principally restricted to *Candida* and *Cryptococcus* spp. However, it needs to be given in combination with amphotericin, since the emergence of drug resistance is very likely when it is used alone. Good concentrations are achieved in the central nervous system and urinary tract, so that infections at these sites are the main indication for use of flucytosine. In view of its myelosuppressive effects, serum drug concentrations should be monitored on a weekly basis, and dosing needs to be reduced in the event of renal impairment.

Of the azole antifungal drugs, ketoconazole and miconazole have been superseded by the newer triazoles fluconazole and itraconazole. Fluconazole has recently received a licence for use in children in the UK. It has good activity in vitro against both *Candida albicans* and *Cryptococcus neoformans* and proven efficacy against these pathogens when they cause systemic infections. Side-effects are infrequent and generally not serious, although when high doses of the drug are given it would be wise to regularly monitor liver function. Pharmacokinetic data are interesting in that in neonates there is prolongation of the half-life, and consequently the dosing interval should be increased; whereas in infants more than 4 weeks old and in children, the half-life is reduced so that higher doses than those used in adults are recommended. Oral administration of the drug achieves comparable serum concentrations to the intravenous route. It should be noted that some of the non-*albicans Candida* species are resistant to fluconazole, including *C. krusei* and *C. glabrata*. For this reason it is important that *Candida* isolates are fully identified to species level and that their antifungal susceptibility is determined when they cause a significant clinical infection.

The use of itraconazole for treatment of systemic fungal infections has been hampered by the fact that there is no preparation of the drug for parenteral administration. When given by the oral route its bioavailability is variable and is dependent on low gastric pH. However, preliminary results with a new cyclodextrin formulation suggest this achieves much improved absorption, although patient compliance may not be so good because of the large volumes of suspension that have to be swallowed. Potentially this drug has a number of important advantages over fluconazole with respect to its antifungal activity. Firstly, it is effective in treatment of aspergillosis which fluconazole is not, and secondly it may be active against strains of *Candida* spp. that are resistant to fluconazole. Although cerebrospinal fluid concentrations of itraconazole are poor it appears that it does achieve therapeutic concentrations in the brain, and anecdotal case reports of successful treatment of fungal brain abscesses appear to support this. While there is no evidence to warrant combining one of these azoles with amphotericin to achieve greater therapeutic effect, at the same time there is no evidence that they would be antagonistic in vivo.

There is considerable interest at present in the therapeutic role of colony stimulating factors (e.g. GCSF, GMCSF) in opportunistic fungal infections, especially in what is probably the most susceptible group, neutropenic children. Even though colony stimulating factors have been shown to reduce the duration of neutropenia after immunosuppressive therapy, there is as yet less conclusive evidence that fungal infections have been reduced in frequency.

Table 18.1 Antifungal drugs

	Amphotericin (Fungizone)	Liposomal amphotericin (Ambisome)	Amphotericin colloidal dispersion (Amphocil)	Fluconazole (Diflucan)	Itraconazole (Sporanox)	Flucytosine (Alcobon)
Preparation	Micellar suspension made with sodium desoxycholate	Amphotericin in liposomal vesicles	Complex of amphotericin and sodium cholesteryl sulphate→disc-shaped particles	Bis-triazole	Dioxolane triazole	Fluorinated pyrimidine
Route of administration	Intravenous	Intravenous	Intravenous	Oral, intravenous	Oral (variable bioavailability)	Oral, intravenous
Kinetics	High protein binding; poor concentration in CSF, eye, urine	High concentrations in liver and spleen; high serum concentrations; low concentrations in kidney	Same as Ambisome but lower serum concentrations	Low protein binding; excellent penetration of of most body sites; > 50% serum concentrations, in CSF; excreted unchanged in high concentrations in urine	High protein binding; low levels in CSF and urine; no adjustment of dose in renal failure	Low protein binding; excellent penetration of body sites including CSF and urine
Toxicity	Immediate: fever, chills* Kidney toxicity Hepatic toxicity	Immediate effects less frequent* Reduced kidney toxicity	Immediate effects less frequent* Reduced kidney toxicity	Low rate of mild side-effects	Low rate of mild side-effects	Myelosuppression; hepatotoxicity

Table 18.1 continued

	Amphotericin (Fungizone)	**Liposomal amphotericin (Ambisome)**	**Amphotericin colloidal dispersion (Amphocil)**	**Fluconazole (Diflucan)**	**Itraconazole (Sporanox)**	**Flucytosine (Alcobon)**
Interactions	Occur with other drugs if mixed in infusion	As for amphotericin	As for amphotericin	Serum levels reduced by rifampicin Phenytoin levels increased by fluconazole	Serum levels reduced by rifampicin	
Dose per day	0.5–1 mg/kg	3–5 mg/kg	3–5 mg/kg	3–6 mg/kg*	2.5–5 mg/kg	100–150 mg/kg*
Antifungal spectrum	*Candida* spp. *Aspergillus* spp. *Cryptococcus neoformans* Dimorphic fungi Wide range of other fungi	Same as amphotericin, plus possibly better activity against: *Mucor* spp. *Fusarium* spp.	Same as amphotericin, plus possibly better activity against: *Mucor* spp. *Fusarium* spp.	*Candida albicans* *C. tropicalis* *Cryptococcus neoformans*	*Candida albicans* Non-*albicans* species *Cryptococcus neoformans* *Aspergillus* spp. Dimorphic fungi *Sporothrix*	*Candida* spp. *Cryptococcus neoformans*

***Rare 'anaphylactoid' reactions have been reported.**
Fluconazole doses need adjustment according to age of child and renal functions.
Flucytosine doses need adjustment in renal cases.
CSF, cerebrospinal fluid.

SPECIFIC FUNGAL INFECTIONS

Systemic candidiasis Intrauterine *Candida* infection is rarely encountered but can result in fetal death. Premature rupture of membranes leading to ascending infection of maternal origin may be the mechanism involved. No particular maternal risk factors have been identified apart from vaginal candidiasis and antibiotic therapy.

Candida spp. are acquired by the newborn from mother's vaginal flora to form part of the normal intestinal flora. The prolonged administration of broad-spectrum antibiotics, especially cephalosporins, is likely to lead to fungal overgrowth as a prelude to invasion of the intestinal mucosa resulting in candidaemia. Babies of very low birth-weight are most at risk of systemic infection in this situation and may develop disseminated disease with deep organ involvement. A factor in this may be immature phagocytic cell responses. Other well-recognized risk factors for candidaemia are the presence of indwelling vascular catheters and parenteral nutrition. The use and need for any or all of these support therapies should be continually reviewed to try to reduce the risk of fungal infection. Studies on neonatal PICUs have shown that the colonizing yeast flora progressively change from *C. albicans* to non-*albicans* species; this may be the result of cross-infection due to transmission between patients of these strains on the hands of unit staff. Systemic candidiasis often has an insidious onset without any specific signs, although once the infection becomes established the infant will be clinically septic. A perineal rash or perioral septic spots may be observed, as may oral thrush. In order to establish the diagnosis it is essential to take repeated blood cultures, as the documentation rate with single or few cultures is poor. A single isolation of a yeast from blood or other sterile site should be regarded as evidence of systemic infection. Overall, documentation rates run at only 50–70% with currently available mycological tests. New molecular tests based on amplification and detection of fungal DNA in blood or other samples should improve these figures once they have been properly validated. What is important is to have a high level of awareness of which infants are most at risk and to consider early empirical antifungal therapy when the presentation requires it. There is a high incidence of meningitis complicating candidal sepsis in neonates such that there should be a readiness to obtain spinal fluid for laboratory examination: features consistent with this diagnosis would be pleocytosis, elevated protein and lowered glucose levels. Culture of the spinal fluid may be positive for *Candida* while blood cultures are sterile. There may be involvement of the brain with abscesses as another feature of this infection, giving a worse prognosis. Also, there is a high incidence of endophthalmitis complicating candidaemia which can be diagnosed by careful examination of the fundi.

A suprapubic urine culture can also help in diagnosis as involvement of the urinary tract occurs in as many as 50% of cases. This may be complicated by renal parenchymal infection and rarely the development of fungus balls obstructing the renal pelvis, a complication that may require urgent surgical intervention. Endocarditis is a rare but well-recognized complication of candidaemia believed to arise most often from seeding off an infected indwelling vascular catheter.

The most important therapeutic considerations in cases of neonatal candidaemia are as follows. When the candidaemia arises as a complication of vascular line sepsis in the absence of obvious organ involvement, will removal of the implicated catheter be sufficient? The answer is no, and the recommendation is to give antifungal therapy. Amphotericin is first choice with a total dose of 15–25 mg/kg. Flucytosine 100 mg/kg per day should be added in all cases of central nervous system infection in view of its excellent penetration across the blood-brain barrier. Serum levels of this drug must be measured at least weekly (and not exceed 80 mg/l) to prevent marrow toxicity. At least 3 weeks' therapy will be required. Fluconazole may become established as an alternative therapy for this indication. Systemic candidiasis in older children may be complicated by pneumonia, meningitis or endocarditis. Endophthalmitis and skin rash are particularly associated with this infection.

Aspergillosis Disseminated aspergillosis, with involvement of vital organs, typically occurs as a complication of prolonged profound neutropenia after leukaemia chemotherapy or bone marrow transplantation. The initial focus of the infection is pulmonary, characterized by single or multiple pulmonary infiltrates; the presence of fungus balls (mycetoma) within cavitary lesions is best detected by computed tomographic scan. At least 25% of cases will have extrapulmonary dissemination to other sites, especially skin, brain, kidneys and heart. Amphotericin or itraconozole are agents of first choice for treatment. Mortality is characteristically more than 90%.

Cryptococcosis For treatment of cryptococcosis the choice of regimen is either amphotericin (with or without flucytosine) or fluconazole for at least 6 weeks. In cases of severe HIV disease life-long suppression with fluconazole is necessary to prevent relapse.

FUNGAL INFECTION IN THE NEUTROPENIC CHILD

In the febrile, neutropenic child, the possibility of a systemic fungal infection due to *Candida*, *Aspergillus* or less commonly *Mucorales* arises when there is a failure to respond to 5–7 days of broad-spectrum antibiotics. The need for empirical antifungal therapy at this point is well accepted. Amphotericin is used (0.5 mg/kg per day) with adjustment according to how the patient's illness progresses. If the fever abates and the patient improves, then amphotericin can be stopped after 7 days. However, when a fungal infection has been documented, treatment should be continued for at least 4–6 weeks, according to the causative agent. As yet, there is no established fungal chemoprophylaxis regimen for neutropenic patients, although itraconazole would be the most appropriate choice in view of its spectrum of activity and oral administration (see also Chapter 17).

THE CHILD WITH HIV INFECTION

19

All HIV infected children and children born to HIV infected women should be reported to the BPA Surveillance Unit (see p. viii).

ORGANISM

The human immunodeficiency virus (HIV) is an enveloped RNA virus of the family Retroviridae. There are two major types: HIV-1 and HIV-2.

EPIDEMIOLOGY

By the year 2000 it is estimated that about 40 million people will have been infected with HIV worldwide, including 10 million children. By mid 1995 over 1 million cases of acquired immune deficiency syndrome (AIDS) had been reported to the World Health Organization (WHO) in persons of all ages, though this is estimated to be less than one-quarter of the global total of over 4.5 million AIDS cases. By early 1995, over 6000 children had been reported with AIDS in WHO's European Region, while similarly over 6000 children had been reported with AIDS in the USA. However, it is estimated that 90% of future paediatric infections will be in developing countries. So far HIV-1 is by far the most prevalent of the two virus types in adults and children. Vertical transmission of HIV-1 is the major route for HIV acquisition in children, contributing over 80% of cases in the USA and Europe. Outbreaks of nosocomial transmission have taken place through poor infection control, for example in Romania and Russia, where some children were infected via blood products. Children continue to be infected through blood transfusions in developing countries where it is not possible always to ensure a safe blood supply. Because of the importance of vertical transmission the epidemiology of paediatric HIV-1 infection reflects patterns of infection in women. In developed countries injecting drug use has been a major risk factor for infection in women in southern Europe and the USA, but this is being overtaken in some areas by acquisition via heterosexual sex, which is the major route of acquisition of maternal infection in developing countries worldwide. In the British Isles, risk factors vary by area. In Edinburgh and Dublin, the major risk factor has been injecting drug use, while in the other high prevalence area, London, the majority of vertically infected children are born to women who acquired their infection in association with time spent in sub-Saharan Africa. By the end of April 1995, a total of 752 babies born to HIV-1 infected women had been reported in the UK of whom 301 were known to be infected; over two-thirds were reported from London and other parts of the Thames regions.* Data from unlinked anonymous monitoring of HIV-1 in neonatal dried blood spots show a continuing rise in the numbers of children being born to

---

***Cases of HIV infection and AIDS seen by paediatricians are reported through the British Paediatric Association Surveillance Unit while cases of HIV infection in pregnant women are reported through the Royal College of Obstetricians and Gynaecologists Survey of HIV in Pregnancy. Reports of both are received by the Department of Epidemiology, Institute of Child Health, Guilford Street, London WC1N 1EH (Tel: 0171-829-8686). Microbiologists detecting new infections of HIV types 1 or 2 should report these to the Director, Communicable Disease Surveillance Centre (Tel: 0181-200-6868) (England, Wales & Northern Ireland) or the Scottish Centre for Infection and Environmental Health (Tel: 0141-946-7120). All reporting is voluntary and confidential.**

HIV-1 infected women in London but that only a small percentage of pregnancies in infected women are recognized as such by the time of birth. The majority of infected children are only recognized when they present with symptoms.

Transmission The most important routes of transmission are vertical (mother to child) and through blood and blood products. Vertical infections can take place in utero, intrapartum or post-natally via breast-feeding. The relative contribution of each of these is unclear, but there is increasing evidence to suggest that most occurs in late pregnancy or at the time of delivery. Vertical transmission rates of HIV-1 infection have been found to vary in different parts of the world; typical values found in prospective studies are 15% to 20% in Europe, 15% to 30% in the USA and 25% to 35% in Africa. Known risk factors which explain some of this variation are shown in Table 19.1. The transmission efficiency of HIV-2 seems considerably less. Risk of vertical and other forms of person-to-person transmission of HIV-1 may be higher (owing to increased viral load) during the primary 'seroconversion illness'.

Cases of 'casual' transmission from an infected child without the possibility of blood-to-blood contact have not been reported. There have been a very few cases of transmission between children within households and in all of these cases there were possibilities for blood-to-blood contact such as sharing of toothbrushes, injection equipment, biting and spillage of blood or other tissue fluids. Transmission from sexual intercourse to children occurs. Heterosexually and homosexually acquired HIV-1 infection is seen among teenagers in the USA and there are some reports of HIV-infected children who have been sexually abused by HIV-1 positive perpetrators.

Table 19.1 Risk factors for vertical transmission

Maternal	HIV disease status (related to virus burden)
	Primary infection*
	Advanced clinical disease*
	Low CD4 count or low CD4/CD8 ratio*
	Presence of other sexually transmitted disease, chorioamnionitis*
Delivery	Mode of delivery (caesarean delivery may reduce risk)
	Prolonged labour/rupture of membranes*
	Premature delivery*
Breast-feeding*	
Other	Viral phenotype
	Genetic factors

***Associated with increased risk of transmission.**

NATURAL HISTORY AND CLINICAL FEATURES

The virus predominantly infects and affects the T4 lymphocyte (CD4, T helper cells); it also affects other cells including macrophages and neuronal and glial cells in the central nervous system. The type 1 virus does not cause any congenital syndrome and infected babies appear normal at birth. Up to twenty-five per cent of infected children develop AIDS or die in the first year (called 'rapid progressors'), while the remainder progress more slowly (slow progressors) and some infected children are now entering their teenage years. Reasons for these differences are unclear but may be related to the timing of HIV-1 acquisition, the infecting dose and virulence of the virus. As disease progresses the level of CD4 cells (CD4 count) declines.

The main manifestations of HIV-1 are shown in Table 19.2. Many are non-specific in young infants and a high index of suspicion is required. The spectrum of disease has been classified by the Centers for Disease Control and Prevention, Atlanta, USA (1987 and 1994). Paediatric AIDS is defined by the appearance of a number of AIDS indicator diseases: opportunistic infections, recurrent severe bacterial infections, failure to thrive, encephalopathy and malignancy (most commonly central nervous system lymphoma). Lymphoid interstitial pneumonitis (LIP) is now recognized to be associated with a better prognosis and should not be included as an indicator of severe disease; however at present it remains an

Table 19.2 Most frequent manifestations of vertically acquired HIV infection in children

AIDS (severe HIV disease)	Approximate percentage of reported first AIDS indicator diseases*
Opportunistic infections	
Pneumocystis carinii pneumonia	30–40
Candidal oesophagitis	5–10
CMV infection	5–10
Atypical mycobacteria	5
Cryptosporidiosis	< 5
Toxoplasmosis	< 2
Cryptococcal infection	< 1
Other manifestations	
Recurrent bacterial infections	20–30
HIV encephalopathy (developmental delay or regression)	10–15
Neoplasms (mainly lymphomas)	< 5
Wasting	10–15

***Note, these estimates are not from prospective series and are not necessarily representative of what can be expected for individual infected children.**

AIDS indicator for purposes of AIDS reporting. The type of indicator disease to an extent predicts survival. Children with opportunistic infections (especially *Pneumocystis carinii* pneumonia and cytomegalovirus disease), encephalopathy and lymphoma have a worse survival than those with LIP and bacterial infections.

AIDS indicator diseases

Opportunistic infections are less likely to be due to reactivation of prior infection than to primary disease in children with vertical HIV-1 infection. In Europe and the USA *Pneumocystis carinii* pneumonia (PCP) is the most commonly reported opportunistic infection. It occurs most frequently at 3–6 months of age, sometimes when the CD4 count is relatively high, and has a high mortality. Cytomegalovirus (CMV) may cause disseminated disease, especially early in life, but retinitis alone (which occurs in adults) is uncommon in children. As in adults, CMV is often cultured from asymptomatic children with or without HIV-1 infection, and difficulty may arise in defining its role in the pathogenesis of symptoms. Cryptosporidiosis and atypical mycobacterial infections are being diagnosed with increasing frequency as children with profound immune deficiency are living longer.

Bacterial infections The organisms most frequently responsible for bacterial infections are polysaccharide encapsulated bacteria such as *Streptococcal pneumoniae*, *Haemophilus influenzae* and *Salmonella* species. Pneumonia is the commonest infection, causing significant morbidity, and children with lymphoid interstitial pneumonitis (see below) are particularly prone to recurrent bacterial lung infections often resulting in bronchiectasis.

Failure to thrive HIV wasting disease is multifactorial. It may occur secondary to infections, poor oral intake or from HIV-1 enteropathy. In older children, poor growth and pubertal development are likely to become increasingly important.

HIV encephalopathy Early encephalopathy often presents with motor developmental delay and progressive motor signs, particularly spastic diplegia. A computed tomographic or magnetic resonance imaging scan may show generalized atrophy and/or basal ganglia calcification. There is an association with concomitant opportunistic infections. Expressive language delay, behavioural abnormalities and memory loss may occur in older children.

Lymphocytic interstitial pneumonitis is found commonly in vertically infected children though it is rare in adults and in children acquiring HIV-1 infection later in childhood. It is often initially asymptomatic and without chest signs and is diagnosed in the second year of life on the basis of persistently abnormal chest X-ray only. Children may have associated parotitis and very high immunoglobulin levels (IgG > 50 U/l). The pathogenesis is unclear but may be due to HIV-1 itself or early acquisition of another virus such as Epstein–Barr virus. The differential diagnosis includes other causes of interstitial pneumonia including tuberculosis. A presumptive diagnosis can usually be made on clinical and radiological grounds without resorting to lung biopsy.

DIAGNOSIS

Children born to HIV-infected mothers all have maternal HIV antibody (anti-HIV) detectable at birth. Therefore testing for anti-HIV will not diagnose an infected infant until maternal antibody has been lost. The median time to loss of maternal antibody is 10 months and all have lost it by 18 months. Children confirmed (on a second specimen) anti-HIV negative can be considered uninfected. A child over 18 months old who has antibody is HIV-infected. Earlier diagnosis of HIV infection can now be made in many centres by detecting HIV by culture, detection of the HIV genome by polymerase chain reaction (PCR) or the presence of viral antigen (P24 antigen). However, as transmission may occur late in pregnancy or at delivery, a negative result in the first weeks (up to 2–3 months) of life does not exclude recent infection. Two positive results on separate specimens using one or a combination of techniques (viral culture, PCR or P24 antigen) are required to confirm infection. High immunoglobulin levels (especially IgG), reversed CD4/CD8 T-lymphocyte ratio or low CD4 levels for age, and clinical signs are other pointers to an infected child.

MANAGEMENT

Therapy for specific infections is discussed under individual diseases in other chapters. The following discussion focuses on prophylaxis and antiretroviral therapy.

PCP prophylaxis

In contrast to adults where a CD4 count below 200/mm^3 is a useful indicator for commencing PCP prophylaxis, the CD4 count is a poor predictor for the development of PCP in infants. Therefore, PCP prophylaxis should commence as soon as a diagnosis of HIV infection is suspected. When follow-up or early diagnosis of infants at risk presents a problem, an alternative strategy is to give PCP prophylaxis to all children born to HIV-positive mothers until diagnosis is certain; then uninfected infants can stop. For HIV-infected infants the use of cotrimoxazole (trimethoprim-sulphamethoxazole, TMP-SMX) prophylaxis 12 mg/kg cotrimoxazole twice a day; may also help to prevent recurrent bacterial infections. Some infants develop sensitivity reactions to cotrimoxazole, these seem to be more common in white children than in black children. Dapsone (1 mg/kg per day) or pentamidine (300 mg, monthly by an inhaler that can deliver a small enough droplet size, for example Respigard II) are second-line drugs, but PCP breakthrough has been documented with both.

Prevention of bacterial infections Immunization against *Haemophilus influenzae* type b and *Streptococcus pneumoniae* is recommended for all children with HIV infection. Monthly intravenous immunoglobulin (IVIG) therapy may help to reduce bacterial infections in some children with recurrent bacterial infections and not responding to cotrimoxazole though this has no effect on other aspects of HIV disease progression, or mortality. Other prophylactic antibiotics may be helpful in children with LIP and recurrent chest infections. In children with severe LIP, a short course of steroids, followed by low-dose maintenance oral or inhaled steroid (with or without a bronchodilator if evidence of bronchospasm exists) may improve lung function.

Immunizations Children infected with HIV should receive all routine immunizations with the exception of BCG, which should be withheld from those with symptomatic disease and where tuberculosis is uncommon. As tuberculosis incidence is low in the UK and most children born to HIV-infected mothers are followed closely, BCG is not usually given to these children at birth. If the child turns out to be uninfected then BCG is given.* Adverse reactions to other live vaccines have not posed a problem. Inactivated polio vaccine (IPV) is recommended because of a possible risk of transmission of live poliovirus to an infected child and other immunocompromised family members. A recent report describes a case of paralytic polio due to vaccine virus in a child who was HIV infected. Immunization should not be delayed, as the immunogenicity of vaccines in children with severe immune suppression is reduced. Normal human immunoglobulin and varicella-zoster immune globulin (VZIG) are recommended after exposure to measles and chickenpox respectively. Booster immunization against measles may be helpful and this approach is under evaluation.

Antiretroviral therapy

Zidovudine (azidothymidine, AZT) is the standard antiretroviral therapy for children with symptomatic disease. No efficacy studies have been performed in children, although some data suggest benefit in those with symptomatic HIV disease, particularly encephalopathy. The timing of initiation of zidovudine in children with early symptoms remains unclear; in adults, the initiation of zidovudine early in HIV infection does not prolong time to development of AIDS or death. However, in vertically infected children, early antiretroviral therapy may have a different effect and a trial of early versus deferred treatment in asymptomatic and mildly symptomatic disease (the PENTA 1 trial) is taking place in Europe. The dose of zidovudine recommended in children has been 600–720 mg/m^2 daily in three or four divided doses. The higher dose should be used in children with HIV encephalopathy to allow adequate central nervous system penetration. In other children, 600 mg/m^2 or even 480 mg/m^2 daily may suffice. Zidovudine can cause a reduction in neutrophil count and haemoglobin concentration particularly in the first weeks of therapy. These side-effects are, however, reversible. Non-haematological side-effects include nausea and headaches. In children, zidovudine has generally been well tolerated, especially early in the course of disease. The incidence of neutropenia due to therapy increases with HIV disease progression.

Didanosine (DDI; 90–135 mg/m^2 orally 12-hourly) is another nucleoside analogue with reverse transcriptase inhibitory activity. The toxicities are peripheral neuropathy (rare at low doses) and pancreatitis (about 5% of children and also dose-related). It is licensed for use in children as a second-line drug for zidovudine intolerance or progression of HIV disease on zidovudine.

Dideoxycytidine (DDC, Zalcitabine; 0.01 mg/kg 8-hourly) is also a nucleoside analogue. Its main toxicity is peripheral neuropathy and it may also cause mouth ulcers and skin rashes. It is not yet licensed for children in Europe. It is inferior to zidovudine as monotherapy in adults, and studies of combination therapy with zidovudine in adults are in progress. A toxicity and tolerability study comparing zidovudine plus DDC syrup with zidovudine plus DDC placebo in zidovudine-naive children (PENTA 3) started in Europe in 1994.

***If, however, the child is shortly returning to a country with a high prevalence of tuberculosis and will not be closely followed, he or she should receive BCG at birth; this is WHO policy for developing countries.**

3TC (2′-deoxy-3-thiacytidine) This nucleoside analogue has been shown, in preliminary studies in adults, to reduce virus load and increase CD4 cell counts when used in combination with zidovudine. It has minimal toxicity and studies are planned for children in Europe who have already been on zidovudine.

Care in the community Children with HIV infection may attend school normally, and the need to know within the school setting should be influenced by the needs of the HIV-infected child and not teachers and other children. Universal precaution guidelines for dealing with blood spillages in schools (see Chapter 27) should be carried out. This also prevents transmission of other blood-borne infections such as hepatitis B.

Social and psychological aspects of management are among the most difficult problems. Issues include testing of children and mothers, telling children their diagnosis, and retaining confidentiality. Infection with HIV carries a stigma in every country, and two (mother and child) or more family members may be sick or dying at the same time. The association with sex and injecting drug use add to the stigma and families are often overwhelmed at the time of diagnosis, especially if the family members only learn of the diagnosis through illness in the child. Social and cultural isolation, and fear of disclosure of the diagnosis are common. Management of the wide range of medical, psychological and social issues requires coordination between disciplines, between hospital and community services and voluntary and statutory sectors, while at the same time allowing the family to maintain control over who knows about the case. In the UK, family clinics are being set up in higher prevalence areas. As the numbers of infected children are still small and the issues are often complex, some centralization of expertise is required. This will also allow children to participate in multicentre treatment protocols. Development of shared care protocols, similar to those set up for shared management of children with cancer and leukaemia, provide models of care. Coordination between adult genitourinary medicine physicians, communicable disease physicians, obstetricians and paediatricians is essential if pregnant women with HIV infection are to benefit from current and future developments to prevent vertical HIV transmission.

PREVENTION OF FURTHER CASES

Reduction of vertical transmission Breast-feeding increases the risk of vertical transmission by about 15%, thereby doubling the risk of transmission in Europe. There is conflicting evidence over whether caesarean section reduces transmission risk, and a mode of delivery trial is planned for Europe. In 1994 results of a randomized, placebo-controlled trial showed that use of zidovudine (given to the mother in pregnancy and during delivery, and to the neonate for the first 6 weeks of life*) reduced vertical HIV-1 transmission risk from 26% in a placebo group to 8% in the treated group. Reported maternal and infant side-effects were balanced

***Trial dosages were: mother—100 mg zidovudine five times daily initiated at 14–34 weeks' gestation and continued throughout pregnancy (a pragmatic alternative is to give the same daily dose, 500 mg, but in three doses). During labour zidovudine given intravenously, 1-hour loading dose of 2 mg/kg followed by a continuous infusion of 1 mg/kg hourly until delivery. Neonate—zidovudine 2 mg/kg every 6 hours for the first 6 weeks of life commencing 8–12 hours after birth.**

between the two groups with the exception of mild anaemia in infants on zidovudine, which resolved on completion of therapy. The possibility of long-term adverse effects on children exposed to zidovudine during fetal life remains, and follow-up of all zidovudine-exposed children is essential. It remains unclear which component of the zidovudine treatment is of most value. Further research is required, and the results of this study can only be extrapolated to women who have never previously taken zidovudine and who are not breast-feeding.

Other suggested interventions to reduce mother-to-child transmission include cleansing of the birth canal (vaginal lavage), and passive and active immunization. Trials of these are in progress or being planned in the USA and in countries in the developing world.

Antenatal HIV testing In most developed countries it is now considered advantageous for an HIV-infected pregnant woman to know her HIV status. Health care needs of the mother herself can be met and she can make informed plans for the future. Information can be given about the risks of mother-to-child transmission, in particular breast-feeding, and the options of taking zidovudine to further reduce transmission, or termination can be considered. The subsequent follow-up of the infant and advantages of early diagnosis can also be discussed.

FURTHER READING

Department of Health (1992) *Children and HIV—Guidance for Local Authorities*, Available from DH Store, Health Publications Unit, No. 2 Site, Manchester Road, Heywood, Lancs OL10 2PZ.

Gibb DM & Walters SW (1994) *Management Guidelines for HIV-1 Infected children*. Available from AVERT, PO Box 91, Horsham, West Sussex RH13 7YR (telephone 01403-210202).

Lwin R, Duggan C & Gibb DM (1994) *HIV and AIDS in Children. A Guide for the Family*. The Hospitals for Sick Children and Institute of Child Health, London.

Mok J & Newell ML, eds (1995) *Practical Management of HIV Infection in Children*. Cambridge University Press, Cambridge.

PREPARATION FOR TRAVEL ABROAD

International travel is increasing: The International Passenger Survey suggests that in 1992 UK residents made more than 33 million trips abroad; more than 13 million trips to countries outside North America and northern and central Europe and nearly a million trips to malarious countries. Children travelling abroad generally fall into one of three major groups: (a) those taking a holiday in Europe, the Mediterranean or further afield; (b) those going to spend an extended period abroad with their parents; and (c) those returning with their parents to their country of origin, of which the Indian subcontinent is the most common, followed by West Africa. This third group is probably most at risk, as the children are likely to be going home to villages where risk of exposure is high; also, their parents frequently do not appreciate that the children are at risk through not having developed immunity from lifelong exposure to pathogens such as malaria, hepatitis A, etc.

The infections to which a child may be exposed include those commoner in less developed countries, many of which are amenable to immunization or chemoprophylaxis (e.g. polio, diphtheria, yellow fever and especially malaria) and also those which remain prevalent in Britain (gastroenteritis, whooping cough, hepatitis A, measles, tuberculosis). With air travel, almost all diseases contracted abroad may be incubating on return. Hence, a history of recent travel must be sought in any child with fever, gastrointestinal or other symptoms suggestive of infection (see Chapter 21).

Health advice for travel is a complex subject and a book can never be up to date. Also, the protection recommended for a holiday may be very different from that needed for an extended stay. This chapter simply outlines the advice most commonly sought and lists the sources which the health care worker or traveller can consult for more detailed and current information.

GENERAL ADVICE

Travel abroad has many potential hazards, not all associated with infection. These include different safety standards, exposure to extremes of climate, and language difficulties compounding ignorance of the local medical system. To a certain extent, parents must exercise their own common sense regarding their child's visit. A family checklist is: appropriate clothing, entertainment for the journey, adequate protection against sunburn, protection against insect bites, medical insurance, immunization prophylaxis and simple medications including malaria prophylaxis where appropriate. These topics are well covered in many popular and professional publications, examples of which are listed at the end of the chapter. Specific guidelines for individual countries are also provided in the Department of Health booklet *Health Information for Overseas Travel* (1995) which is updated biannually.

SIMPLE PRECAUTIONS

Water-borne and food-borne infections Most holiday-acquired infections (mostly the various forms of gastroenteritis) are water-borne and/or food-borne, and though they are not preventable by immunization, simple precautions will help to protect all family members. Some guidelines are given below. The extent to which they are followed will depend on local conditions and family preference. However, it is wise to emphasize to parents that diarrhoea is a common cause of a spoilt holiday and may be a serious risk.

- Pay scrupulous attention to hand hygiene, especially after using the toilet, or changing a baby's napkin, and before meals. Soap and toilet paper may be unavailable locally.
- Where the water supply is of uncertain quality (that is, most countries outside northern Europe, North America, New Zealand, Australia and urban South Africa), the traveller should not drink water from taps or other sources unless it is known to be purified. Hot, bottled or canned drinks with well-known brand names are safest. Alternatively, water can be treated. If visible matter is present, the water should first be strained through a closely woven cloth. Sterilization is achieved by boiling for 5 minutes or disinfecting. Appropriate disinfectants are chlorine and iodine (either liquid bleach, tincture of iodine or 'sterilizing' tablets). Iodine is preferable as chlorine is less effective. All tablets have maker's instructions. Tincture of iodine (2%) should be used at a concentration of 4 drops to 1 litre of water; the water is then allowed to stand for 30 minutes before use. The above ingredients are available from some chemists, travel clinics and by mail order from the Medical Advisory Services for Travellers Abroad (MASTA—address at end of chapter).
- In countries where water precautions are advised, the following should be avoided: uncooked vegetables, salads, unpeeled fruit, uncooked shellfish, cream, ice-cream, underdone meat or fish, uncooked or cold precooked food, and ice cubes. Similarly, unpasteurized milk (unless boiled) and cheese apart from that known to be made from pasteurized milk may also carry infection.
- Families preparing their own food should cook meat well. Fruit and vegetables should be washed thoroughly in clean, soapy water. If they are not then being cooked, they should be soaked for half an hour in treated water at three times the concentration of disinfectant used for purifying drinking water (see above).
- In case a child develops gastroenteritis, the family need to pack some oral rehydration mixture (e.g. Dioralyte); care must be taken over reconstitution so as not to provide too concentrated a solution. One cupful for each loose stool is a memorable dosage, but parents must seek medical help if excessive vomiting, severe diarrhoea, drowsiness, or other signs of dehydration occur, especially in a young baby (see Chapter 6).
- Children (and adults) should not play on beaches or swim in water visibly polluted with sewage; this also applies in European countries including the UK.

Insect bites Another important source of ill-health is insect bites which can result in a spectrum of problems from mild irritation to death from malaria. Hence protection against insect bites is highly advisable. Insect repellents can be effective against flying and crawling insects, though their effectiveness varies according to constituents. Those containing diethyltoluamide (known as 'deet'), ethylhexanediol or dimethyl phthalate are effective. These are non-toxic to children if used according to the manufacturer's instructions (which require avoiding excessive applications in babies and small children) and should be put on the skin before going out, especially in the evening when biting is most common. Insect bites can also be reduced by keeping arms and legs covered when out after sunset. Where night-biting flying insects present a hazard and bedrooms are not air-conditioned, use of a 'knock-down' insect spray is advisable. A mosquito net will give additional protection but must be well tucked in around the end of the bed and without holes. Nets can be made much more effective if impregnated with permethrin (which must be repeated 6-monthly), and families spending extended periods in malarious countries will often invest in their own nets (special nets are available for cots).

Animal bites Rabies is endemic in most developing countries and the Mediterranean (see Chapter 21). Even though the risks from a single bite or scratch of a dog, cat or wild animal are small, they are a considerable source of anxiety and parents need to educate their children against approaching animals on holiday. Families going to rabies-endemic areas should know how to treat a bite and may need pre-exposure immunization (see Chapter 82).

SPECIFIC ADVICE FOR PARTICULAR COUNTRIES AND DISEASES

Because the specific advice can change so frequently, it is best for the traveller or the professional to consult regularly updated publications or to contact designated information centres. Suitable publications are the pamphlet *Health Information for Overseas Travel*, the World Health Organization booklet *International Travel and Health—Vaccination Requirements and Health Advice* and the medical newspaper *Pulse* (table and chart updated monthly). These list the advice and requirements by country. However, the advice is not always consistent. Requirements tend to lag behind the times, local officials at times operate their own rules, and protection in addition to the formal requirements is very often advisable. Also, what is necessary for a trip to a country's main city may be radically different from the protection appropriate for an extended stay up-country. The main information centres are listed at the end of this chapter. Parents taking children abroad would normally consult their family doctor or practice nurse for advice in the first instance, who would use one of the sources above. When a complicated tour or extended trip is planned MASTA in London is useful (see below for details). It tailors a personalized health brief to the specific journey and medical history. It does charge a fee. Family application forms are available directly from MASTA and some pharmacists.

ROUTINE IMMUNIZATIONS FOR TRAVEL

Poliomyelitis There have recently been cases in the UK of poliomyelitis in the children of African and Asian immigrant parents. Although born in Britain, these children had either not started or not completed their immunization before being taken on visits to the home country where they acquired their infection. Some parents do not realize the need for continuing the course. Such high-risk babies must be fully protected before they leave, by starting in the neonatal period if necessary. It is equally important to advise that children of any age visiting an endemic area (for practical purposes all less developed countries) should be fully immunized against polio. Adults accompanying them should have boosters if they have had none in the preceding 10 years.

Diphtheria and measles are both common in the Indian subcontinent, Africa and parts of the Middle East including Turkey, and an epidemic of toxigenic pharyngeal diphtheria has existed in the countries of the former Soviet Union since 1991. All children visiting these areas should be protected by ensuring their immunization is up to date, while those travelling to an endemic area should consider a booster if they have not had an immunization in the prior 10 years, especially if they are going to mix closely with the local population such as on school exchanges. Children going to the USA (and some other countries) and entering school or registered day-care will be required by law to produce documentary proof of immunization.

Tuberculosis Children at risk are those making extended visits to developing countries. If the child has not had BCG as a neonate, the vaccine must be given before the child visits an endemic area for a month or more. Forward planning is needed, as a tuberculin (Heaf or Mantoux) test must be used first if the child is over 3 months of age, and 6 weeks should elapse between giving BCG and departure.

Tetanus Whatever and wherever the holiday, the consultation for advice should include ensuring up-to-date tetanus vaccination (note—not more frequently than 10-yearly after the primary course) (see Chapter 93).

ADDITIONAL IMMUNIZATIONS AND CHEMOPROPHYLAXIS COMMONLY RECOMMENDED FOR TRAVEL

Hepatitis A Protection can be given by passive immunization with immunoglobulin which should be given as close as possible to departure and will normally afford up to 6 months' protection. An effective vaccine is available (see Chapter 55), but it requires two doses 1 month apart for children (in adults a single dose and a booster 6–12 months later). It is also expensive. It is generally only used by those travelling frequently and though there is a junior version it is not licensed for use in children under 1 year old. Immunization is thought to give protection for at least a year and probably longer; its exact duration is unknown, but a booster produces some years of protection. It needs to be remembered that hepatitis A is best prevented by good hygiene and observing food and water precautions (see above), and that the greatest risk is to older members of the family as the disease is most severe beyond childhood.

Typhoid There are 100–200 notifications of typhoid in the UK each year, the majority of cases acquired overseas, chiefly in the Indian subcontinent. Prevention is most effectively achieved by good standards of personal hygiene and avoidance of contaminated food and water. The risk of infection in children under 1 year old is low. A range of typhoid vaccines is available but these are only moderately protective (see Chapter 97), and not all specialists recommend their routine use in short-term travellers to countries where risk is low.

Cholera is endemic in most developing countries (see Chapter 21). A handful of cases occur annually in the UK, all acquired abroad. As for typhoid, good hygiene is the best prevention and the vaccine is of very limited effectiveness (see Chapter 41). It is no longer recommended, but a certificate of vaccination or exemption from vaccination may be needed to satisfy some border authorities.

Yellow fever occurs in two endemic zones, central Africa and the northern zone of South America, with cases occurring in both urban and rural settings. Cases are almost unheard-of in Britain, but travellers to these countries are certainly at risk and must be protected. Yellow fever immunization is mandatory for entry to some countries in the endemic zone for *all* travellers over 9 months old. For other countries travellers *direct* from the UK do not have to show a yellow fever certificate, but those travelling from infected areas must do so. Listings for these two types of countries are published in the sources of further reading. Immunization is always advised (whether mandatory or not) for travel to rural areas within the endemic zones. Many general practices are now registered as yellow fever centres offering immunization, and the Department of Health booklet *Health Information for Overseas Travel* (1995) contains a current list. For a description of the disease, see Chapter 102.

Malaria Around 2000 cases of malaria are imported annually into the UK. In 1994 there were 1877 cases reported (including 11 fatalities), 228 in children under 15 years old. Malarious countries include almost all African countries, most of the Middle East, south and south-east Asia, Oceania and Latin America. Protection against malaria infection and severe disease is based on three strategies: prevention of bites (see above), chemoprophylaxis and prompt diagnosis.

Chemoprophylaxis is highly effective when the recommended regimens are taken properly; even when breakthrough infections occur, its use will almost always prevent the most severe sequelae. Two essential points must be made to families:

- Medication must be taken throughout the trip and continue for 4 weeks after return.
- If a febrile illness develops it may be malaria—medical assistance must be sought immediately and the doctor informed about the travel abroad (see Chapter 21).

The choice of chemoprophylaxis is a complex subject and recommendations differ with the area in the world, patterns of resistance to antimalarials and experience of new medications. A general guide is contained in Chapter 68, and the most authoritative source of guidance for the UK at the time of this publication is the article by Bradley and Warhurst (see Further Reading). Current guidance can be sought from the latest published material or expert sources of advice (see below). A general move has been to recommend weekly mefloquine for travellers to Africa and Oceania, though at the time of writing this drug is not recommended for children under 2 years old, for pregnant women in the first trimester or during breast-feeding, while the more traditional daily proguanil (Paludrine) and weekly chloroquine regimen remain effective.

Japanese B encephalitis Cases are rare but have been reported in persons travelling from the UK to South and South East Asia. The disease is caused by a flavivirus transmitted by a night flying culicene mosquito from animals (e.g. pigs) to man. The risk is greatest in those travelling to rural areas of India, Bangladesh, Lower Nepal, Sri Lanka and all of South East Asia. Prevention is by physical protection against mosquitos (see Malaria, above). Vaccination with an inactivated vaccine is recommended for trips of two weeks or more to rural areas. Vaccine is unlicensed, available on a named patient basis at British Airways Travel Clinics or to practitioners from Cambridge Diagnostics Ltd (Tel: 0191 261 5950). A short course consists of two doses separated by one to two weeks. This gives 3 months protection in most people. A course of three doses (separated by 2 and 4 weeks) gives 2–4 years protection. Under age 3 years the dose is 0.5 ml, over 3 years, 1 ml.

Tick borne encephalitis Cases are reported in persons being bitten by ticks in rural parts of Central and Eastern Europe (especially Austria). An inactivated, unlicensed vaccine is available on a named patient basis from Immuno Limited (Tel: 01732 458101) and is recommended for those going walking and camping.

The primary course consists of three doses given subcutaneously or intramuscularly separated by one month and nine months. This gives three years protection. A regimen of two doses separated by two weeks gives 12 months protection. No lower age limit is stated but the vaccine is not usually given before the first birthday.

Conventional protection against insect bites are recommended for protection against Japanese B and tick borne encephalitis.

FURTHER READING

Bradley DJ & Warhurst DC (1995) On behalf of a meeting convened by the Malaria Reference Laboratory. Malaria prophylaxis—guidelines for travellers from Britain. *British Medical Journal* **310**: 709–14.

Dawood R (1992) *Travellers Health—How to Stay Healthy Abroad*. Oxford Paperbacks.*†

Health Information for Overseas Travel (1995) HMSO, London (updated, annually and available on Prestel).

World Health Organization (1995) *International Travel and Health—Vaccination Requirements and Health Advice*. WHO, Geneva*† (updated annually).

ADVICE SERVICES

Note—this information was correct in February 1995 but changes are frequent.

Birmingham Department of Infection and Tropical Medicine. Telephone 0121-766-6611 (extension 4403/4382/4535).*

Liverpool School of Tropical Medicine. Telephone 0151-708-9393.*

Manchester Department of Infectious Diseases and Tropical Medicine, Monsall Hospital. Telephone 0161-720-2267.†

London Hospital for Tropical Diseases has a payline for the public: 0839 337733.†

Medical Advisory Services for Travellers Abroad (MASTA), Keppel Street, London WC1E 7HT. Telephone 0171-631-4408. Mail order service and provides individual health briefs (telephone payline 0891-224100); charges a fee.*†

Oxford John Warin Ward, Churchill Hospital. Telephone 01865-225214.*

National British Airways Travel Clinics are in many cities and prescribe medicine and vaccines. Details of the nearest clinic can be obtained by telephoning 0171-831-5333, but no advice can be given over the telephone.†

Communicable Disease Surveillance Centre. Telephone 0181-200-6868 (open to enquiries by health professionals, does not give advice on individual cases but is happy to advise on policy which is applicable to a particular circumstance).*

Malaria Reference Laboratory. Telephone (for doctors) 0171-927-2437;* (for the public) 0891-600350 (payline) or 0171-636-3924 (9:30–10:30 a.m. and 2–3 p.m.).†

Scottish Centre for Infection and Environmental Health. Telephone 0141-946-7120 (policy on individual cases as for CDSC).*

***Services giving advice for doctors, nurses and pharmacists.**
†Suitable for enquiries by members of the public.

MANAGEMENT OF THE CHILD WITH AN INFECTION CONTRACTED ABROAD

THE SIZE AND NATURE OF THE PROBLEM

There are no studies specifically looking at the incidence of infectious diseases in children who have returned from travelling abroad. Some surveys have included children, but it is often difficult to separate out them, and their problems, from the greater number of adults. This is important because the risks and consequences of travel-related illnesses are very different in children from those in adults. Children are at little risk of acquiring hepatitis B and human immunodeficiency virus (HIV) infections while on holiday, as these are predominantly spread by sexual intercourse. On the other hand they are more likely to contract hepatitis A, as immunity in young children from developed countries is low. However, the consequences of the disease are rarely serious in children, whereas it can be fatal in adults.

An extensive survey of travellers from Scotland showed that 33.5% of children aged 0–9 years experienced an episode of illness compared with 41% of those aged 10–19 years, 48% aged 20–29 years, 38% aged 30–39 years and only 20% of those aged over 60 years. One imagines that the main explanation for this pattern is the behaviour of the travellers.

Table 21.1 shows the risk of illness and use of medical resources in relation to travel. Most of the illnesses are trivial and many are no different from those acquired at home. However, in 1993 there were 253 cases of imported malaria in children in the UK and in 1994 a child died of diphtheria acquired on a visit to Pakistan. As a generalization, the risk of developing a travel-related illness increases the further south and east the destination; however, there are illnesses found in parts of Europe that are exceedingly rare in the UK. Examples include tick-borne encephalitis in some parts of Austria, Germany and Scandinavia; diphtheria in the countries of the former USSR; and rabies in many parts of Europe. Remember that some illnesses, e.g. malaria and schistosomiasis, may not become apparent until months or even years after exposure. Some travellers return from sojourns abroad with more than one acquired infection. It is therefore important not to assume that all a patient's symptoms may be explained by the first infection diagnosed.

IMPORTANCE OF DIAGNOSIS

It is important to make a diagnosis for a number of reasons:

- Urgent treatment may be life-saving, e.g. for malaria.
- Unrecognized cases may act as a source of an outbreak, e.g. gastrointestinal diseases.
- The condition may be notifiable.

TRAVELLERS' DIARRHOEA

The most common illness acquired abroad is travellers' diarrhoea which occurs in up to a third of tourists. Causative organisms include bacteria (enterotoxigenic *Escherichia coli*, *Shigella*, *Salmonella*, *Campylobacter* and *Vibrio* species), viruses (especially rotavirus) and parasites (*Giardia lamblia*, *Entamoeba histolytica* and *Cryptosporidium parvum*). The diagnosis is made on the basis of history and stool

Table 21.1 Estimated monthly incidence of health problems per 100 000 travellers (all ages) to tropical areas

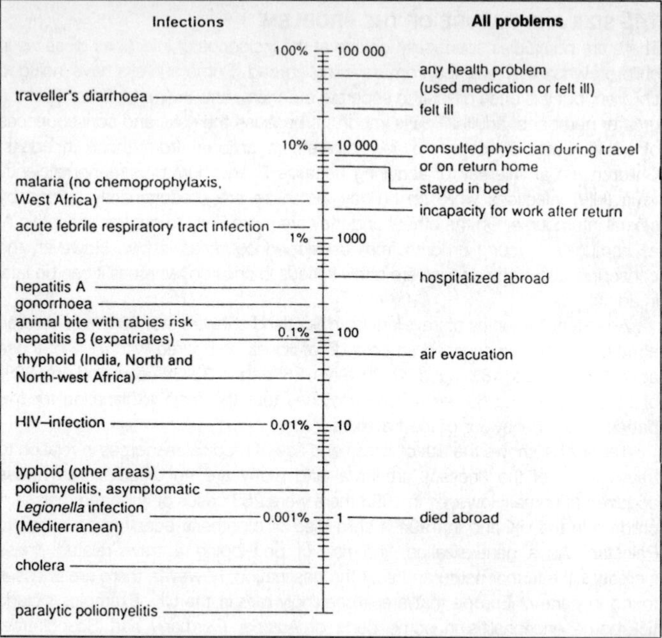

Source: Steffen R, Lobel HO. Traveller's diseases. In: Cook GC, edn., *Manson's tropical diseases*, 20th edn. London, WB Saunders, in press.

examination. Treatment should concentrate on rehydration and, as the condition is usually self-limiting, antimicrobial chemotherapy is not usually indicated. Moderate to severe diarrhoea has been treated successfully with trimethoprim or ciprofloxacin. Remember that malaria may present with diarrhoea as a prominent feature.

OTHER INFECTIONS

Other infections typically present as a fever. If the itinerary has included any country where malaria is endemic, it is essential that this diagnosis is excluded by a blood film. This applies even if appropriate chemoprophylaxis has been taken. Resistance is common and increasing. Falciparum malaria can be rapidly fatal and is often not considered. Having excluded malaria, the history should include:

- Medical conditions antedating travel.
- Nature and time of onset of symptoms.
- The countries visited.

- Living conditions and eating arrangements.
- Activities pursued, including bathing in fresh-water lakes and rivers, and forest walking.
- Illness in travelling companions.
- Details of immunizations and malaria prophylaxis.

A complete physical examination is important and should include careful examination of the skin.

All the usual 'home' causes of a fever should be considered as well as more exotic explanations. Combinations of symptoms with a fever may give a clue to the underlying cause. A *sore throat* (with or without skin lesions) raises the possibility of diphtheria and, rarely, Lassa fever. *Jaundice* may be due to hepatitis (most commonly hepatitis A) or haemolysis, e.g. malaria. *Neurological symptoms* may be due to tick-borne diseases (e.g. Lyme disease, tick-borne encephalitis and Japanese B encephalitis), typhoid, malaria and meningitis (including poliomyelitis). *Respiratory symptoms* may be caused by tuberculosis, legionellosis, pneumonic plague, anthrax, acute respiratory distress syndrome due to falciparum malaria, typhus, typhoid, Q fever, *Entamoeba histolytica* infection and tropical pulmonary eosinophilia. *Arthritis* may be present in a number of infections including Lyme disease, brucellosis, Reiter's syndrome, salmonellosis, yersiniosis and many of the arbovirus infections. A marked *lymphadenopathy* should raise the possibility of visceral leishmaniasis, tuberculosis, trypanosomiasis, typhus or bubonic plague. *Hepatosplenomegaly* is found in malaria, typhoid, visceral leishmaniasis, Q fever, brucellosis and the Katayama syndrome of schistosomiasis. *Rashes* may give a clue to the nature of an infection:

- A macular rash is found in typhus, typhoid, dengue and other arbovirus infections.
- A haemorrhagic rash occurs with yellow fever and the viral haemorrhagic fevers.
- Circinate erythema is found in early trypanosomiasis.
- Erythema migrans may be present with Lyme disease.
- Eschars are found in typhus and cutaneous anthrax.

A full blood count, and urine and stool microscopy and culture are essential in all returning travellers with an undiagnosed fever of more than a few days duration. An eosinophilia is a common finding (5–10%) and in approximately 50% will be due to a parasite. This is commonly intestinal, but may be due to other conditions such as schistosomiasis. Haematuria may be the only indication of schistosomiasis. The index of suspicion should be high if the child has been in fresh water in an endemic area (mainly Africa but also in some parts of South America, south-east Asia and the Middle East). A schistosoma enzyme-linked immunosorbent assay (ELISA) should be performed and, if positive, further definitive tests will be necessary.

Further investigations will be dictated by the history and physical findings (see also Chapter 15). The following section gives an indication of the most likely infectious diseases depending on the itinerary. It must be used with caution, as not all possible infections are listed and some of those that are listed do not occur in all parts of the region. For features of the specific infections, reference should be made to Part Two of this book or to a specialized textbook.

NORTHERN AFRICA

Algeria, Egypt, Libya, Morocco and Tunisia

Arthropod-borne diseases are unusual but can occur. The main manifestation is fever possibly accompanied by neurological symptoms. *Diarrhoeal diseases* and *hepatitis A* are common as is *typhoid fever* in some areas. *Schistosomiasis* occurs mainly in close proximity to the Nile. *Trachoma*, *rabies* and *poliomyelitis* are other potential hazards.

SUB-SAHARAN AFRICA

Angola, Benin, Burkina Faso, Burundi, Cameroon, Cape Verde, Central African Republic, Chad, Comoros, Congo, Côte d'Ivoire, Djibouti, Equatorial Guinea, Eritrea, Ethiopia, Gabon, Gambia, Ghana, Guinea, Guinea-Bissau, Kenya, Liberia, Madagascar, Malawi, Mali, Mauritania, Mozambique, Niger, Nigeria, Réunion, Rwanda, São Tomé and Principe, Senegal, Seychelles, Sierra Leone, Somalia, Sudan, Togo, Uganda, Tanzania, Zaïre, Zambia and Zimbabwe

Arthropod-borne diseases are common. *Falciparum malaria* and *filariasis* occur in most areas. *Leishmaniasis*, *relapsing fever*, *typhus* and forms of *haemorrhagic fever* can be found in many areas. Outbreaks of *yellow fever* happen periodically. *Diarrhoeal diseases* such as the *dysenteries* and *giardiasis* are common. *Cholera* is found in many areas. *Hepatitis A, B and E* are widespread. *Polio*, *rabies* and *schistosomiasis* are found in most parts of the region. The *haemorrhagic fevers* (Lassa, Marburg and Ebola), although present, are uncommon. Epidemics of *meningococcal disease* occur in the tropical savanna areas during the dry season.

SOUTHERN AFRICA

Botswana, Lesotho, Namibia, St Helena, South Africa and Swaziland

Malaria is only significant in certain areas. Other *arthropod-borne diseases*, although reported, are not a major problem to travellers. *Amoebiasis* and *typhoid fever* are common as is *hepatitis B*. The area is *polio* free but *schistosomiasis* is common in many areas.

NORTH AMERICA

Bermuda, Canada, Greenland, St Pierre and Miquelon, and USA

Plague, *rabies*, *Rocky Mountain spotted fever* and *arthropod-borne encephalitides* occur, but are uncommon. In the north-eastern USA and the upper Midwest *Lyme disease* is endemic.

MAINLAND MIDDLE AMERICA

Belize, Costa Rica, El Salvador, Guatemala, Honduras, Mexico, Nicaragua and Panama

Cutaneous and mucocutaneous leishmaniasis and *malaria* are found in all countries, but the latter's distribution is limited in Mexico, Costa Rica and Panama. *Chagas' disease* (*American trypanosomiasis*) is found in localized rural areas. *Visceral leishmaniasis*, *onchocerciasis*, *filariasis*, *dengue fever* and *Venezuelan equine encephalitis* are found to varying degrees in the region. *Amoebic and bacillary dysentery*, *typhoid fever*, *helminth infections* and *animal rabies* are common. *Hepatitis A* is common and *cholera* occurs in all countries.

CARIBBEAN MIDDLE AMERICA

Antigua and Barbuda, Aruba, Bahamas, Barbados, Cayman Islands, Cuba, Dominica, Dominican Republic, Grenada, Guadeloupe, Haiti, Jamaica, Martinique, Montserrat, Netherlands Antilles, Puerto Rico, St Kitts and Nevis, St Lucia, St Vincent and the Grenadines, Trinidad and Tobago, Turks and Caicos Islands, and the Virgin Islands (USA)

Malaria occurs only in Haiti and parts of the Dominican Republic. *Cutaneous leishmaniasis*, *filariasis*, *human fascioliasis* and *tularaemia* are found in small pockets. *Dengue fever* is also present. *Bacillary and amoebic dysentery*, and *hepatitis A* are common.

TROPICAL SOUTH AMERICA

Bolivia, Brazil, Colombia, Ecuador, French Guiana, Guyana, Paraguay, Peru, Surinam, and Venezuela

Malaria (falciparum, vivax and malariae), *American trypanosomiasis* (*Chagas' disease*), and *cutaneous and mucocutaneous leishmaniasis* occur throughout the area. *Yellow fever* is found in forest areas of all countries except Paraguay and areas east of the Andes. *Visceral leishmaniasis*, *onchocerciasis*, *filariasis*, *plague*, *dengue fever*, *viral encephalitis*, *bartonellosis* and *louse-borne typhus* may be found in some parts. *Amoebiasis*, *diarrhoeal diseases*, *helminth infections*, *hepatitis A* and *brucellosis* are common. *Cholera* occurs in some countries. *Hepatitis B and D* are common in the Amazon basin. *Schistosomiasis*, *rabies* and *hydatid disease* are found in some countries. *Epidemic meningococcal meningitis* can be a major health hazard in Brazil.

TEMPERATE SOUTH AMERICA

Argentina, Chile, Falkland Islands (Malvinas) and Uruguay

American trypanosomiasis is widespread. *Cutaneous leishmaniasis* occurs in north-eastern Argentina and *malaria* in the north-west of the country. *Salmonellosis*, *hepatitis A* and *intestinal parasitosis* are common in Argentina. *Cholera* and *typhoid* are not common in Argentina. Tapeworm, *typhoid*, *viral hepatitis* and *hydatid disease* are found in the other countries of the area.

EAST ASIA

China, Hong Kong, Japan, Macao, Mongolia, North and South Korea

Malaria is found only in China. *Filariasis*, *visceral and cutaneous leishmaniasis* and *plague* may also be found in some areas of the country. *Hantavirus*, *dengue fever*, *Japanese encephalitis* and *scrub typhus* occur in many areas. *Diarrhoeal diseases*, *hepatitis E* and *brucellosis* are common in China. The *oriental liver fluke* (*clonorchiasis*) and *oriental lung fluke* (*paragonimiasis*) are reported in most countries. *Hepatitis B* is common whereas *schistosomiasis* is found mainly in the Yangtze river basin of China. *Polio*, *trachoma* and *leptospirosis* also occur in China.

EASTERN SOUTH ASIA

Brunei Darussalam, Cambodia, Indonesia, Laos, Malaysia, Myanmar, Philippines, Singapore, Thailand and Vietnam

Filariasis occurs in all countries and *typhus* in most. *Malaria* is endemic in all but Brunei, Darussalam and Singapore. *Plague* and *melioidosis* are found in Myanmar, Malaysia and Vietnam. *Dengue fever* occurs in epidemics. *Cholera*, *amoebic and bacillary dysentery*, *typhoid fever*, and *hepatitis A and E* are found in all countries. The giant intestinal fluke (*fasciolopsiasis*) and oriental lung fluke (*paragonimiasis*) are found in most countries, whereas the oriental liver fluke (*clonorchiasis*) and the cat liver fluke (*opisthorchiasis*) are found mainly in the Indochina peninsula. *Schistosomiasis*, *polio* and *trachoma* are found in some areas. *Hepatitis B* is common. *Rabies* is a potential hazard.

MIDDLE SOUTH ASIA

Afghanistan, Armenia, Azerbaijan, Bangladesh, Bhutan, Georgia, India, Iran, Kazakhstan, Kirgizstan, Maldives, Nepal, Pakistan, Sri Lanka, Tadzhikistan, Turkmenistan and Uzbekistan

Malaria is found in all countries except the Maldives. *Filariasis*, *leishmaniasis*, *relapsing fever*, *typhus*, *dengue fever*, *Japanese encephalitis* and various *haemorrhagic fevers* are found in many countries of the area. *Cholera*, *dysentery*, *typhoid fever*, *hepatitis A and E*, and *helminth infections* are common. *Brucellosis* and *hydatid disease* are found in many countries. There are pockets of *dracunculiasis* in India and Pakistan. *Hepatitis B* and *animal rabies* are found in most countries. *Urinary schistosomiasis* is found in the south-west of Iran and meningococcal meningitis in India and Nepal. *Polio* is found all countries throughout the region, except for Bhutan and the Maldives.

WESTERN SOUTH ASIA

Bahrain, Cyprus, Iraq, Israel, Jordan, Kuwait, Lebanon, Oman, Qatar, Saudi Arabia, Syria, Turkey, United Arab Emirates and Yemen

Malaria is found in the rural parts of many countries of the area. *Typhus* and *relapsing fever* are present in some countries as is *visceral leishmaniasis*. *Cutaneous leishmaniasis* is common. *Typhoid fever*, *hepatitis A* and *brucellosis* occur in most countries. Tapeworm and *dracunculiasis* are present in most countries. *Hydatid disease*, *trachoma*, *animal rabies* and *polio* occur in some countries.

NORTHERN EUROPE

Belarus, Belgium, Channel Islands, Czech Republic, Denmark, Estonia, Faroe Islands, Finland, Germany, Iceland, Ireland, the Isle of Man, Latvia, Lithuania, Luxembourg, Moldova, Netherlands, Norway, Poland, Russian Federation, Slovakia, Sweden, Ukraine and the United Kingdom

Malaria is not a problem. *Tick-borne encephalitis*, *Lyme disease* and *Crimean–Congo haemorrhagic fever* occur in the north. *Hantavirus disease* is present throughout the area. Infection with Tapeworm, *Trichinella*, *Diphyllobothrium* and *Fasciola hepatica* and *hepatitis A* may occur in some areas. *Diphtheria* is a problem in some countries, especially in the former USSR. *Polio* is found in the Russian Federation and the Ukraine. *Animal rabies* is found in the rural parts of northern Europe except Finland, Iceland, Norway, Sweden and the UK.

SOUTHERN EUROPE

Albania, Andorra, Austria, Azores, Bosnia-Hercegovina, Bulgaria, Canary Islands, Croatia, France, Gibraltar, Greece, Hungary, Italy, Liechtenstein, Madeira, Malta, Monaco, Portugal, Romania, San Marino, Slovenia, Spain, Switzerland, and Yugoslavia

Tick-borne encephalitis, *Lyme disease* and *hantavirus disease* are found in the south and east. *Typhus, West Nile fever, cutaneous and visceral leishmaniasis* and *sandfly fever* are found in countries bordering the Mediterranean. *Bacillary dysentery* and *typhoid fever* are common in the south-eastern and south-western parts of the area, where brucellosis may also be found. *Hydatid disease* occurs in the south-east. *Hepatitis A* and *Fasciola hepatica infection* are a problem in some parts of the area. *Polio* is present in parts of the former Yugoslavia. *Hepatitis B* is endemic in Albania, Bulgaria and Romania. *Animal rabies* is found in all countries of the area apart from Gibraltar, Malta, Monaco and Portugal.

AUSTRALIA, NEW ZEALAND AND THE ANTARCTIC

Communicable diseases are rarely more hazardous to tourists than in their country of origin. Mosquito-borne *epidemic polyarthritis* and *viral encephalitis*, and *amoebic meningoencephalitis* have been reported.

MELANESIA AND MICRONESIA-POLYNESIA

American Samoa, Cook Islands, Easter Island, Fiji, French Polynesia, Guam, Kiribati, Marshall Islands, Micronesia, Nauru, New Caledonia, Niue, Palau, Papua New Guinea, Samoa, Solomon Islands, Tokelau, Tonga, Trust Territory of the Pacific Islands, Tuvalu, Vanuatu, and the Wallis and Furtuna Islands

Malaria is endemic in some of the islands and *dengue fever* can occur in epidemics in most. *Filariasis* is widespread. *Typhus* has been found in Papua New Guinea. *Typhoid fever*, *hepatitis A* and *helminth infections* are common. *Hepatitis B* is endemic throughout the area. *Trachoma* is found in parts of Melanesia and *polio* in Papua New Guinea.

22 REFUGEES AND INTERNATIONALLY ADOPTED CHILDREN

POSSIBLE PROBLEMS

Refugees and children being adopted from abroad may have similar medical problems. Many of these will relate to lack of routine child health surveillance in the countries of origin, e.g. undetected defects of vision, hearing and speech, and omission of routine immunizations, whereas others will be infections acquired from the child's country of origin. The risk and type of infection depends upon the country from which the child has come. Children from the USA, western Europe and Australasia will be subject to the same level of care as in the UK and will suffer, broadly speaking, the same infectious diseases (some arthropod-borne diseases may be more common in these countries). Children from some countries of eastern Europe may be at increased risk of diphtheria and tuberculosis. Enteric infections are also more common. Children who have lived in orphanages or received blood transfusions may have acquired human immunodeficiency virus (HIV) and/or hepatitis B infection, especially in Romania. Children from Africa, the Indian subcontinent and some parts of South America may have been exposed to numerous diseases not usually encountered in the West. Treatment for diagnosed diseases may have been suboptimal, suppressing the illness rather than eliminating the infection. Many infections may be asymptomatic at the time of entry to the country and some (e.g. schistosomiasis and liver flukes) may take years to become apparent. Recurrent fever due to chronic malaria is accepted as the norm in many countries.

MANAGEMENT AND SCREENING

In this section the management of asymptomatic children only is considered. The management of a child from abroad who has a fever or other symptoms is considered in Chapter 21 and relevant chapters in Part 2. For children being adopted from abroad an inter-country adoption form should be completed. This includes a thorough history and examination. All other children coming from abroad should, at least, answer a health questionnaire. Any omissions in routine child health surveillance or immunizations should be rectified. Whether or not to screen asymptomatic children from abroad for infections is unclear. In 1991, a study at the Hospital for Tropical Diseases, London, screened 1029 asymptomatic individuals (135 less than 14 years old) returning from a prolonged stay abroad. It was difficult to estimate in how many people the abnormalities that were found related to their stay abroad. Urine analysis of 830 cases showed abnormalities in 116. In none of these was the abnormality related to the stay abroad. Stool microscopy for cysts, ova and parasites showed abnormalities in 207 of 995 (20.8%). The most common finding was the presence of cysts of *Entamoeba histolytica* or *Giardia lamblia*. Almost all were treated, in spite of being asymptomatic. Out of 852 blood samples, 67 (7.9%) showed an eosinophilia. In 26 people this was associated with parasitosis (schistosomiasis in 18). The authors concluded that screening for tropical disease can be efficiently carried out by an informed health professional using structured history taking and relevant laboratory tests. A survey of health authorities and boards in the UK, published in 1990, showed a wide variation in policy of screening children from abroad. The

Table 22.1 Immunization of children with unknown immunization status†

Age	Primary immunizations required	Booster immunizations required
Under 1 year	DTP × 3 OPV × 3 Hib × 3 MMR × 1	DT + OPV at age 31/2 years Td + OPV at age 15 years
1–4 years	DTP × 3 OPV × 3 Hib × 1 MMR × 1	DT + OPV at age 3 years Td + OPV at age 15 years
4–10 years	DTP × 3 OPV × 3 MMR × 1	Td + OPV after 15 years Td + OPV at age 25 years
10–15 years	Td × 3 OPV × 3 MMR × 1	Td + OPV after 3 years Td + OPV at age 25 years

†BCG should be given according to local policy.
Key: DTP, diphtheria/tetanus/pertussis; OPV, oral polio vaccine; Hib, *Haemophilus influenzae* type b; MMR, measles/mumps/rubella; Td, tetanus/low dose diphtheria.

authors suggested the following procedure for children entering the educational systems in the UK after spending more than 8 weeks in Asia, the Far East, Africa and South America.

- The school nurse should interview the family before the child starts school and review the child's health. A Heaf test should be performed, and if negative, BCG given. Children already in school should be interviewed as soon as possible.
- If asymptomatic, the child can start school as soon as the interview has been completed.
- Immunizations should be completed* (Table 22.1).
- If the child does not already have a general practitioner, advice should be given on registering.

In the absence of evidence to the contrary, the above procedure is recommended. Consideration should also be given to voluntary confidential testing for children and adults from high-risk areas for HIV and hepatitis B infection. Screening for infectious diseases other than these and for tuberculosis cannot be justified.

***Unfortunately, immunization schedules vary enormously between different countries, even in western Europe. They also vary from time to time and it is not possible to publish a guide to them as it would rapidly be out of date.**

23 ZOONOSES

Zoonoses are infections that are naturally transmissible between vertebrate animals and humans. Many of the human communicable diseases described in detail in Part Two of this manual are zoonoses or, in the case of some of the infections, may be transmitted zoonotically from animals to humans. The zoonoses are a highly varied group of diseases and constitute an important public health problem. The organisms responsible may be bacteria, viruses, protozoa, helminths, chlamydiae or rickettsiae. Some are fortunately rare, while others such as the food-borne infections are all too common. Some may cause serious disease in humans, while others produce apparently mild, non-specific symptoms in some people, but severe effects in others; others may cause no apparent signs or symptoms at all. Rabies, for example, is a life-threatening and usually fatal illness. Toxocariasis and toxoplasmosis, on the other hand, are usually asymptomatic, although in some circumstances can cause severe disablement in affected humans. Cryptosporidiosis is generally an acute self-limiting illness in healthy individuals, whereas in an immunocompromised patient the same infection may prove fatal. Other gastrointestinal zoonotic organisms such as salmonellae can cause extensive morbidity; such human zoonotic infections may occur as local clusters or outbreaks that may be geographically widespread, both nationally and internationally, affecting large numbers of people. Other zoonoses more often occur as single, apparently sporadic cases, such as hydatid disease. There are many zoonotic infections that are found in Britain, while others are only likely to be encountered overseas.

The variety of vertebrate animals from which humans may inadvertently acquire infections is as broad as the range of zoonotic infections themselves (Table 23.1). The animal types may be characterized within one of three groups; first, the domestic pets (or companion animals as now described by the veterinary profession) such as cats and dogs. These live in close proximity to their owners and may transmit gastrointestinal and skin infections as well as toxoplasmosis and toxocariasis. Rabbits have been known to transmit yersiniosis. The second group includes all livestock and infections that may be acquired either through direct contact with infected live animals, dead carcasses or the consumption of infected or contaminated meat. Examples include skin and gastrointestinal infections such as cowpox and orf viruses, cryptosporidiosis and salmonellosis as well as toxoplasmosis. The last group comprises all wild or exotic animals. Some of these may come into the first group: for example psittacine birds such as parrots are kept as pets and are known to transmit psittacosis, turtles may transmit salmonellosis and tropical fish may transmit *Mycobacterium marinum* infections. Other diseases usually associated with wild or exotic animals include imported infections such as leishmaniasis.

The transmission characteristics of human zoonotic infections are an interesting feature in the epidemiology of these infections. Zoonoses may be transmitted via direct or indirect means, and there may be several routes within each of these.

Direct transmission includes the consumption or ingestion of undercooked or raw meat or other food derived from animals that may contain pathogenic organisms; for example, *Salmonella* in poultry, fresh eggs and untreated milk.

Table 23.1 Some of the zoonotic infections that may be acquired by children in Britain and other parts of Europe

Disease/infection	Causative organism/ common species	Common animal sources	Mode of spread/vector	Human epidemiology (England and Wales)*
GASTROINTESTINAL INFECTIONS				
Campylobacteriosis†	*Campylobacter jejuni*, *C. coli* *C. lardis*	Cattle, poultry, pigs, sheep, birds, rodents, puppies and kittens	Ingestion of water contaminated by animal faeces; consumption of undercooked chicken, unpasteurized milk or contaminated foods; by the faecal–oral route direct from animals or person-to-person	There are over 40 000 indigenous and imported laboratory reported infections annually; about 20% of these occur in children. A major proportion of the infections are probably food-borne
Cryptosporidiosis†	*Cryptosporidium parvum*	Sheep, cattle, deer, goats, puppies and kittents	By the faecal–oral route direct from animals, or via contaminated water; consumption of contaminated milk; or person-to-person	There are around 5000 indigenous and imported laboratory reported cases each year; nearly two-thirds are in children
Giardiasis†	*Giardia lamblia*	Various wild and domestic animals	Direct by the faecal–oral route from animals or person-to-person; or ingestion of contaminated water	There are around 6000 indigenous and imported laboratory reported infections each year; over a quarter are in children. Travel-associated cases and water-borne outbreaks have been reported

Table 23.1 continued

Disease/infection	Causative organism/ common species	Common animal sources	Mode of spread/vector	Human epidemiology (England and Wales)*
Haemolytic uraemic syndrome (HUS) haemorrhagic colitis†	*Escherichia coli* 0157 (verotoxin-producing *E. coli*, VTEC) Entero-haemorrhagic *E. coli* (EHEC)	Cattle	Consumption of raw inadequately cooked beef, milk, unwashed fruit and vegetables contaminated with animal faeces, other contaminated foods; by the faecal–oral route direct from animals or person-to-person	Around 400 isolates of VTEC are confirmed annually; nearly half are in children. Several food-borne incidents have been recorded. Not all develop HUS
Hymenolepiasis (dwarf and rat tapeworm infections)	*Hymenolepis nana*, *H. diminuta*	*H. nana*: house-mice; dogs, cats and their fleas, beetles *H. diminuta*: rats, fleas, beetles	*H. nana*: direct ingestion of eggs passed in animal faeces, or by the faecal–route from person to person *H. diminuta*; inadvertent ingestion of the infected insect	There are around 100 laboratory reports of human *H. nana* infections each year; over half are in children. *H. diminuta* infections are very rare
Salmonellosis†	*Salmonella* spp. (excluding *S. typhi* and *S. paratyphi*)	Poultry, cattle, sheep and pigs	Consumption of raw or inadequately cooked food from animals; raw milk; cross-contamination of cooked foods; by the faecal–oral route from animals or person-to-person	There are around 30 000 indigenous and imported cases confirmed each year; nearly 30% are in children. Most are probably associated with food consumption

Yersiniosis†	*Yersinia pseudotuberculosis* and *Y. enterocolitica*	Wild and domestic animals	Infections may be food-borne, water-borne, or possibly acquired by the faecal–oral route from animals or person-to-person	There are around 250 laboratory-reported infections each year; a quarter of these are in children. Food-borne infections from unpasteurized milk and cheese, for example, have occurred, as has an outbreak attributed to contact with an infected rabbit
SKIN INFECTIONS				
Cowpox†	Parapox virus	Cats and other felines, cattle and rodents	Direct contact between infected animals and abraded human skin	There are only a few laboratory reports each year in both children and adults (see Chapter 80)
Dermatophytosis or ringworm†	*Trichophyton* spp., *Microsporum* spp.	Dogs, cats, cattle and horses	Direct skin contact with animals or through abrasions or cuts; transmission from the environment contaminated with fungal spores; or person-to-person	No data available but probably a common infection particularly among farmers, veterinarians, slaughterhouse workers and those who work with horses

Table 23.1 continued

Disease/infection	Causative organism/ common species	Common animal sources	Mode of spread/vector	Human epidemiology (England and Wales)*
Mycobacteriosis†	*Mycobacterium marinum*	Fish and marine mammals	Direct transmission from infected fish, contaminated aquaria or marine mammal bites	Between 20 and 30 laboratory-reported infections each year, mostly amongst tropical fish keepers
Orf viurs infections†	Orf-paravaccinia virus	Sheep and goats	Direct abraded skin contact with animal lesions, infected wool or hides, or contaminated pastures	There are around 20 laboratory reports each year including a few infections in children. It is probably an occupational hazard affecting mainly shepherds, veterinarians, slaughterhouse workers and butchers
Pasteurellosis	*Pasteurella multocida* and *P. haemolytica*	Dogs and cats	Direct transmission via animal bites, scratches and licks	There are over 200 laboratory-reported infections each year but only a small proportion occur in children

RESPIRATORY TRACT INFECTIONS				
Q fever	*Coxiella burnetii*	Sheep, cattle, goats and ticks	Inhalation of dust contaminated by placental tissue and fluids; direct contact with animals or animal products; consumption of contaminated milk; or possibly tick bites	About 100 laboratory reports of indigenous and imported infections each year, but very rarely in children. Cases have been reported in farmers, veterinarians, and slaughterhouse and tannery workers
Chlamydiosis, ornithosis or psittacosis	*Chlamydia psittaci*	Avian strain: psittacine and other birds including ducks, turkeys, pigeons Ovine strain: sheep and possibly goats and cattle	Avian strain: inhalation of aerosols or dust contaminated by infected bird faeces or nasal discharges Ovine strain: inhalation of aerosol or dust contaminated by the products of gestation or abortion	There are on average 400 laboratory reported indigenous and imported infections annually but very few occur in children. Cases have occurred in poultry processing, aviary, quarantine station and pet shop workers, bird keepers and veterinarians
SYSTEMIC/OTHER INFECTIONS				
Capnocytophaga canimorsus infection	*Capnocytophaga canimorsus* (CDC group DF-2)	Dogs	Direct transmission via bites or ticks	Reports of this infection are rare and occur infrequently in children
Cat-scratch disease	Uncertain—*Bartonella henselae*	Cats	Direct transmission via scratches, bites and ticks	There are very few reported cases

Table 23.1 continued

Disease/infection	Causative organism/ common species	Common animal sources	Mode of spread/vector	Human epidemiology (England and Wales)*
Hydatid disease (echinococcosis)	*Echinococcus granulosus*	Dogs and sheep	Ingestion of tapeworm eggs that are passed in infected dog faeces from the contaminated environment, dog hairs or unwashed salads/vegetables	There are around 20 laboratory reports each year but rarely in children. Many infections are probably acquired overseas
Leishmaniasis (cutaneous and visceral)†	*Leishmania* spp.	Wild animals such as rodents and canines, and domestic dogs	Transmitted by sandfly bites from infected animals or from human to human	Between 10 and 20 laboratory reports of imported infections occur annually, occasionally in children
Leptospirosis, including Weil's disease	*Leptospira interrogans* serovars *hardjo* and *icterohaemorrhagiae* (Weil's disease)	*L. hardjo*: cattle *L. ictero-haemorrhagiae*: rats and other rodents	Organisms are excreted in animals' urine and transmission may occur through inhalation of aerosols, or through abrasions, wounds or mucous membranes	30–50 cases of leptospirosis, mainly in adults, are confirmed each year although there is likely to be underdiagnosis of *L. hardjo* infections. An average of 15 cases of Weil's disease are confirmed annually. Mostly in farmers and those in contact with inland waters

Listeriosis†	*Listeria monocytogenes*	Various domestic and wild animals	Direct transmission from animals; ingestion of contaminated food; or direct from mother to the unborn infant in utero, or during birth	Around 100 infections are reported each year and about 25% are associated with pregnancy. A variety of foods such as cheese have been implicated as the source of infection in some cases
Lyme disease†	*Borrelia burgdorferi*	Deer, wild rodents and ticks	Tick bites	There are around 40 reported indigenous and imported infections each year, mostly in adults. More are clinically diagnosed and treated without recourse to laboratory confirmation. Those at risk include foresters, deer farmers and residents in or visitors to endemic areas
Rabies†	Rabies virus	Wild and domestic animals such as dogs, foxes or bats	Transmission via saliva through bites, scratches or abrasions; person-to-person spread via corneal transplants has been recorded	Reports are rare in both adults and children; the last recorded imported case was in England and Wales in 1988

Table 23.1 continued

Disease/infection	Causative organism/ common species	Common animal sources	Mode of spread/vector	Human epidemiology (England and Wales)*
Toxocariasis†	*Toxocara canis*, *T. cati*	Dogs, foxes and cats	Ingestion of worm eggs from the environment contaminated with infected animal faeces	There are on average 40 annual laboratory reports, around half of which are in children; many more infections probably go unrecognized or undetected
Toxoplasmosis†	*Toxoplasma gondii*	Cats, rodents or birds; sheep, pigs, cattle and goats	Ingestion of cysts from soil or water contaminated with infected cat faeces; ingestion of tissue cysts in raw or undercooked meat or goats' milk; through transplantation of organs or blood from an infected person; or transplacental from mother to fetus	Around 750 infections are reported on average annually; many more probably go unrecognized or undiagnosed. About 10% of the infections are in children

†See Part Two for a more detailed discussion.

***Sources of data: laboratory reports to the Public Health Laboratory Service (PHLS) Communicable Disease Surveillance Centre and cases confirmed by the PHLS Reference Laboratories.**

Other direct means of transmission are via the faecal–oral route; for example, cryptosporidiosis is a common infection in calves and lambs suffering from diarrhoea, and may be transmitted to humans following direct contact. Similarly, *Campylobacter* enteritis may be acquired directly from infected puppies. The inhalation of organisms in respiratory aerosols is another direct route of transmission; the cattle form of leptospirosis (*Leptospira interrogans* var. *hardjo*) or psittacosis may be acquired by this route. Finally, transplacental or vertical transmission of infections from a pregnant mother to her fetus may occur with some zoonoses such as toxoplasmosis.

Indirect routes of transmission include the consumption of food, or ingestion or contact with water that has been contaminated by zoonotic organisms; for example, there have been food-borne outbreaks of *Campylobacter* infection, water-borne incidents of cryptosporidiosis, and Weil's disease (*Leptospira interrogans* var. *icterohaemorrhagiae*) transmitted through contact with natural waters contaminated with infected rats' urine. Psittacosis may be acquired through the inhalation of dust contaminated by discharges from infected birds, or the ovine form of this disease may be acquired from clothing contaminated by the products of gestation from aborting sheep suffering from enzootic abortion of ewes. Finally, certain zoonoses may be transmitted to humans by other, non-vertebrate animals, e.g. Lyme disease (*Borrelia burgdorferi*) which is acquired from infected animals via tick bites. However, it must be remembered that this relatively simple classification of transmission routes for zoonotic infections may be complicated by diseases that may be acquired via more than one route, some of which may not necessarily be zoonotic. For example, cryptosporidiosis may be transmitted directly by the faecal–oral route from infected farm animals to humans, by the consumption of raw milk from infected animals, or by ingestion of contaminated water. Alternatively, it may also be transmitted between humans by the faecal–oral route such as during outbreaks amongst nursery school children. Another example is toxoplasmosis, which may be acquired by the consumption of undercooked meat such as lamb containing *Toxoplasma* cysts; the inadvertent ingestion of oocysts excreted by infected felines; inadequate washing of salads and vegetables contaminated by infected cat faeces; or by direct transmission from infected pregnant women to their fetuses which may result in symptomatic congenital toxoplasmosis. There are other examples of zoonotic diseases which have more than one route of transmission, such as salmonellosis and listeriosis, although it is often difficult to determine the relative importance of each with respect to prevention and control of infections.

ZOONOSES IN CHILDREN

Some zoonotic infections, particularly those associated with occupational exposure are rare in children. For example, certain streptococcal infections such as *Streptococcus suis* meningitis and bacteraemia are usually found in butchers, abattoir workers and pig farmers. However, many children are raised on farms or in rural environments, and many more have contact with household pets, with whom they invariably have close contact. Children playing in parks and other public areas are also at some risk from acquiring infections from animals either through direct contact or from the contaminated environment. Objects from gardens, parks and elsewhere may be picked up, handled and sucked by infants, children often put dirty fingers in their mouths, and pica may result in the transmission of zoonotic infections. Hand-washing and drying may be infrequent and inadequate, and usually requires adult supervision. Schoolchildren are increasingly likely to visit zoos, farms and other sites of recreational and educational interest where they are often encouraged to make close contact with the animals, and participate in grooming, feeding and other such activities. Some children who live in or visit rural areas may be more likely to encounter zoonotic infections such as Lyme disease, usually endemic where deer are present, or hydatid disease, associated with sheep farming areas, although such indigenous infections in children appear to be rare. Children may be bitten or scratched by animals and thus acquire infections such as pasteurellosis. Many now travel overseas with their parents, sometimes to exotic places, and may be exposed to a wide range of infections for which there is no preventative measure apart from avoidance of direct contact with certain animals, the consumption of undercooked or raw meat, untreated water and unwashed salads or vegetables, and the adoption of general hygienic precautions.

PREVENTION

The zoonoses are a complex and intriguing group of diseases. They have received much media and public health attention in recent years and it seems unlikely that the current interest will wane. However, there are many unanswered questions in the epidemiology of these infections, and further research is required if progress is to be made in their prevention, treatment and control. Those working in public health as well as the general public should be kept informed, but not alarmed, about the possible risks of acquiring infection from animals, whether at home or abroad. Simple hygienic measures such as the careful washing and drying of hands before eating and drinking, the adequate cleansing of wounds inflicted by animals, and the covering of cuts and abrasions, are all important measures in preventing the acquisition of many zoonotic infections. The likelihood of acquiring a serious infection from animals needs to be put into perspective. Education is an important factor in the prevention and control of zoonoses, and it should be remembered that contact with animals can be as beneficial to an individual's health as it may be harmful.

FURTHER READING

Bell JC, Palmer SR & Payne JM (1988) *The Zoonoses. Infections Transmitted from Animals to Man*. Edward Arnold, London.

LABORATORY DIAGNOSIS OF INFECTION

The laboratory diagnosis of infection is entirely dependent on the clinical acumen of the paediatrician in recognizing the possibility that the child might be infected. Laboratory tests are not a substitute for clinical diagnosis but a necessary adjunct to confirm the diagnosis, to identify the micro-organism and to aid treatment. In order for this to be maximally efficient there must be good communication between clinician and laboratory and it is essential that well-taken, appropriate samples are sent, together with as much relevant information as possible. In general the procedures available for diagnosis of infection are (a) non-specific tests to help to determine whether infection is present and (b) specific tests which will determine the nature and antimicrobial susceptibility of the pathogen (Table 24.1).

NON-SPECIFIC TESTS

Non-specific tests will only act as pointers to or confirmation of the presence of an infection. They are neither completely sensitive nor completely specific.

White cell count In general the peripheral white cell count will be raised with a neutrophilia, often with a left shift in bacterial infection and lymphocytosis in viral infection. Severe bacterial infection may also induce thrombocytopenia. Exceptions to this include neutropenia in severe bacterial infection (e.g. meningococcal septicaemia and particularly in sepsis neonatorum) and lymphocytosis in pertussis. A very high neutrophil count usually indicates a collection of pus.

Acute phase proteins During acute infection due to bacteria or fungi the liver produces a variety of acute phase proteins which result in an increased plasma viscosity and raised erythrocyte sedimentation rate. Perhaps the most useful measurement is of C-reactive protein (CRP). Levels can be estimated in blood or in cerebrospinal fluid (CSF). During acute bacterial infection levels rise from less than 1 mg/l to 100 mg/l or more, and remain raised for several days. Viral infection does not lead to a large rise in CRP levels.

Cytokines The cytokines tumour necrosis factor (TNF), interleukin-1 (IL-1) and interleukin 6 (IL-6) are produced in particular by macrophages, neutrophils and monocytes in response to bacterial infection; indeed, they contribute to the pathogenesis of sepsis. The value of measuring these cytokines as markers of infection has still to be completely evaluated.

Endotoxin is an integral constituent of the outer membrane of Gram-negative bacteria. It is released either spontaneously (e.g. by meningococci) or when the bacteria die. Its measurement in blood is difficult but can provide evidence of infection by Gram-negative bacteria.

SPECIFIC TESTS

Rapid

To be of most value in management of infection, tests should be sensitive, specific and (if possible) rapid.

Direct visualization Organisms can be directly visualized by light microscopy using stained or unstained material. In general the sensitivity of this method is a

Table 24.1 Laboratory tests for infection

NON-SPECIFIC TESTS: IS INFECTION PRESENT?

White cell count and differential (nitroblue tetrazolium test)
Acute phase proteins (ESR, C-reactive protein, orosomucoid, α-antitrypsin)
Cytokines (tumour necrosis factor, interleukins 1, 6)
Endotoxin (*Limulus* lysate for Gram-negative bacteria)
CSF lactate, protein and glucose estimations

SPECIFIC TESTS: WHAT IS THE PATHOGEN?

- **RAPID (20 min–4 h)**

Visualization

Light microscopy
Electron microscopy
Immunofluorescence microscopy

Antigen detection

Enzyme-linked immunosorbent assay (ELISA)
Latex particle agglutination (LPA)
Radioimmunoassay (RIA)
Counterimmunoelectrophoresis (CIE)

Genome detection

DNA hybridization
Polymerase chain amplification

Toxin detection

Vibrio cholerae heat labile toxin
Clostridium difficile toxin

- **CONVENTIONAL (slower: minimum of 18 h)**

Viral culture (not available for all viruses, expensive)
Bacterial culture (most pathogenic bacteria are cultivable within 24 h)
Fungal culture (can take up to 1 week depending on fungus)
Antimicrobial susceptibility (by culture takes about 18 h usually)

- **ANTIBODY DETECTION**

Except for certain infections (e.g. hepatitis A) serological tests are of greater value for epidemiological rather than diagnostic purposes

minimum of 10^3–10^4 organisms per millilitre. It is simple and rapid to carry out and is useful for detecting (for example) protozoa (*Cryptosporidium*, *Giardia*) in faeces, bacteria in CSF or pathogens in wounds. It is less useful for detecting bacteria in blood (the numbers are too small) or for detecting bacterial pathogens where there is a rich normal flora (i.e. stool samples).

Negative stain electron microscopy is a rapid and specific test and is used primarily to detect viral enteropathogens in stool or virus in skin lesions, although it has also been used to detect viruses in respiratory secretions. To be visualized, there needs to be a minimum of 10^6 virus particles per millilitre in a sample.

The above methodologies are 'catch-all' techniques that will detect the pathogen no matter what it is. The remaining rapid techniques are all directed to detecting an individual pathogen and thus if there are five potential pathogens for a particular infection, five separate tests must be carried out.

Immunofluorescence antigen detection using the indirect fluorescent antibody test (IFAT) employs fluorochrome-tagged antibodies against, for example, respiratory viruses. Since such tests detect viral antigens on infected cells it is important that the sample (usually a nasopharyngeal aspirate) is transported to the laboratory as quickly as possible, or if there is a delay on ice. Using this technique it is possible to detect measles, respiratory syncytial, influenza or parainfluenza virus infections, with relatively high sensitivity and specificity.

Antigen detection A variety of antigen detection tests employing diverse technologies such as enzyme-linked immunosorbent assay (ELISA), latex particle agglutination (LPA), radioimmunoassay and counterimmunoelectrophoresis (CIE) have been developed. Their speed of operation, sensitivity and specificity depend upon the sample tested and the technology used. Examples include detection of bacterial antigens such as capsular polysaccharides of meningococci, pneumococci and *Haemophilus influenzae* type b (Hib), viral antigens such as rotavirus, respiratory syncytial virus and Norwalk agent, and fungal antigens such as the capsular antigen of *Cryptococcus neoformans*. The use of urinary antigen detection in diagnosis remains unclear, especially since it is known for example that urinary excretion of *H. influenzae* type b capsular antigen can be detected in throat carriers or following Hib immunization.

Genome detection Potentially the most sensitive diagnostic tests are those for genome detection. For example, theoretically it is possible through genome amplification using the polymerase chain reaction to detect just one infective particle. This high sensitivity can be a disadvantage by producing false positives. Such techniques are not yet in routine use but it is envisaged that they will be of greatest value in detecting pathogens that are difficult or slow to grow and which have predictable antimicrobial susceptibility.

Antibody detection For the most part antibody detection is not useful for the immediate diagnosis of infection since as well as acute samples it usually also requires convalescent samples to be taken approximately 2 weeks later. However, there are some sensitive specific IgM assays (e.g. for hepatitis A) which will provide diagnosis at clinical presentation.

Conventional

Conventional tests involve culture of samples from infected sites; this requires that the micro-organisms remain viable until they can be cultured (i.e. samples should be taken to the laboratory as quickly as possible). Some samples may require transport media, for example samples for virological culture are placed in iso-osmotic media containing protein and antibiotics (to prevent bacterial overgrowth). For interpretation of bacteriological culture it is necessary to know what is normal and what is abnormal at a particular site. The major disadvantage of cultural techniques is the time taken—most aerobic bacteria will require 18–24 hours of incubation for colonies to appear, and some anaerobes will take longer. The major

Table 24.2 Normal flora

Sites normally colonized (no. of bacteria)	Sites normally sterile
Mouth and nose (about 10^{8-9}/ml)	Trachea and lungs
Pharynx (about 10^{6-8}/ml)	Blood
Oesophagus and stomach (10^{2-3}/ml)	Cerebrospinal fluid
Small intestine (10^2/ml)	Bone and joints
Large intestine (10^{10-12}/ml)	Urinary tract above anterior urethra
Vagina (10^8/ml)	Liver, gallbladder and peritoneal cavity
Skin (10–10^4/cm^2)	Pleural space
Anterior urethra (10^{2-3}/cm^2)	Middle ear and sinuses

advantages are that the organism is available for determination of antimicrobial susceptibility, and for epidemiological and medicolegal purposes.

Normal flora

Of the 10^{14} cells in the human body only 10^{13} or 10% are actually human. The remainder (9×10^{13}) constitute the normal flora. The normal flora are composed of bacteria, fungi and some protozoa and multicellular organisms. In addition some viruses are 'normally' present within the body and excreted from body surfaces. The colonization is not uniform throughout the body (Table 24.2): for example, the respiratory tract below the vocal cords is normally sterile whereas the oropharynx and gastrointestinal tract have a rich and varied normal flora. It is important to know which sites have a normal flora and which micro-organisms can be found at a particular site in order to interpret the results of laboratory tests.

Viruses Following initial infection each of the human herpesviruses (HHV-1 to HHV-7) remains with the host for life. All except varicella-zoster virus (HHV-3) are excreted asymptomatically for the rest of the individual's lifetime. Adenovirus (in particular type 1) tends to persistently infect lymphoid tissue and can be excreted for long periods in saliva and faeces. Other viruses—human immunodeficiency virus (HIV), hepatitis B and C viruses—persist for long periods asymptomatically but may eventually cause symptomatic disease.

Bacteria The vast majority of the normal flora is composed of bacteria. Thus the large intestine contains large numbers (about 10^{12}/ml) of anaerobic bacteria (Bacteroides, Clostridia, Eubacteria, Fusobacteria spp.) and lesser numbers of aerobic bacteria such as *Escherichia coli* (10^7/ml) and *Staphylococcus epidermidis* (10^3/ml). The naso-oropharynx has a rich normal flora and potential respiratory or meningeal pathogens (*Streptococcus pneumoniae* in 20–40%, *Haemophilus influenzae* in 40–80%, *Staphylococcus pyogenes* in 5–10%, *Staphylococcus aureus* in 10–20% and *Neisseria meningitidis* in 5–20% of individuals) can be found. Thus isolation of these organisms from a throat swab or nasopharyngeal aspirate does not necessarily mean that they are causing disease. In contrast, detection of bacteria in normally sterile areas (providing the sample has been taken correctly) indicates infection.

Fungi Yeasts such as *Pityrosporon ovale* can be readily detected on skin, and *Candida albicans* is part of the normal flora of the mouth, large intestine and vagina. Dermatophytes may be found on the skin in the absence of overt infection.

Parasites Protozoa such as *Entamoeba coli*, *Endolimax nana* and even *Giardia lamblia* and *Entamoeba histolytica* can be present in the intestine in the absence of disease. Infestation with the adult worms of *Taenia solium* or *T. saginata* is rarely symptomatic, as is that of the whipworm (*Trichuris trichuria*). Finally, a large proportion of the population will harbour the arthropod *Demodex folliculorum* (follicle mite) especially in the hair follicles and sebaceous glands of the face.

The potential pathogens, samples required, precautions of transport and time taken for detection of agents causing infection by organ system are shown in Tables 24.3–24.10.

Table 24.3 Laboratory investigation of central nervous system infection

	Potential pathogens	Samples required	Transport	Non-specific tests	Specific tests	Time taken
Meningitis in neonate	*E. coli*, group B streptococci, *Listeria*, other Gram-negative bacilli	CSF, blood (for culture)	Rapid	CSF: protein, WCC glucose, CRP Blood: WCC, CRP	CSF Gram film, antigen-detection (group B streptococcus, *E. coli* K1)	1–24 h
	Herpes simplex virus	CSF, saliva, blood	VTM		Virus culture, PCR	24–36 h
Meningitis in older child	*Neisseria meningitidis*, *Streptococcus pneumoniae*, *Haemophilus influenzae* type b, *Mycobacterium tuberculosis*	CSF, blood (for culture Throat swab	Rapid BTM	CSF: protein, WCC, glucose, CRP Blood: WCC, CRP	CSF: Gram film, antigen detection, culture Blood: culture, antigen detection	1–24 h
	Enteroviruses, mumps virus	CSF, throat swab Faeces Serum	VTM		Virus culture, PCR Serology: CSF, serum	24–48 h
Meningoencephalitis	Mumps virus Enteroviruses Herpes simplex virus Lymphocytic choriomeningitis virus	CSF, throat swab, faeces	Rapid VTM Serum	Blood: WCC, CRP CSF: WCC, protein, CRP	Viral culture, PCR Serology: blood, CSF	24–48 h
Cerebral or spinal abscess	*Staphylococcus aureus* *S. milleri* *Streptococcus pneumoniae* Oral anaerobes (Bacteroides, Fusobacteria) *Haemophilus influenzae*	Pus Blood for culture	Rapid BTM (put some pus in blood culture bottle)	Blood: WCC, CRP	Gram-stained film, culture	18–72 h

Key: BTM, bacterial transport medium; CRP, C-reactive protein; CSF, cerebrospinal fluid; PCR, polymerase chain reaction; VTM, viral transport medium; WCC, white cell count.

Table 24.4 Laboratory investigations of gastrointestinal infection

	Pathogens	Samples	Transport	Non-specific tests	Specific tests	Time taken
Hepatitis	Hepatitis A virus Hepatitis B virus Hepatitis C virus Hepatitis D virus Hepatitis E virus	Serum	No special precautions except to prevent infection of hospital staff	Liver function tests	HAV IgM ELISA HBsAg, HBeAg, HBcAb (IgM) HCVAb, HCV genome (RT/PCR) HDVAb HEV IgM, IgG	1–4 h, but since tests are expensive, batched
Gastritis	*Helicobacter pylori*	Gastric biopsy serum Saliva	Rapid BTM		Histology ('gold standard') Rapid urease Culture Serology (serum and saliva)	5–7 d
Diarrhoeal disease	Viruses: Rotavirus, astrovirus, adenovirus 40/41, calicivirus, Norwalk agent	Faeces, vomit	No special precautions		Electron microscopy, ELISA, LPA	1–8 h
	Bacteria: *Salmonella*, *Shigella* *Campylobacter*, *E. coli*,		Rapid	Stool pus cells	Culture	24–48 h
	Protozoa: *Cryptosporidium*, *Giardia*, *Cyclospora* *Entamoeba histolytica*		No special precautions		Microscopy of stained smears	1–2h

Key: Ab, antibody; Ag, antigen; BTM, bacterial transport medium; ELISA, enzyme-linked immunosorbent assay; Ig, immunoglobulin; LPA, latex particle agglutination; PCR, polymerase chain reaction; RT, reverse transcriptase.

Table 24.5 Respiratory tract infection

	Pathogens	Samples	Transport	Non-specific tests	Specific tests	Time taken
Otitis media, sinusitis	*Haemophilus influenzae* *Streptococcus pneumoniae* *Moraxella catarrhalis* Anaerobes	Pus from cavity Blood culture	Rapid BTM	Blood: WCC, CRP	Gram film, antigen detection, culture	18–48 h
Tonsillitis, pharyngitis	Viruses (most common) e.g. adenovirus, EBV *Streptococcus pyogenes* (A or C) *Corynebacterium diphtheriae*	Throat swab, serum Throat swab	VTM BTM	Blood: WCC and film for EBV	Virus culture, serology Gram film, culture	1–3 d 18–24 h
Epiglottitis	*Haemophilus influenzae* type b	Blood culture Swab (with care) once intubated Urine	BTM	Blood: WCC, CRP	Culture Antigen detection in urine	18–24 h
Laryngotracheo-bronchitis, croup	Parainfluenza viruses 1–4 Influenza viruses A,B,C, Respiratory syncytial virus Adenovirus	Nasopharyngeal aspirate Serum	Rapid, on ice		IFAT Virus culture Serology	< 8 h 24–72 h
Tracheitis	Staphylococcus aureus	Swab	BTM	Blood: WCC, CRP	Culture	18–24h

Pneumonia	Viruses: Parainfluenza virus RSV Influenza virus Adenovirus Measles virus	Nasopharyngeal aspirate Serum	Rapid or on ice		IFAT Virus culture Serology	8–48 h
	Bacteria: *Streptococcus pneumoniae* *Haemophilus influenzae* type b *Staphylococcus aureus* *Mycoplasm pneumoniae* *Chlamydia psittaci* *C. pneumoniae* *L. pneumophila*	Blood (for culture) Sputum Transtracheal aspirate Evoked sputum (if possible) Serum, urine	Rapid	Blood: WCC, CRP	Blood culture Sputum and aspirate: Gram film, culture, antigen detection Urine: antigen detection	18–24 h
Pertussis	*Bordetella pertussis* *B. parapertussis*	Pernasal swab Serum, saliva	BTM rapid	WCC—lymphocytosis	Bacterial culture Serology	24–48 h
	Adenovirus	Nasopharyngeal aspirate Serum	VTM		Virus culture Serology	24–48 h

Key: BTM, bacterial transport medium; CRP, C-reactive protein; EBV, Epstein–Barr virus; IFAT, indirect fluorescent antibody test; VTM, viral transport medium; WCC, white cell count.

Table 24.6 Laboratory diagnosis of exanthems and enanthems

	Pathogens	Samples	Transport	Specific tests	Time taken
Maculopapular erythematous rash	Viruses: Measles virus Enteroviruses EBV Parvovirus Rubella virus HHV-6	Throat swab NPA Serum	VTM	Virus culture IFAT Serology IgM, rise in titre	4–72 h
	Bacteria: *Neisseria meningitidis* (septicaemia) *Streptococcus pyogenes*	Blood culture Throat swab	BTM rapid	Blood culture Serum antigen	18–24 h
Petechial purpuric rash	Viruses: Enteroviruses Adenoviruses	Throat swab Faeces, serum	VTM	Virus culture, serology	24–72 h
	Bacteria: *Neisseria meningitidis* Other Gram-negative bacteria	Blood culture Lesion scraping	BTM	Gram film, culture	18–24 h

Vesicular or pustular rash	Viruses: HSV-1 and 2 Varicella-zoster virus Enterovirus (hand, foot & mouth)	Vesicle fluid Serum Throat swab, faeces	VTM	Electron microscopy Virus culture Serology	1–72 h
	Bacteria: *Staphylococcus aureus* (impetigo)	Lesion swab or pus	BTM	Gram film Bacterial culture	18–24 h
Nodules	Papillomavirus Molluscum contagiosum virus Cowpox, parapox virus	Needle sample of lesion	No special precautions	Electron microscopy	1 h

Key: BTM, bacterial transport medium; EBV, Epstein–Barr virus; HHV, human herpesvirus; HSV, herpes simplex virus; IFAT, indirect fluorescent antibody test; IgM, immunoglobulin M; NPA, nasopharyngeal aspirate; VTM, viral transport medium.

Table 24.7 Laboratory diagnosis of genitourinary tract infection

	Pathogen	Sample	Transport	Non-specific tests	Specific tests	Time taken
Urinary tract	*E. coli*	MSU/clean catch urine	Rapid or keep cool	Blood: WCC, CRP	Quantitative bacterial culture	18–24 h
	Proteus			Urine: WCC (>10/mm^3)	(>10^5 cfu/ml in pure culture)	
	Klebsiella spp.	Suprapubic aspirate			(catheter or suprapubic	
	Staphylococcus epidermidis	*Catheter specimen*			aspirate should be sterile unless	
	Pseudomonas aeruginosa	Bag (least useful)			there is infection)	
Genital tract	Vulvovaginitis:					
	Candida albicans	Swab or better still discharge	Rapid		Gram film	18–24 h
	GpB streptococci		BTM		Culture	
	Enterobius vermicularis	*Sellotape slide*			Examination of slide for ova	1 h
	Sexually transmitted disease:					
	Herpes simplex virus	Discharge swab	VTM		Virus culture	1–24 h
	Human papillomavirus	Sample of wart			Electron microscopy	
	Neisseria gonorrhoeae	Discharge swab	BTM		Bacterial culture	18–48 h
	Chlamydia trachomatis		Rapid		Cell culture, ELISA, IFAT	6–72 h
	Treponema pallidum	Blood for serology			Dark-ground microscopy	1–4 h
					Serological tests for syphilis	
	Trichomonas vaginalis				Culture and microscopy	18–24 h

Key: MSU, midstream urine; BTM, bacterial transport medium; CRP, C-reactive protein; ELISA, enzyme-linked immunosorbent assay; IFAT, indirect fluorescent antibody test; VTM, viral transport medium; WCC, white cell count.

Table 24.8 Laboratory diagnosis of skin and soft tissue infections

	Pathogens	Samples	Transport	Non-specific tests	Specific tests	Time taken
Skin						
Carbuncle, furuncle	*Staphylococcus aureus*	Pus	2–3 h		Gram film, culture	18–24 h
Vesicle	HHV-1, 2 or 3 Enterovirus	Vesicle fluid	Rapid		Electron microscopy, culture	2–24 h
Impetigo	*Staphylococcus aureus* *S. pyogenes*	Pus, vesicle fluid or crust	2–3 h		Gram film, culture	18–24 h
Nodules	Molluscum contagiosum virus Papillomavirus (warts) Cowpox, orf viruses	Sample of nodules	2–3 h		Electron microscopy (culture)	2–24 h
Granuloma	*Mycobacterium tuberculosis*, *M. marinum*	Sample of tissue	2–3 h		Histology, acid-fast stain culture	2 h–6 wk
Cellulitis	*Staphylococcus pyogenes* *Haemophilus influenzae* b Anaerobes (necrotizing fasciitis)	Samples of tissue or exudate	Rapid		Gram film, culture	2–48 h
Ringworm	*Microsporum* *Trichophyton* *Epidermophyton*	Skin, nail scraping, hair		Wood's light	Microscopy (KOH), culture	2 h–5 d

Table 24.8 Laboratory diagnosis of skin and soft tissue infections

	Pathogens	Samples	Transport	Non-specific tests	Specific tests	Time taken
Intertrigo	*Candida* spp.	Sample of lesion			Gram film culture	2–24 h
Scabies	*Sarcoptes scabiei*	Clinical or sample from burrow			Microscopy	2 h
Lice	*Pediculus capitis*	Hair			Microscopic examination (nit = egg)	2 h
Lymph gland						
Lymphadenitis	*Streptococcus pyogenes* *Mycobacterium tuberculosis* *M. avium/intracellulare* *Bartonella henselae* (cat-scratch disease)	Pus from gland			Gram or acid-fast film culture	2 h–6 wk
Eyes						
Conjunctivitis	Adenovirus (3, 7, 8, 19) Enterovirus (70) Coxsackie virus (A24) Herpes simplex virus	Swab from conjunctivae	VTM Rapid		Electron microscopy Virus culture Immunofluorescence PCR	18–48 h
	Haemophilus influenzae *Streptococcus pneumoniae* *Neisseria meningitidis* *N. gonorrhoeae* *Chlamydia trachomatis*	Swab of pus and conjunctivae	BTM Rapid Chlamytic transport		Gram film culture Giemsa (poor) ELISA, IFAT Culture	18–24 h 4–72 h
Orbital cellulitis	*Haemophilus influenzae* b	Samples from lesion Blood culture	Rapid		Bacterial culture	18–24 h

Key: BTM, bacterial transport medium; ELISA, enzyme-linked immunosorbent assay; HHV, human herpesvirus; IFAT, indirect fluorescent antibody test; PCR, polymerase chain reaction; VTM, viral transport medium.

Table 24.9 Laboratory diagnosis of infections of bone, joint and muscle

	Pathogen	Samples	Transport	Non-specific tests	Specific tests	Time taken
Bone						
Acute osteomyelitis	*Staphylococcus aureus* *Haemophilus influenzae*	Blood culture Pus from bone	Rapid	WCC, CRP	Gram film Culture	18–24 h
Chronic osteomyelitis	*Mycobacterium tuberculosis* *Pseudomonas aeruginosa* coliforms	Pus Pus		WCC, CRP WCC, CRP	Acid-fast film, culture Gram film, culture	2 h–6 wk 18–24 h
Joint						
Acute arthritis	*Staphylococcus aureus* *Haemophilus influenzae* *Salmonella* spp. *Neisseria meningitidis* *N. gonorrhoeae*	Joint fluid Blood culture	BTM Rapid	WCC, CRP	Gram film Culture	2–24 h

Table 24.9 continued

	Pathogen	Samples	Transport	Non-specific tests	Specific tests	Time taken
Reactive arthritis	Immune reaction to: *Neisseria meningitidis* *N. gonorrhoeae* *Chlamydia trachomatis* *Salmonella* spp. *Campylobacter* spp.	Blood Joint fluid		WCC, CRP HLA typing (HLA-B27)	Culture (should be -ve) PCR (is +ve)	
Muscle						
Pyomyositis	*Staphylococcus aureus* (tropical) *S. pyogenes*	Pus Tissue Blood culture	BTM Rapid	WCC, CRP	Histology, Gram film Culture	2–24 h
Gas gangrene	*Clostridium perfringens* *Streptococcus*	Tissue Blood culture	BTM Rapid	WCC, CRP	Histology, Gram film Culture	2–48 h
Necrotizing fasciitis	*Staphylococcus pyogenes*	Tissue	BTM		Gram film, culture	18–24 h
Synergistic gangrene	*Staphylococcus aureus* and anaerobes	Tissue	BTM Rapid		Gram film, culture	18–72 h

Key: BTM, bacterial transport medium; CRP, C-reactive protein; PCR, polymerase chain reaction; WCC, white cell count.

Table 24.10 Infection of the cardiovascular system

	Pathogen	Sample	Transport	Non-specific tests	Specific tests	Time taken
Infective endocarditis	Viridans streptococci Coagulase-negative staphylococci *Haemophilus aphrophilus* *Enterococcus* spp. *Candida* spp. *Aspergillus* spp. *Coxiella burnetii* *Salmonella* spp. *Staphylococcus aureus* (acute)	Blood culture (4 or 5 samples)		WCC, CRP	Culture	18–72 h (may be much longer)
Pericarditis	Coxsackie virus B	Faeces Pericardial fluid Blood	VTM Rapid	WCC, CRP	Virus culture Serology PCR	24–72 h
	Haemophilus influenzae *Streptococcus pneumoniae* *S. pyogenes* *Staphylococcus aureus* *Neisseria meningitidis* *Mycobacterium tuberculosis*	Blood culture Pericardial fluid	BTM	WCC, CRP	Gram film Culture	18–24 h
Myocarditis	Coxsackie viruses A & B Echovirus Mumps virus	Faeces, throat swab Blood	VTM Rapid	WCC, CRP	Virus culture Serology	24–72 h
	Neisseria meningitidis *Staphylococcus aureus* *S. pyogenes*	Blood culture		WCC, CRP	Culture	24–48 h

Key: BTM, bacterial transport medium; CRP, C-reactive protein; ECG, electrocardiogram; PCR, polymerase chain reaction; VTM, viral transport medium; WCC, white cell count.

25

THE USE OF ANTIBIOTICS

Antibiotics or antimicrobials are one of the few examples of drugs administered to a patient not for their direct effect on the patient (although this does occur as a consequence of their action) but in order to kill infecting micro-organisms. Antibiotics are the most frequently used and arguably the most frequently abused agents in the pharmacopoeia.

In designing a new antibiotic the aim is to produce an agent that is maximally toxic for the micro-organisms and minimally toxic to the patient. This is achieved by targeting sites or pathways that are unique to the bacterium. Unfortunately this is not always successful, and all antibiotics produce human toxicity to varying degrees. The therapeutic index (maximum tolerated dose divided by minimum effective dose) provides a numeric expression of this. Some antibiotics such as penicillins are very safe and thus have a very high therapeutic index. Others such as gentamicin have a low maximum tolerated dose and thus a therapeutic index which is low. A further complication is that bacteria which under optimal conditions have a doubling time of 20 minutes have boundless opportunities to mutate to circumvent an antibiotic's activity. Furthermore, the genes for antibiotic resistance may be disseminated promiscuously among bacterial genera by means of plasmids and transposons ('jumping genes'). The production of new antimicrobials is only just exceeding the development of resistance.

An unwanted side-effect of antimicrobials is the alteration of the host's normal flora (see Chapter 24). Some antibiotics, e.g. ampicillin, erythromycin and co-amoxiclav, are excreted back into the gastrointestinal tract (others are poorly absorbed) and affect the predominantly anaerobic normal flora of the large bowel. This may result in antibiotic-associated diarrhoea or, at worst, promote colonization by toxin producing *Clostridium difficile* resulting in pseudomembranous colitis. The intestinal flora may also act as a sink for development and dissemination of antibiotic resistance genes.

Antibiotics can be bactericidal (actively kill dividing bacteria) or bacteriostatic (prevent bacteria dividing). Although these divisions are not immutable (e.g. chloramphenicol is bactericidal for meningococci but bacteriostatic for *Escherichia coli*), in general it is better to use bactericidal antibiotics for life-threatening infection, especially if the host is immunoincompromised.

Antimicrobial agents can act at various sites within the micro-organisms (Table 25.1).

CELL WALL REPLICATION

By possessing a thick peptidoglycan cell wall, bacteria are able to survive both severe changes in osmotic pressure and many host degradative enzymes. This represents a target unique to bacteria and antibiotics acting at this site should thus theoretically be less toxic to humans.

Bacitracin is a very toxic antibiotic obtained from a strain of *Bacillus licheniformis* isolated from a wound of a patient named Tracy. It is not absorbed orally and when given parenterally is highly nephrotoxic. Its main use is as a topical agent in combination with other antibiotics. Although there are generally few problems when it is applied topically, hypersensitivity reactions are possible, and if it is applied to extensive areas of inflammation, significant absorption can occur. Bacitracin is active against most Gram-positive bacteria.

Table 25.1 Antibiotics by mode of action

Inhibition of	Spectrum of activity	Bactericidal	Routes of administration	Volume of distribution (l/kg)	Toxicity	Need to monitor levels	How excreted	Used in neonates
DNA replication								
Flucytosine	Fungi	+	PO, IV	0.7–1	M,* GI	+	U	+
Griseofulvin	Fungi	–	PO, IV	1.2–1.4	Mild	–	H	–
Metronidazole	Anaerobes, protozoa	–	PO, IV	0.76–1.02	Mild	–	H	+
Nitrofurantoin	GNB	+	PO	0.6	Mild	–	U	–
Quinolones	Bacteria (broad)	+	PO, IV	1–2.5	Mild	–	U	NL
Sulphonamides	Bacteria (broad)	+	PO, IV	0.2–0.8	D,* M,* S,* R*	–	H, U	–
Trimethoprim	Bacteria (broad)	+	PO, IV	1–1.5	Mild	–	U	+
Co-trimoxazole	Bacteria (broad), fungi, *Pneumocystis*	+	PO, IV	–	Principally due to sulphonamide	–	U	–
Para-aminosalicylic acid	Mycobacteria	+	PO, IV	0.8	Mild, S	–	U	–
Transcription								
Rifampicin	Bacteria (broad) Mycobacteria	+	PO, IV	1	L, S*	–	H	–
Translation								
Aminoglycosides	Bacteria (broad)	+	IV, topical	0.2–0.3	R,* O*	+	U	+
Chloramphenicol	Bacteria (broad)	+ & –	PO, IV	0.25–1.99	M*	+	H	–
Fusidic acid	GPB	+	PO, IV, topical	0.2	L, GI	–	H	+
Macrolides	GPB, mycobacteria	–	PO, IV, topical	0.75	L,* S,* O	–	H	+
Tetracyclines	Bacteria (broad)	–	PO, IV, topical	1.3	Teeth	–	H	–

Table 25.1 Continued

Inhibition of	Spectrum of activity	Bactericidal	Routes of administration	Volume of distribution (l/kg)	Toxicity	Need to monitor levels	How excreted	Used in neonates
Cell wall replication								
Bacitracin	GPB	+	Topical	NA	R,* S*	–	NA	+
Beta-lactams	Bacteria (broad)	+	PO, IV	0.2–0.7	S (rare)	–	U	+
Glycopeptides	GPB	+	IV	0.6	S,* R (rare)	+	U	+
Cycloserine	GPB, mycobacteria	+	PO, topical	0.8	N, P	–	U	–
Cell membranes								
Amphotericin	Fungi	+	IV, topical	4	R,* M	–	U	+
Nitroimidazoles	Fungi	–	PO, IV, topical	0.3–0.5	H*	-	H	+
Nystatin	Fungi	+	Topical	NA	Rare	–	NA	+
Polymyxins	GNB	+	Topical	NA	R,* S	–	NA	+
Isoniazid	Mycobacteria	+	PO	0.6–0.8	L* (rare), N	–	U	–
Ethambutol	Mycobacteria	–	PO	3.9	Optic neuritis	–	U	–

Key: PO, oral; IV, intravenous; M, marrow suppression; GI, gastrointestinal disturbance; D, dermatological; S, hypersensitivity; R, renal; L, liver; N, neurotoxic; P, psychiatric; O, ototoxicity; H, hepatic metabolism; U, urinary excretion; GPB, Gram-positive bacteria; GNB, Gram-negative bacteria; NA, not applicable; NL, not licensed in UK but used.
***Severe toxicity.**

Glycopeptides Vancomycin and teicoplanin are both glycopeptide antibiotics and are active against most Gram-positive bacteria, principally staphylococci. They are not absorbed when given orally. Vancomycin is given by a slow intravenous infusion or intraventricularly; teicoplanin can be given as a bolus. Glycopeptides are occasionally nephrotoxic. The major problem is of hypersensitivity and allergic reactions, in particular the 'red man' syndrome. This apparently occurs less readily with teicoplanin, is more likely to occur if the infusion is too rapid and can be managed with antihistamines. Vancomycin is indicated for severe infections due to multidrug-resistant Gram-positive bacteria in neonates or older children. Levels should be monitored.

Beta-lactams The largest and most widely used group of antibiotics is the beta-lactams. Within this group there are three major subdivisions: the penicillins, the cephalosporins and the monobactams. Each has a β-lactam ring as the active moiety and inhibits transpeptidation, the final stage in assembly of peptidoglycan.

Benzylpenicillin, the first penicillin to be used therapeutically, is still effective against streptococci, pneumococci and meningococci, although varying prevalences of resistance occur in many parts of the world. *Staphylococcus aureus* is resistant by virtue of producing β-lactamase enzymes. The penicillinase-resistant penicillins flucloxacillin (for oral administration) and cloxacillin (for IV administration) were developed to counter this problem. Staphylococci resistant to these agents (methicillin-resistant *Staphylococcus aureus*, MRSA) have now emerged (permeability mutants). Ampicillin was developed to broaden the spectrum to cover Gram-negative as well as Gram-positive bacteria. Now, however, many enterobacteria produce β-lactamases that render them resistant to ampicillin. Clavulanic acid, a β-lactamase inhibitor, is added to ampicillin (co-amoxiclav) to overcome this problem. New β-lactamases not susceptible to inhibition by clavulanic acid have already emerged. The ureidopenicillins such as azlocillin were developed to extend the spectrum to cover *Pseudomonas aeruginosa*. The penicillins are among the safest antibiotics available. Hypersensitivity reactions ranging from skin rashes to anaphylactic shock are the main—but rare—side-effects. Their incidence seems to be overestimated. There is a 10% chance that a penicillin-allergic patient will also be cephalosporin-allergic.

Cephaloridine was the first cephalosporin; it should not be used now since it is toxic and is easily hydrolysed by Gram-positive and Gram-negative β-lactamases. In general the second-generation cephalosporins such as cephradine, cefuroxime and cefaclor have a broad spectrum of activity. Cefaclor and cefuroxime have useful activity against *Haemophilus influenzae* but no cephalosporin is active against *Listeria monocytogenes*. They are likely to be hydrolysed by Gram-negative β-lactamases. The third-generation cephalosporins such as ceftazidime, cefotaxime and ceftriaxone must be given parenterally, have high intrinsic activity, are less likely to be inactivated by Gram-negative β-lactamases but are less likely to be active against *Staphylococcus aureus*. Enterococci are resistant to third-generation cephalosporins. and production of extended-spectrum β-lactamases by *Proteus*, *Serratia* and *Enterobacter* spp. has now appeared in *E. coli* and *Salmonella* spp. The cephamycins cefoxitin and moxalactam are also active against most anaerobic bacteria. Their use should be avoided in neonates since they interfere with vitamin K metabolism.

Aztreonam is the only monobactam available for clinical use. It is active only against Gram-negative bacteria, must be administered parenterally and has been little used in paediatric practice.

The new carbapenems such as imipenem, which have a very broad spectrum of activity, have been used in children with cystic fibrosis; their use in neonates has still to be fully evaluated.

The β-lactams are a very useful and non-toxic group of antibiotics. Their use will depend upon the particular infection and prevalence of resistance in the locality.

CELL MEMBRANE DISRUPTION

Amphotericin is the principal antifungal drug available for treating systemic mycoses. It is fungicidal for yeasts (*Candida*, *Cryptococcus*), dimorphic fungi (*Histoplasma*, *Blastomyces*, *Coccidioides*), dermatophytes (*Trichophyton*, *Microsporum*, *Epidermophyton*) and moulds (*Aspergillus*, *Penicillium*). Fungal resistance is not yet a problem. The drug is not absorbed through skin or mucous membranes when given topically. For systemic mycoses it must be given as a slow infusion. The main side-effects are hypotensive reactions and nephrotoxicity, the earliest sign of which is hypokalaemia. A test dose should be given. Liposomally entrapped amphotericin is less toxic. Combination with flucytosine is useful.

Nystatin is a polyene antifungal drug. It is fungicidal for a variety of fungi but is used most often in candidiasis. It is applied topically and must not be given parenterally since it is particulate and not a solution. Development of resistance is rare. Both nystatin (discovered in New York State) and amphotericin chelate sterols in the fungal membrane.

Nitroimidazoles inhibit the production of ergosterol in the fungal cell membrane. In general they are fungistatic. They are absorbed well orally. Miconazole is given orally or topically, and ketoconazole (which is hepatotoxic) can also be given intravenously. Both affect a wide spectrum of fungi, but are excreted poorly in urine. The newer imidazoles, fluconazole and itraconazole, are fungicidal and have been used in place of amphotericin for systemic mycoses, although there are no paediatric trial data.

Polymyxins bind to the lipid A portion of lipopolysaccharide of Gram-negative bacteria and cause membrane disruption. Most Gram-negative bacteria (except *Proteus*, *Neisseria* and *Brucella*) are susceptible, but the main use of polymyxins has been in treating severe *Pseudomonas* infections. Polymyxin B and colistin (polymyxin E) can be given intravenously, but both have been superseded to a large extent by less toxic antibiotics. They cause nephrotoxicity, neurotoxicity and hypersensitivity. When used topically, it is usually in combination with other antibacterials for superficial infections.

DNA REPLICATION

Most micro-organisms are rapidly and continually replicating and thus need a continuous supply of nucleic acids for chromosomal replication.

Flucytosine is a nucleoside analogue used for treating systemic fungal infections (*Candida*, *Cryptococcus*, *Torulopsis*). It can be given by the oral or intravenous route. Resistance develops rapidly both in vitro and in vivo and flucytosine is often combined with amphotericin with synergistic effects. High dosage (peak serum levels greater than 100 mg/l) is associated with bone marrow toxicity with reversible thrombocytopenia and leukopenia. It can be used in neonates providing levels are monitored.

Griseofulvin is an antifungal drug that inhibits mitosis by affecting microtubules. It is fungistatic for common dermatophytes (*Microsporum*, *Epidermophyton*, *Trichophyton*). It is given orally, is concentrated in keratinized tissue and is thus used for treating ringworm, onychomycosis and tinea capitis. It is generally non-toxic but is contraindicated in neonates and should only be used for specific childhood infections.

Metronidazole is active against obligate anaerobes and some protozoa (*Trichomonas*, *Entamoeba*, *Giardia*). Under anaerobic conditions it is converted to a nitrosamine which causes DNA fragmentation and inhibits DNA synthesis. It can be administered orally, rectally or intravenously. Although mutagenic for bacteria it is not associated with carcinogenesis. It has a disulfiram-like effect and high doses may cause central nervous system effects and peripheral neuropathy. It is used prophylactically in large intestinal surgery.

Nitrofurantoin is used for treating urinary tract infections due to Gram-negative bacteria. It causes DNA fragmentation in *E. coli*, but resistance can develop readily. It is administered orally and can be used for both therapy and prophylaxis. It is inactive under alkaline conditions and is not useful for treating urinary tract infection due to *Proteus* spp. The most serious side-effect is an allergic pneumonitis, which is fortunately rare. In patients with glucose-6-phosphate dehydrogenase (G6PD) deficiency, nitrofurantoin produces haemolytic episodes. It should not be used in neonates.

Quinolones prevent DNA replication by inhibiting bacterial DNA gyrase. The first quinolone, nalidixic acid, is used solely for the treatment or prophylaxis of urinary tract infection and is administered orally. It is active only against Gram-negative bacteria and resistance develops easily. It should not be used in infants under 3 months old nor in G6PD deficiency. Currently the 'newer' quinolones such as ciprofloxacin or ofloxacin are not licensed for use in patients under 18 years old, since these compounds induce cartilage damage in weight-bearing joints of young beagle dogs. The quinolones are very useful agents: they have a large volume of distribution, a broad spectrum of activity and are bactericidal. For these reasons they have been used in paediatric practice for severe infection including those in neonates and patients with cystic fibrosis. They are also used in the chemoprophylaxis of meningococcal disease. Serious reactions (anaphylactoid) are rare, but these drugs should not be administered with theophylline since quinolones inhibit the metabolism of methylxanthines. Resistance to these quinolones is developing slowly but is not plasmid-encoded. The drugs can be administered orally or intravenously.

Sulphonamides are structural analogues of para-aminobenzoic acid and competitively inhibit the bacterial synthesis of folic acid. Bacteria have an absolute requirement for folic acid to produce new nucleotides. Because of relatively high prevalence of resistance (which can be plasmid-encoded) and of side-effects, sulphonamides are little used in paediatric practice. Sulphonamides are a frequent cause of rashes and can cause Stevens–Johnson syndrome. They may also cause crystalluria and renal failure, bone marrow suppression, and haemolytic anaemia in G6PD deficiency. They may precipitate kernicterus in neonates. Some sulphonamides (e.g. silver sulphadiazine) are used topically in the treatment and prophylaxis of infection in patients with burns.

Trimethoprim inhibits bacterial dihydrofolinic acid reductase and this prevents conversion of folic to folinic acid. It has a broad spectrum of antibacterial activity, is bactericidal and has a large volume of distribution. High-level resistance to trimethoprim (>1000 mg/l) is increasing and is usually plasmid-encoded. The drug can be administered by the oral or intravenous routes. It is generally well tolerated with no serious side-effects. If administered to neonates, folate supplementation may be necessary.

Co-trimoxazole is a combination of sulphamethoxazole and trimethoprim. It was considered that this combination by blocking two steps on the same pathway might prevent the development of resistance. This expectation has not been realized. Most of the toxicity of co-trimoxazole results from the sulphamethoxazole. Absolute indications for the use of co-trimoxazole (rather than trimethoprim) are for *Pneumocystis carinii* pneumonia, brucellosis and nocardiasis.

TRANSCRIPTION

Rifampicin is a rifamycin, the only class of antibiotics to inhibit DNA-dependent RNA polymerase. It can be administered orally or intravenously. It has a broad spectrum of antibacterial activity, a large volume of distribution, and is bactericidal. Unfortunately resistance (a one-step event) develops readily. The main indications for use are for treating tuberculosis, leprosy and atypical mycobacteria, and in prophylaxis of meningococcal or *Haemophilus influenzae* type b disease. It has also been used (usually in combination) to treat brucellosis and severe or multiresistant staphylococcal (coagulase positive or negative) infections including endocarditis and central nervous system shunt infection. Rifampicin should not be given to patients with liver damage. The most severe side-effect is hypersensitivity. It induces liver microsomal enzymes and may decrease the efficacy of drugs (e.g. corticosteroids, oral contraceptives or warfarin) that are conjugated by such enzymes. It colours urine and tears pink or red.

TRANSLATION

Aminoglycosides prevent binding of peptidyl transfer RNA to polysomes and inhibit protein synthesis. They are derived from *Streptomyces* spp. (names ending '-mycin') or *Micromonospora* spp. (names ending '-micin'). They are rapidly bactericidal broad-spectrum antibacterials; they have no activity against anaerobes, streptococci or intracellular pathogens. There are varying prevalences of resistance to the individual aminoglycosides among aerobic Gram-negative bacilli (least frequently to amikacin). This resistance is frequently plasmid-encoded. Aminoglycosides are poorly absorbed orally and thus must be given intravenously—some (e.g. gentamicin) can be given intrathecally. Penetration into cerebrospinal fluid (CSF) or bronchial secretions is poor. These compounds are most useful for treating septicaemia in children or neonates, complicated urinary tract infection and bacterial endocarditis. They are also used prophylactically for abdominal surgery. They have a low therapeutic index and levels must be monitored. Toxicity is particularly associated with prolonged high trough levels.

The aminoglycosides are ototoxic (tinnitus, deafness and vestibular disturbances), nephrotoxic (usually reversible) and may promote neuromuscular blockade. Diuretics (such as frusemide) and cephaloridine interact with aminoglycosides to potentiate nephrotoxicity. Some aminoglycosides are used topically (e.g. neomycin) in combination with other antibiotics in eye-drops, ear-drops and ointments. Aminoglycosides have also been administered by nebulization to children with cystic fibrosis.

Chloramphenicol inhibits peptide bond formation and mitochondrial NADH oxidase. It is administered orally, intravenously or topically in ointments and eye-drops. It is bactericidal for *Haemophilus influenzae*, *Neisseria meningitidis* and *Streptococcus pneumoniae*, and bacteristatic for aerobic Gram-negative bacilli such as *E. coli*, salmonellae and *Klebsiella pneumoniae*. It has a wide volume of distribution and penetrates well into CSF. It used to be the mainstay of treatment for bacterial meningitis and still is in developing countries. Because of concerns over toxicity, bacterial resistance and efficacy it has largely been superseded by third-generation cephalosporins such as cefotaxime or ceftriaxone. It is still indicated for initial empiric treatment of brain abscesses, melioidosis and rickettsial infection (e.g. Rocky Mountain spotted fever) where tetracycline cannot be used. Chloramphenicol can produce dose-related marrow suppression and a rarer, dose-independent, irreversible aplastic anaemia. It should not be used in neonates because of the risk of 'grey baby' syndrome (pale cyanotic skin, hypotension and metabolic acidosis, followed by cardiovascular collapse).

Tetracyclines prevent access of aminoacyl tRNA to acceptor sites on the messenger RNA–ribosome complex. They are broad-spectrum, bacteriostatic antibiotics with a large volume of distribution. They should not be used in children under 8 years old or in pregnant women, because they are deposited in immature teeth, which may become soft and discoloured, and in bone. They may be indicated for treatment of infection due to erythromycin-resistant strains of *Chlamydia psittaci*, *Rickettsia* spp., *Mycoplasma* spp., *Ureaplasma* spp. and in relapsing fever (*Borrelia recurrentis*) and Lyme disease (*Borrelia burgdorferi*). They may be administered intravenously, orally (absorption may be unpredictable) or topically. The topical administration is usually for conjunctivitis or infected eczema.

Macrolides are a group of antibiotics that affect bacterial peptide chain initiation. They are bacteriostatic or bactericidal for anaerobic and aerobic Gram-positive bacteria, *Mycoplasma* spp. and *Chlamydia* spp., depending on the organism, the macrolide and the dosage. Erythromycin may be given orally or intravenously and is the most frequently used macrolide. It penetrates most sites except for brain and CSF. The newer macrolides azithromycin and clarithromycin have much higher potency. Macrolides are indicated for the treatment of infection due to *Chlamydia* spp., *Mycoplasma* spp., atypical mycobacteria and Gram-positive bacteria, and for prophylaxis of bacterial endocarditis in patients who are allergic to penicillin. Erythromycin has been used to eliminate carriage of *Bordetella pertussis* and is the drug of choice for legionellosis. Clindamycin is used for treating deep staphylococcal sepsis. Erythromycin can cause hepatotoxicity and rarely Stevens–Johnson syndrome. Lincomycin should not be given to neonates, and clindamycin can induce ventricular fibrillation. Spiramycin is used for prevention of transmission of toxoplasmosis from mother to fetus and treatment of congenitally infected infants. It has also been used for treating cryptosporidiosis in immunocompromised children but controlled trials have not demonstrated efficacy.

Fusidic acid prevents binding of aminoacyl tRNA to the ribosome. It is bactericidal for both aerobic and anaerobic Gram-positive bacteria, but is used principally to treat staphylococcal (coagulase positive and negative) infections. It penetrates well into bone, joints and burn crusts, but poorly into CSF. It can be administered orally, intravenously or topically, but resistance develops readily both in vitro and in vivo. Its main indications for use are in osteomyelitis, arthritis and endocarditis; it is often used in combination with other antistaphylococcal antibiotics. Fusidic acid produces phlebitis when given into peripheral veins and should be given through a central line. It is generally a safe drug but can cause hyperbilirubinaemia and jaundice.

CLINICAL USAGE

The decision on which antibiotics to use will depend upon the likely pathogen, the current resistance patterns of the pathogen, the site of infection and the toxicity of the agent. Some pathogens have remained predictably sensitive to antibiotics (e.g. in the UK all meningococci are sensitive to penicillin or cefotaxime). For others the situation is much more fluid. For example, Gram-negative enteric bacteria such as *E. coli*, *Klebsiella* spp. and *Salmonella* spp. are able to acquire plasmids conferring resistance to aminoglycosides and third-generation cephalosporins with great ease. The incidence of such resistance varies from hospital to hospital and even from ward to ward. It is thus of great importance for units such as neonatal intensive care or oncology units to have information on their local antibiotic resistance patterns.

Antibiotics may be used prophylactically or therapeutically.

Prophylactic use There are few absolute indications for the prophylactic use of antimicrobials and this is one area where misuse is common. Examples of indications for prophylaxis include rifampicin or ciprofloxacin for close contacts of cases of invasive meningococcal or *Haemophilus influenzae* type b disease (the latter only in children less than 5 years old);[†] metronidazole and gentamicin prior to colonic surgery; and amoxycillin (or erythromycin) prior to dental treatment in children with cardiac valvular defects. Examples of misuse include giving antibiotics to children with viral respiratory tract infections to prevent bacterial superinfection, or giving antibiotics to prevent infection in children with urinary catheters.

Therapeutic use In general antibiotics may be administered when:

- Infection is suspected but not proven on clinical grounds (pre-emptive).
- Infection is proven, pathogen suspected or unknown (empiric).
- Infection is proven, pathogen and antimicrobial susceptibility known.

In paediatric practice the first two situations are the most commonly encountered

[†] **Strictly speaking this is treatment of carriage rather than prophylaxis.**

and the last applies 24–48 hours after initial administration of antibiotics. At this stage the antimicrobial chemotherapy should be reviewed and rationalized. For initiation of pre-emptive therapy there will be varying levels of suspicion which trigger its administration. For example, in premature neonates the signs of infection are so non-specific and the results of infection so potentially catastrophic that therapy with broad-spectrum antibiotics is frequently initiated. On subsequent review infection is actually present in only about 10% of such episodes. Hence rationalization of therapy after 48–72 hours is important. For empiric therapy there will be good evidence that an infection is present and it may be possible to predict likely pathogens and even their antimicrobial sensitivity. For example, urinary tract infection is usually caused by *E. coli*, which is usually susceptible to trimethoprim, cephradine or co-amoxiclav. Again, it will be possible to rationalize the therapy according to the microbiology results. Paediatricians should not be afraid to change therapy to optimize chances of recovery from infection. All hospitals will have local guidelines to aid treatment which will be based on local patterns of infection and antibiotic resistance.

26

INFECTION CONTROL IN THE HOSPITAL

Nosocomial or hospital-associated infections are those infections that occur as a result of the patient being admitted to hospital or visits to the out-patients departments. The pathogens are acquired during the hospital stay and may present during hospitalization or after discharge to home. In contrast, community-acquired infections are due to pathogens acquired outside hospital. Nosocomial infections have been targeted as one of several potentially preventable health problems.

THE SIZE OF THE PROBLEM

Most of the data on the incidence of paediatric nosocomial infection come from North America. It is not possible to extrapolate data from surveys of adult nosocomial infection to paediatric populations. Paediatric infection rates from North America range from 1.2 to 10.3 per 100 discharges. The reported rate is higher in children's hospitals (mean 4.1 per 100 discharges, range 2.8–10.3) than in paediatric wards within general hospitals (mean 1.2 per 100 discharges, range 1.2–5.5). A prevalence survey undertaken in 1980 in 43 district general hospitals in the UK indicated that 22% of paediatric patients had community-acquired infection and 6.3% had hospital-acquired infection. In contrast, 16.8% of patients in neonatal intensive care units (NICUs) had hospital-acquired infection.

There are no specific data on the overall morbidity, mortality and financial costs of paediatric nosocomial infection. However, in 1987 in the USA it was estimated that nosocomial infection, taking all age groups, resulted, on average in 4 days extra stay in hospital per infected patient, caused an estimated 30 000 deaths each year and added an extra 3–10 billion dollars to hospital costs. Clearly, there are major benefits in decreasing hospital-associated infection. In order to do this there must be an understanding of the major sites of infection, the pathogens involved, their pathogenesis, and which services are most likely to experience nosocomial infection.

WHICH PATIENTS AND WHICH SERVICES?

In most paediatric surveys the majority of nosocomial infections present in NICUs, haematology and oncology wards, and, after neonatal surgery. This is not surprising since patients on these wards are the most likely to be immunocompromised and are exposed to the greatest risk. A Canadian study showed that nosocomial infection rates for NICUs, infant neurosurgery, haematology/oncology, neonatal surgery and paediatric ICUs were 14.0%, 12.3%, 11.7%, 9.1% and 6.0% respectively. In contrast, infection rates in ophthalmology, isolation and orthopaedic wards were 0.2%, 1.3% and 2.9% respectively. In general, the younger the child the higher the nosocomial infection rate (NIR). Thus those younger than 23 months had an NIR of 11.5%, those aged 2–4 years had an NIR of 3.6% and those older than 5 years had an NIR of 2.6%. The patterns of infection also changed with age.

SITES OF INFECTION

Although there are wide differences between different surveys, respiratory tract infections (16–24% of infections), gastrointestinal tract infections (17–35%) and bacteraemia (10–21%) are the three most frequent nosocomial infections. This contrasts with adult nosocomial infection, where urinary tract infection is the most common. In paediatric hospitals urinary tract infection accounts for 6–9% of nosocomial infection. It has been shown that the median lengths of stay in hospital prior to the development of nosocomial infections were 8.4 days, 10.7 days, 12 days, 19 days and 24.9 days for meningitis, wound infection, gastrointestinal infection, urinary tract infection and bacteraemia respectively. This may be an underestimate if patients discharged home subsequently developed a hospital-associated infection.

PATHOGENS INVOLVED

Another area of difference from adult nosocomial infection is the type of pathogen. Children are at greater risk of viral infection, and surveys of paediatric nosocomial infection that do not include viruses will underestimate rates. Outbreaks of nosocomial respiratory tract infection due to respiratory syncytial virus (RSV) and adenovirus, of gastrointestinal tract infection due to rotavirus and hepatitis A virus and of varicella-zoster in NICUs are well described. In most surveys bacteria account for 65–70% (Gram-positive about 50%, Gram-negative about 18%) of paediatric nosocomial infection, viruses for up to 25% (mostly gastrointestinal infection) and fungi for 5%. The distribution of pathogens varies according to the paediatric service, the age of the patient and site of infection. For example, coagulase-negative staphylococci (e.g. *Staphylococcus epidermidis*) are particularly associated with implant infections (most often intravascular catheters) and infections related to intravascular catheters are responsible for 5–6% of paediatric nosocomial infection.

PATHOGENESIS OF NOSOCOMIAL INFECTION

Nosocomial infections can occur as outbreaks or epidemics or as sporadic cases. Although the outbreaks of infection are the most highly visible and worrying, sporadic infections numerically are far more important. In order to prevent both epidemic and sporadic nosocomial infection it is necessary to understand the pathogenesis of infection, modes of transmission and portals of entry.

Infections can be divided into exogenous and endogenous. In exogenous infection the pathogen gains direct access to the patient from the environment (animate or inanimate) and initiates disease. Endogenous infections are derived from the patient's own microflora (see Chapter 24). Endogenous infections may be subdivided into primary endogenous infections in which the pathogen is derived from the patient's own normal flora, and secondary endogenous infections in which the pathogen colonizes the patient, becoming part of the 'normal' flora and subsequently causes infection. Examples of exogenous infection are secondary cases of bronchiolitis due to RSV and of gastroenteritis due to *Salmonella* spp. or rotavirus. Exogenous nosocomial infections can be sporadic but have a propensity to result in outbreaks. Examples of primary endogenous infections include abdominal abscesses due to *Streptococcus milleri* following appendicectomy or CSF shunt infections due to *Staphylococcus epidermidis*. Primary endogenous infections are always sporadic. Secondary endogenous infection can appear either sporadically or in outbreaks, examples include cases of multidrug-resistant *Klebsiella aerogenes* colonizing neonates in NICUs, resulting in septicaemia and meningitis in a proportion of those colonized. It can be seen that different methods are needed to control exogenous and primary and secondary endogenous infections.

MODES OF SPREAD

Although there are numerous possibilities for spreading potential pathogens in hospital, in general nosocomial infections are transmitted by contact, vehicles, air or vectors. Of the above, person-to-person transmission by hands of hospital staff or even patients is undoubtedly the most important. The incidence of nosocomial infections rises when staffing levels are inadequate, since this leads to a decrease in hand-washing by overburdened staff, and staff have contact with an increased number of patients. It has been shown that hands are an important mode of spread even of respiratory pathogens such as RSV and adenovirus which were previously considered to be spread by air. Overcrowding on wards also increases the likelihood of transmission of pathogens by air or by contact.

Vehicles of transmission of nosocomial infection could be food (e.g. *Salmonella* spp.), water (e.g. *Cryptosporidium*), contaminated intravenous solutions (e.g. *Klebsiella*, *Serratia* or *Enterobacter* spp.) or blood and blood products (e.g. hepatitis B or C virus, human immunodeficiency virus, cytomegalovirus). Of equal importance are items of medical equipment; for example, there have been outbreaks of infection due to contaminated rectal thermometers (*Salmonella eimsbuettel*), breast milk pumps (*Klebsiella pneumonia*) and gastroscopes (*Helicobacter pylori*).

Air-borne spread of pathogens can occur; examples include varicella-zoster virus in neonatal units, and *Aspergillus* spp. in oncology units. Nevertheless, this is of secondary importance in comparison with hand transmission. Although rodents and cockroaches can be found in hospitals, there is little evidence that they are important vectors of infection.

HOST FACTORS

The variations in hospital-associated infection rates in the different paediatric services are to a large extent a reflection of the immunocompetence and thus susceptibility to infection of the patients. Patients in NICUs have defects in non-specific immunity (poor temperature control, no established normal flora, poor inflammatory response, impaired phagocytosis) and in specific immunity (IgG reflecting maternal IgG levels, no IgA, low IgM levels, depressed T-cell function), which are more evident the more premature the neonate. In haematology and oncology wards patients are immunosuppressed both by their disease and by chemotherapy or radiotherapy.

CONTROLLING NOSOCOMIAL INFECTIONS

From the foregoing it is apparent that controlling nosocomial infections is of major importance. It is also apparent that the interactions between micro-organisms in patients, hospital staff and the hospital environment that result in nosocomial infection are complex, and that infection control measures must extend into many facets of the paediatric hospital or ward. The aims of effective infection control are:

- To prevent patients from acquiring infection in hospital.
- To provide adequate hospital care for patients entering hospital with a community-acquired infection while preventing its dissemination to others.
- To prevent transmission of infection to or from hospital staff and visitors.
- To prevent nosocomial infections being disseminated in the community.

In order to do this it is essential that each hospital should have an infection control team.

Role of the infection control team The infection control team (ICT) normally consists of the infection control doctor (ICD), infection control nurses, a medical microbiologist (who may be the ICD) and a representative of the hospital management team. This team should report to an infection control committee (ICC) which should comprise the ICD, the consultant in communicable disease control (CCDC), occupational health physician, a paediatrician or a physician with an interest in infectious diseases, surgeon and a nurse manager, The committee may co-opt as necessary representatives from the central sterile supply department, laundry services, building services, catering, pest control, pharmacy and the operating theatres. The ICT should be responsible for the day-to-day control of nosocomial infection. It will be responsible for formulation and application of infection control policies (including involvement in formulation of policies on antibiotic usage, isolation, immunization, disinfection and sterilization, commissioning and decommissioning theatres and medical equipment). It will be responsible for surveillance of nosocomial infection and providing regular reports to the ICC. It will be responsible for liaising with the community over problems of infection. Finally—and most importantly—the ICT has an educative role for hospital staff to present information on how nosocomial infection occurs and how best to prevent it. Such education will require repeated reinforcement. In addition to general infection control the ICT will be responsible for initiating the correct responses for notification, investigation and curtailment of outbreaks of infection. Each hospital should have structures (policies and action group) to manage major or minor outbreaks of infection.

Methods for infection control It is beyond the scope of this chapter to give a detailed description of infection control policies. Each hospital and under certain circumstances each ward (e.g. NICU and PICU) will need to draw up its own policy taking into account local problems and facilities. The policy will need to encompass areas such as preadmission infection screening (for booked admissions), precautions to be taken with infected patients, methods and degrees of patient isolation and hand-washing between handling patients. Isolation policies should balance the risk of transmission of infection with the difficulty of treating patients in isolation and the psychological problems posed to a child by isolation. Examples of types of isolation and precautions are shown in the Table 26.1.

The NICU and PICU are areas of particular risk for development of nosocomial infection. Extra attention focused on them can yield great benefit. As in other areas, hand-washing is of prime importance in preventing transmission of micro-organisms that can cause either exogenous or secondary endogenous infection. Unlike in most other areas, the inanimate environment may also be a source of infection—for example, outbreaks of bacteraemia and meningitis have been associated with strains of *Klebsiella aerogenes* colonizing blood gas analysers and breast-milk pumps. It is, therefore, advisable to wash hands prior to handling as well as after handling the patients, or their intravenous lines or ventilators. There is no evidence that gowning prevents infection unless the patient is to be directly handled. Masks are usually used only for special procedures such as siting catheters. Gloves are used when handling infants with diarrhoea or draining wounds. They do not replace hand-washing. The use of overshoes is to be

Table 26.1 Examples of isolation and precautions for infection control

	Examples of diseases or pathogens	Methods
Strict isolation	Diphtheria, plague, rabies	Single room. Gown, gloves, mask. Strict hand-washing prior to leaving room. Contaminated articles bagged, labelled and decontaminated or incinerated
Contact isolation	Conjunctivitis, impetigo, IMRSA	Single room. Masks for close contact, gowns if soiling likely, gloves if touching infected area. Strict hand-washing. Contaminated article bagged, labelled, and decontaminated or incinerated
Respiratory isolation	Bronchiolitis (RSV), measles, meningococcal disease, whooping cough	Single room (cohorting for RSV), measles immunization for close contact. Gloves not indicated. Strict hand-washing. Contaminated articles bagged, labelled, decontaminated or incinerated.
Enteric isolation	Rotavirus, shigellosis, cryptosporidiosis. All patients with diarrhoea unless proved to be non-infective	Single room (?cohort for rotavirus). No masks, gown if soiling likely, gloves if handling infective material. Strict hand-washing. Contaminated articles bagged, labelled, and decontaminated or incinerated
Blood and body fluid precautions	Hepatitis B, HIV	Isolation not indicated. No masks. Gloves for handling blood or body fluid. Gowns if soiling likely. Contaminated articles bagged, labelled and decontaminated or incinerated. Avoid needle-stick or sharps injury. Clean spills with 0.5% sodium hypochlorite
Protective isolation	Immunosuppressed patients (e.g. bone marrow transplant)	Single room, positive pressure ventilation. Gowns, gloves, masks. Sterilized food and drink. Aim is to prevent access of potential pathogen to patient

Key: HIV, human immunodeficiency virus; MRSA, methicillin-resistant *Staphylococcus aureus*; RSV, respiratory syncytial virus.

discouraged: it is an ideal way of transferring micro-organisms from shoes to hands.

Control of infection in hospital requires an enthusiastic, able and vigilant team who are prepared to educate and convince hospital staff that nosocomial infection is important and that its impact can be lessened by application of effective methods.

FURTHER READING

Hospital Infection Working Group of the Department of Health and Public Health Laboratory Service (1995) *Hospital Infection Control: Guidance on the Control of Infection in Hospitals*. London: Department of Health available from BAPS Health Publication Unit, DSS Distribution Centre, Heywood Stores, Manchester Road, Heywood Lancashire.

Garner JJ & Simmons BP (1983) CDC Guidelines for isolation precautions in hospitals. *Infection Control* **4**: 245–325.

Wenzel RP (1992) *Prevention and Control of Nosocomial Infection*, 2nd edn. Williams & Wilkins, Baltimore.

27

INFECTION CONTROL IN THE COMMUNITY

PRIMARY PREVENTIVE PRACTICES

The following practices are recommended to reduce the incidence and transmission of infection in the day-care, nursery primary school, and other settings. Many of the practices are applicable elsewhere and will also reduce disease incidence and transmission in the home.

Reducing risks of faecal–oral transmission of infection

- Day-care facilities should have written policies for preventing and managing child and staff illness, with appropriate input from the medical microbiologist and consultant in communicable disease control.
- Toilets and toilet training equipment should be well maintained and cleaned daily. Surfaces used for napkin changing should be non-porous and cleaned between use. If disposable paper coverings are used they must be discarded after each use and the surface underneath cleaned if damp or soiled.
- Soiled disposable napkins or soiled wiping cloths should be discarded in a secure, plastic-lined container operated by a foot pedal so that hand contact can be minimized.
- Faeces should be placed in a toilet. Napkins should not be rinsed in sinks but may be placed to soak prior to washing in a sterilizing solution such as Napisan.
- Napkin changing areas should never be located in, or directly open onto food preparation areas; similarly, napkin changing should never take place where food is prepared.
- The use of child-sized toilets, or access to steps and modified toilet seats, should be encouraged as early as practical. The use of 'potties' should be discouraged. When they have to be used, for example with younger toddlers, they should be emptied into a toilet, cleaned in a sink (not used for food preparation), and disinfected after each use. Potties, flush toilets and changing areas should be cleaned with a freshly prepared solution of household bleach.
- Written procedures for hand-washing in day-care, nursery and primary school facilities should be established and enforced. Hand-washing sinks should be adjacent to each napkin changing and toileting area. These sinks should be washed and disinfected at least daily and when soiled; they must not be used for food preparation or for rinsing soiled clothing or cleaning potties.
- Children should have access to sinks, soap dispensers, and disposable paper towels at appropriate heights.
- Spills of vomit, urine and faeces should be cleaned using a bleach-containing commercial cleaner. Gloves should always be worn when handling bleach.
- Optimally, toys that are placed in children's mouths or otherwise contaminated by body secretions should be cleaned with water and detergent, disinfected and rinsed before handling by another child. All frequently touched toys in rooms that house infants and toddlers should be cleaned and disinfected daily. Toys in rooms for older children (no napkin users) should be cleaned weekly and when soiled. The use of shared soft, non-washable toys in infant and toddler areas of child care programmes should be discouraged.

- Food should be handled in a safe and careful manner to prevent the growth of micro-organisms. Tables and counter tops used for food preparation and food service should be cleaned between uses, and before and after eating. No one who has signs or symptoms of illness (especially vomiting and diarrhoea), who has infectious skin lesions that cannot be covered, or who is infected with potential food-borne pathogens, should be responsible for food handling. Hands should be washed using soap and water before handling food. Staff who work with children wearing napkins, whenever possible, should not prepare food. Carers who prepare food for infants should be especially aware of the importance of careful hand-washing.
- Unpasteurized milk or milk products should not be served.
- Food should be well cooked, particularly chicken and comminuted meat products (beefburgers, sausages, etc.); eggs should not be used without cooking or pasteurization (for example in cake icing, fillings or mayonnaise).
- Hands must be washed after touching an infected child or possibly contaminated material (e.g. napkins, soiled bedding).
- Articles contaminated by vomitus or faecal material should be discarded (if disposable) immediately into a plastic bag or placed in a secure container before washing.
- Disposable gloves may be used for touching infected articles in institutional settings (e.g. day-care centres) where infectious illnesses are concerned. Masks and gowns are not normally used outside hospital.

Persons at higher risk of causing faecal-oral transmission Certain persons are considered to pose a special risk of spreading infection. These can be considered in four groups. Group 1, food handlers whose work involves touching unwrapped foods to be consumed raw or without further cooking. Group 2, health care, nursery and other staff who have direct contact through serving food or direct contact with susceptible patients. Group 3, children aged less than five years attending nurseries, playgroups etc. Group 4, older children and adults who are unable to implement good standards of hygiene. (Source: see Department of Health 1994 in Further Reading).

Universal precautions for preventing transmission of blood-borne infection Written hygiene policies and procedures should include cleaning and disinfecting floors, play tables, and spills of blood, body fluids, and wound or tissue exudates.

For spills of blood or blood-containing body fluid, and of wound and tissue exudates, the procedures are as follows:

- Hands, skin or mucous membranes exposed to another person's fluids should be washed promptly and thoroughly.
- Disposable gloves are to be used throughout and any cuts, abrasions or inflamed areas kept covered by waterproof plasters. Gloves should be securely disposed of afterwards.
- The spill should be cleaned with freshly diluted household bleach (1 in 10 dilution, i.e. 1 part of bleach 10% sodium hypochlorite, to 9 parts water). Gloves must be worn. The bleach should be poured gently over the spill and covered with paper towels. If possible the bleach should be left then for 30 minutes before wiping up with more paper towels. More solid spillages

contaminated with body fluids, such as bloody vomit or faeces can be scooped up into a bucket of hot soapy water and the scoop cleaned or disposed of as contaminated waste.

- Contaminated materials and gloves should be discarded in a sealed bag.
- Hands should be washed afterwards.

Toothbrushes and flannels should not be shared.

When a child with a blood-borne infection* is cared for at home, carers should be supplied with disposable gloves and cleaning fluids.

Preventing exposure to zoonoses Pets should be kept in enclosed spaces which should be kept clean of waste. All animals should be handled by children only under close staff supervision. Hands should be washed under supervision after handling animals or animal wastes. Dogs and cats should be kept away from child play areas.

Immunization status

- Those responsible for the health care of the child in the centre, school or nursery should have access to and must update the child's immunization records. If any child is underimmunized, this should be rectified at the earliest opportunity.
- The health status of all employees must be checked before they begin work, with special attention to screening for pulmonary tuberculosis and immunization status.

Making parents aware

- Upon a child's entry to the school or nursery parents must be made aware of the need to share information about illness, which can be of a communicable nature, in the child or in any member of the immediate household.
- When children are known to have been exposed to an important communicable disease, for example meningococcal infection, the head of the centre, nursery or school should, following consultation with medical advisors, inform parents, preferably in writing, of any action to be taken.

CONSULTATION

The circumstances when consultation should occur cannot be strictly defined; however, Table 27.1 lists conditions for which consultation and action may be required if they occur, or if they are strongly suspected in a child, the family of a child, or in a staff member. If in doubt it is always safer to consult the relevant local health authorities, i.e. the medical officer for the centre, nursery or school, the CCDC, and the environmental health department, who should be notified promptly about cases of communicable diseases involving children or care providers in the child care setting. Action that may need to be taken is detailed under the sections for individual conditions in Part Two. Some recommendations for exclusion periods are contained in Appendix V; however, it is important that these should not be interpreted rigidly but following consultation.

***For example, a child who is hepatitis B antigen-positive, infected with human immunodeficiency virus (HIV) or of HIV indeterminate status.**

Table 27.1 Infectious conditions requiring urgent medical consultation should they appear in the children, staff or families of children in a day nursery or school

Campylobacter infection
Cryptosporidiosis
Diphtheria†
E. coli infection
Food poisoning
Giardiasis
Haemophilus influenzae type b infection
Hepatitis A or B
Impetigo
Measles
Meningococcal disease
Pertussis
Polio†
Ringworm (tinea)
Rotavirus and other viral gastroenteritis
Rubella
Salmonellosis
Shigellosis
Tuberculosis
Typhoid and paratyphoid fevers

†**Rare, but very important when it occurs.**

OUTBREAK CONTROL

Definition An outbreak of infection may be defined either as two or more linked cases of the same illness, or as the situation when the observed number of cases exceeds the expected number.

Objectives of control The objectives in controlling an outbreak are:

- To reduce to a minimum the number of primary cases of illness. This involves the prompt recognition of the outbreak, and identification and control of the source of the infection or contamination.
- To reduce to a minimum the number of secondary cases of infection, by identifying cases and taking appropriate action to prevent any spread.
- To prevent further episodes of illness by identifying continuing hazards and eliminating them or minimizing the risk they pose.

While outbreaks in schools and day-care centres pose the greatest risk because of the potential for rapid and large-scale transmission of infection, it needs to be remembered that transmission within the family is responsible for the majority of outbreaks. Most cases of infection seen in schools or nurseries will represent household or community transmission rather than transmission in the institution itself. However, this does not remove the responsibility of staff and their medical advisers in preventing secondary transmission occurring in the school.

In the UK, the role of the consultants in communicable disease control is crucial. Their remit is the surveillance, prevention and control of all communicable disease among the population of the district. As such they work closely with microbiologists, other medical specialists including paediatricians, and environmental health officers employed by the local authority. Coordinated outbreak control plans should have been drawn up by health and local authorities in consultation with the CCDC, the chief environmental health officer, the Family Health Service Agency (may be part of the health authority), the Public Health Laboratory Service (PHLS), local health service trusts and other bodies (e.g. water companies) as appropriate. These plans can be adapted to different types of outbreaks and are put into operation when the disease poses a health hazard to the local population, there are a large number of cases or the disease is unusual or poses a particular hazard. When an outbreak of any size or importance occurs or is suspected to have occurred, the PHLS Communicable Disease Surveillance Centre (telephone 0181-200-6868) or the Scottish Centre for Infection and Environmental Health (telephone 0141-946-7120) should be informed. Both provide advice on a 24-hour basis and can provide personnel if invited.

FURTHER READING

Department of Health (1994) *Management of Outbreaks of Foodborne Illness*. HMSO, London.

Public Health Medicine Environmental Group (1995) *Guidelines on Control of Infection in Residential and Nursing Homes*. PHMEG, UK. Copies are available by sending a $3\frac{1}{2}$ inch computer disk to Dr Donal O'Sullivan, Consultant in Communicable Disease Control, Lambeth, Southwark and Lewisham, 1, Lower Marsh, London SE1 7NT.

Public Health Laboratory Service Salmonella Committee (1995) Communicable Disease Report (Supplement 1). Notes on the control of human sources of gastrointestinal infections, infestations and bacterial infections in the UK.

PART 2 – Specific Infections

28 **Amoebiasis**

29 **Arboviruses**

30 **Ascaris (Roundworm)**

31 **Aspergillosis**

32 **Botulism (Food-Borne and Infant Botulism)**

33 **Brucellosis**

34 ***Campylobacter* Infection**

35 **Candidiasis**

36 **Cat-Scratch Disease**

37 **Chickenpox and Herpes Zoster (Varicella-Zoster)**

38 ***Chlamydia Pneumoniae* Infection**

39 ***Chlamydia Psittaci* Infection**

40 ***Chlamydia Trachomatis* Infection**

41 **Cholera**

42 **Conjunctivitis**

43 **Cryptosporidiosis**

44 **Cytomegalovirus Infection**

45 **Dermatophytoses: Tinea Capitis, Corporis, Pedis and Unguium**

46 **Diphtheria**

47 **Enterovirus Infection**

48 ***Escherichia Coli* Diarrhoea**

49 **Giardiasis**

50 **Gonococcal Infection**

51 **Haemolytic Uraemic Syndrome**

52 ***Haemophilus Influenzae* Infection**

53 Hand, Foot and Mouth Disease

54 *Helicobacter Pylori* Infection

55 Hepatitis A

56 Hepatitis B

57 Hepatitis C

58 Hepatitis E

59 Herpes Infections

60 Infectious Mononucleosis (Glandular Fever)

61 Influenza

62 Invasive Helminthiasis Causing Multisystem Disease

63 Kawasaki Disease

64 Legionnaires' Disease

65 Leishmaniasis: Visceral (Kala-Azar) and Cutaneous Leishmaniasis

66 Listeriosis

67 Lyme Disease

68 Malaria

69 Measles

70 Meningococcal Disease

71 Mumps

72 Mycobacterial Infection (Atypical)

73 *Mycoplasma* Infections

74 Nits and Head Lice

75 Parvovirus Infection: Fifth Disease (Erythema Infectiosum or Slapped Cheek Disease)

76 Pertussis (Whooping Cough)

77 Plague

78 *Pneumocystis Carinii* Pneumonia

79 **Poliomyelitis**

80 **Poxvirus Infection (including Molluscum Contagiosum)**

81 **Prion Disease (Spongiform Encephalopathies)**

82 **Rabies**

83 **Respiratory Syncytial Virus Infection**

84 **Roseola Infantum, Exanthema Subitum or Sixth Disease (Human Herpesvirus 6/7 Infection)**

85 **Rotavirus and Other Viral Enteropathogens**

86 **Rubella**

87 **Salmonellosis**

88 **Scabies**

89 **Shigellosis**

90 **Staphylococcal Infections**

91 **Streptococcal Infections**

92 **Syphilis (Congenital and Acquired) and Non-Venereal Treponematoses**

93 **Tetanus**

94 **Threadworms**

95 **Toxocariasis**

96 **Toxoplasmosis**

97 **Tuberculosis**

98 **Typhoid and Paratyphoid Fever**

99 **Typhus**

100 **Viral Haemorrhagic Fevers**

101 **Warts and Verrucae**

102 **Yellow Fever**

103 **Yersiniosis**

28

AMOEBIASIS

Notifiable if dysenteric

ORGANISM

Amoebiasis is caused by a protozoan parasite *Entamoeba histolytica*, which exists as potentially invasive trophozoites and a hardy infective cyst. There are pathogenic and non-pathogenic strains identifiable by different isozymes (zymodemes).

EPIDEMIOLOGY

The organism is found worldwide, the major host being humans. Prevalence is higher where sanitation is poor. The parasite can act as a commensal or it may invade from the gut, but most infections are asymptomatic. Infection is unusual in preschool children, especially infants.

Transmission is by contaminated water, the faecal–oral route and by raw fruit and vegetables exposed to contaminated water. Adults can have chronic infection and pass cysts for years, though usually this is confined to non-pathogenic strains.

Incubation period is usually 4 weeks, but can seemingly extend to years.

NATURAL HISTORY AND CLINICAL FEATURES

Most infection is asymptomatic. Symptoms can be mild with constipation or loose stools and abdominal distension, though amoebiasis is an unusual cause of such presentations in children. Severe disease can be dysenteric or non-dysenteric. The dysenteric form (acute amoebic colitis) presents with fever, abdominal pain and diarrhoea with blood and mucus, and can proceed to peritonitis. Non-dysenteric amoebiasis is milder, with intermittent diarrhoea and abdominal pain. Invasion of the liver occurs rarely.

Diagnosis Fresh stool specimens (or specimens preserved in 10% formalin) will reveal trophozoites or cysts on microscopic examination in colonic disease. A single specimen may be insufficient to detect infection. Where there is diagnostic difficulty a rectal biopsy may be useful. Extraintestinal amoebiasis may be difficult to detect or diagnose. Specialist advice should be sought and serology (fluorescent antibody test) is often helpful. Liver abscess may be identified by ultrasound or computed tomographic scan.

MANAGEMENT

Asymptomatic carriage is treated with diloxonide furoate. Amoebic dysentery is treated with oral metronidazole, as is extragastrointestinal amoebiasis where tinidazole can also be used. Rehydration may be required.

PREVENTION OF FURTHER CASES

Water supplies should be treated to remove or kill cysts. Enteric precautions (Chapters 26 and 27) are indicated for patients with symptomatic or asymptomatic infection.

ARBOVIRUSES

29

ORGANISM

There are several hundred arthropod-borne viruses.

EPIDEMIOLOGY

Infections occur worldwide. 'Louping ill' characterized by encephalitis is a rare infection in the UK. Tick-borne encephalitis is seen in central and eastern Europe.

Transmission is usually from mosquitoes or ticks.

Incubation period is anything from 1 day to 15 days.

NATURAL HISTORY AND CLINICAL FEATURES

There are four main types of illness:

- An encephalopathy which in severe cases is fatal.
- A fever of short duration with or without a rash. This may progress to an encephalitis.
- Haemorrhagic fevers which may be fatal and can be associated with hepatitis (see Chapter 100).
- Arthritis or arthralgia and rash, sometimes with fever. This may be a chronic illness.

Diagnosis is by serology, or viral isolation from the blood in some cases.

MANAGEMENT

Management is supportive.

IMMUNIZATION

Immunization is available for yellow fever, tick-borne encephalitis and Japanese B encephalitis (see Chapter 20).

ASCARIS (Roundworm)

30

ORGANISM

Ascaris lumbricoides is a large roundworm. *Ascaris suum* may also infect humans.

EPIDEMIOLOGY

Roundworms are found in moist temperate and tropical climates. They are uncommon in the UK.

Transmission is via the faecal–oral route.

Incubation period is of the order of 4–8 weeks.

NATURAL HISTORY AND CLINICAL FEATURES

Ova are ingested in infected soil or in uncooked meat contaminated with infected soil. The eggs hatch in the small intestine and the larvae migrate through the gut wall to reach the lungs via the circulation. They then pass into the alveoli and proceed up the respiratory tract until they are swallowed and return to the small intestine. Here they mature, mate and produce eggs about 45–60 days after the initial ingestion. In 80% of infestations the only manifestation is the passage of ova or adult worms in the stool. In a small proportion of cases pulmonary or gastrointestinal symptoms may arise. Löffler's syndrome (larval pneumonitis) is caused by the larval migration through the lungs. Cough, fever, wheezing and breathlessness are the most common presenting features. An urticarial rash may be present, and crackles and wheezes may be heard in the chest. Examination reveals rhonchi and crepitations. A heavy infestation in the bowel may cause obstruction. Where nutrition is inadequate the worms may cause malnutrition.

Diagnosis There is usually an eosinophilia. Chest X-ray may show diffuse, mottled opacities with pneumonitis. Larvae may be found in the sputum and stool microscopy will often reveal ova.

MANAGEMENT

Piperazine (75 mg/kg up to a maximum of 4 g on two successive evenings) is effective in eliminating worms from the bowel. In children sensitive to piperazine, mebendazole (100 mg twice daily for 3 days) is equally effective, but mebendazole should not be given to children under 2 years old. There is no specific treatment for the pulmonary effects.

PREVENTION OF FURTHER CASES

Simple hygienic measures (see Chapter 27) prevent the acquisition of infection.

31

ASPERGILLOSIS

ORGANISM

Aspergillus fumigatus, *A. flavus* and other *Aspergillus* species are spore-bearing fungi.

EPIDEMIOLOGY

Aspergillus species are ubiquitous in the environment. Spores in the atmosphere seem to be particularly prevalent at the sites of building works. Invasive *Aspergillus* infections almost exclusively affect immunocomprised individuals. Low-grade infection in sinuses and in the external auditory canal may occur in healthy individuals. Allergic bronchopulmonary aspergillosis is particularly likely to affect atopic individuals.

Transmission is by inhalation of spores. Individuals undergoing severe immunosuppression, as in bone marrow transplantation, may also develop aspergillosis associated with invasion of the organism from previously colonized sinuses.

Incubation period is unknown

NATURAL HISTORY AND CLINICAL FEATURES

Allergic bronchopulmonary aspergillosis affects mainly atopic individuals and particularly asthmatic patients. It is relatively rare in childhood. There is episodic wheezing and sometimes low-grade fever. Chest X-ray shows flitting opacities particularly in the perihilar regions.

Invasive aspergillosis affects patients with prolonged myelosuppression, for instance patients undergoing intensive cytotoxic chemotherapy or bone marrow transplantation. It also occurs in patients with neutrophil function disorders such as chronic granulomatous disease. The infection usually enters through the lung and pneumonia may be evident. Invasion of the blood stream results in disseminated infection which may affect the brain, bones, liver, kidneys, etc. Mortality is extremely high in disseminated disease. *Aspergillus* species may also occasionally grow as a fungal ball in lung cysts or cavities in patients without underlying immunosuppression.

Diagnosis depends on demonstration of the characteristic fungal hyphae in tissue specimens, with or without culture of the organism in Sabouraud agar or other suitable medium. Antibody tests have proved disappointing in the diagnosis, possibly because patients with significant disease are immunocompromised. In bronchopulmonary aspergillosis there is usually a marked eosinophilia in the blood with raised levels of IgE—both total and *Aspergillus*-specific.

MANAGEMENT

Allergic bronchopulmonary aspergillosis is treated with systemic corticosteroids. Maintenance inhaled corticosteroids may be required. Invasive aspergillosis should be treated with systemic antifungal drugs and the treatment of choice is amphotericin (see Chapter 18). In view of the difficulties in confirming a diagnosis of invasive fungal infection, early empirical treatment with antifungal agents is often initiated in immune-suppressed patients who develop fever with or without pneumonitis.

PREVENTION OF FURTHER CASES

Patients undergoing prolonged myelosuppressive treatment should, where possible, be cared for in facilities with filtered air to reduce spore exposure. This is particularly important if building works are nearby. In older children who are to undergo bone marrow transplantation, it is important to check for evidence of chronic sinus infection which might harbour *Aspergillus* species. Prophylactic regimens either with low-dose systemic amphotericin or with the newer oral agent itraconazole are promising approaches to reducing this problem in immunocompromised children.

BOTULISM (FOOD-BORNE AND INFANT BOTULISM) 32

ORGANISM

Clostridium botulinum is an anaerobic, spore-forming bacillus which produces neurotoxins. On the basis of the serological characteristics of the toxins there are seven types (A to G). The bacterium and its toxins are sensitive to boiling but some spores require higher temperatures to ensure their destruction. The toxin irreversibly binds to the synaptic membrane of cholinergic nerves, preventing the release of acetylcholine and blocking neuromuscular transmission. This results in flaccid paralysis and autonomic dysfunction.

EPIDEMIOLOGY

It is important to distinguish between three types of botulism: *food-borne botulism*, *infant botulism* and *wound botulism*. Food-borne botulism is a form of food poisoning or intoxication due to ingestion of food in which *Clostridium botulinum* has produced toxin. Infant botulism is due to the ingestion of *C. botulinum* or its spores leading to colonization of the gut and local production of neurotoxin (the young infant's gut is peculiarly susceptible to such colonization). Wound botulism is due to the local production of toxin by the organism growing in wounds. Most cases of infant botulism are due to neurotoxin type A or B, while food-borne botulism is usually due to toxins type A, B or E, and occasionally type F or G.

Clostridium botulinum is ubiquitous in the environment because it has a spore-forming stage. Spores can be found in dust, soil, untreated water, the digestive tracts of animals and fish and occasionally in a number of foods. However, food-borne botulism does not occur unless circumstances permit the growth of organisms and production of toxins. All three types of botulism are uncommon in industrialized countries, and wound botulism is exceptionally rare and has not been reported in the UK. Cases of food-borne botulism often occur as outbreaks and have occurred sometimes through large-scale contamination of foodstuffs. An important source of cases in the USA is from inadequately performed home preserving of meats, fish and vegetables, but this has not been a recent source of cases in the UK where there have been 32 cases (all ages), including three deaths since 1977. Over 1000 cases of infant botulism have been reported worldwide but only 5 cases were in the UK. Ninety per cent of cases are in infants less than 6 months old and 50% in infants under 3 months old. Honey has been implicated as the dietary source in some cases in the USA, where spores have been found occasionally in honey. However, no spores of *C. botulinum* were found in a survey of commercial honey in the UK.

Transmission Food-borne botulism arises from ingestion of preformed toxin in contaminated food, while infant botulism is due to the ingestion of spores or bacteria. Person-to-person spread has not been recorded for any form of the infection.

Incubation period In food-borne botulism symptoms appear rapidly, within 12–36 hours, if toxin levels are high. Longer periods have been described (up to a week) when intoxication is light. In infant botulism there may be a period of between 3 days and 2 weeks between colonization and symptoms appearing.

NATURAL HISTORY AND CLINICAL FEATURES

Food-borne botulism Clinical features are mostly due to toxin affecting the nervous system. In older children and adults cranial nerve palsies predominate, causing (among other bulbar signs) dysphonia, ptosis and double vision. Mental function and sensation are generally well preserved. Vomiting, diarrhoea or constipation and abdominal cramps may be features. A generalized weakness and a descending paralysis is ominous, and death may occur at all ages due to respiratory failure or superinfection.

Infant botulism Signs of intoxication in infants are non-specific. The first sign is usually constipation which is followed by lethargy, poor feeding, drooling, hypotonia and general weakness. There is often a descending symmetrical weakness starting in the muscles innervated by the bulbar centres, leading to a number of signs including decreased cry, poor suck and gag reflexes and loss of facial expression and eye control followed by loss of deep tendon reflexes.

Sudden apnoea and respiratory failure are the major life-threatening complications. However, with meticulous care prognosis is good, though recovery is slow as it requires sprouting of new terminal motor neurones to renervate muscle fibres. Infant botulism is a rare but important differential diagnosis for the 'floppy baby' syndrome. It has also been implicated as a rare cause of sudden infant death syndrome.

In both food-borne and infant botulism the condition may last for 6–8 months. However, the condition is potentially self-limiting and with meticulous supportive care a complete recovery can be achieved.

Diagnosis Because of the non-specific clinical features, demonstration of toxin (from food, serum and faeces) or culture of the organism (from food) is essential for diagnosis. Stool specimens may be difficult to obtain because of constipation in which case a rectal wash-out may be justified. Once the diagnosis is suggested clinicians and microbiologists should take specialist advice and refer specimens for testing.* All samples, including the suspect food, should be sent urgently if the diagnosis of botulism is considered likely.

MANAGEMENT

The course of both infant and food-borne botulism is often prolonged. Specialist advice is essential, with all but the mildest cases being managed in intensive care until the severity of intoxication can be ascertained. Much of the treatment is supportive and includes careful attention to respiratory status, hydration and nutrition. In infant botulism, elective ventilation is preferable to awaiting the development of apnoea and ventilatory failure.

In food-borne botulism an equine-based antitoxin is available and its use should be considered for symptomatic cases, at an early stage as application of antitoxin is ineffective after the toxin has fixed to tissues.† However, antitoxin should be given with great care because of the high incidence of adverse reactions produced by the equine-based serum. Antibiotics are only used to treat secondary infection.

In infant botulism antibiotics are also only used to treat secondary infections, for example pneumonias. Antitoxin is not recommended for infant botulism because of the high incidence of adverse reactions and the lack of evidence of any efficacy in the face of ongoing toxin release.

PREVENTION OF FURTHER CASES

Prevention of botulism is by meticulous attention to instructions in food preparation, especially in homepreserving. All toxin is inactivated by heating at 80 °C for 30 minutes and spores are destroyed by heating to over 120 °C for 2 minutes. However, not all foodstuffs are suitable for such treatment. Once a case of infant or food-borne botulism is suspected, the consultant in communicable disease control or the director of public health must be contacted immediately so

---

***In the UK the Food Hygiene Laboratory, Central Public Health Laboratory, 61 Colindale Avenue, London NW9 5HT (telephone 0181-200-4400) provides specialist testing and advice.**

†Small stocks of the antitoxin are held at centres around the country. Details of current centres are available from the Food Hygiene Laboratory (see footnote above).

that other persons who have shared the food can be identified, along with other food which may also be contaminated. The Communicable Disease Surveillance Centre and the Food Hygiene Laboratory, Central Public Health Laboratory must also be informed and the latter will assist in diagnosis.*

FURTHER READING

Brett M (1994) Infant botulism. Quarterly Communicable Disease Review. *Journal Public Health Medicine* **16**: 361–363.

33

BRUCELLOSIS

ORGANISM

Causative organisms of brucellosis are Gram-negative coccobacilli and include *Brucella melitensis*, *B. suis*, *B. abortus* and *B. canis*.

EPIDEMIOLOGY

Infection occurs in cattle, sheep, goats and humans. Few cases are seen in the UK and most of these have been acquired in the Mediterranean and Middle East.

Transmission Person-to-person infection does not occur. Although infection in adults usually results from occupational exposure (slaughterhouses) the disease does occasionally occur in children as a result of ingestion of infected milk.

Incubation period is difficult to determine, but is thought to be 2–3 months.

NATURAL HISTORY AND CLINICAL FEATURES

Brucellosis is often a mild infection, particularly when caused by *Brucella abortus*. A more serious illness is caused by *B. melitensis*, with fever, chills, weight loss and arthralgia. Clinical signs include hepatomegaly and splenomegaly. Occasionally meningoencephalitis is present.

Diagnosis is by culture of blood, bone marrow or urine. Prolonged culture is needed and serological tests are available.

MANAGEMENT

Tetracycline 30–40 mg/kg daily in four doses for 3–6 weeks is the treatment of choice in older children. With severe disease, gentamicin 7.5 mg/kg per day should be added to tetracycline. In children under 9 years old, trimethoprim-sulphamethoxazole is an alternative, given for 3–6 weeks (trimethoprim 10 mg/kg daily, maximum 480 mg per day; sulphamethoxazole 50 mg/kg daily, maximum 2.4 g per day).

PREVENTION OF FURTHER CASES

Eradication of brucellosis in cattle, swine and other animals and avoidance of unpasteurized milk should prevent the disease. The local consultant in communicable disease control and the veterinary officials should be alerted to any cases.

***Central Public Health Laboratory, 61 Colindale Avenue, London NW9 5HT (telephone 0181-200-4400).**

CAMPYLOBACTER INFECTION

ORGANISM

Infection is mainly with *Campylobacter jejuni*, a Gram-negative bacillus. Some other campylobacters—*C. fetus*, *C. laridis* and *C. coli*—also cause diarrhoea.

EPIDEMIOLOGY

The main reservoir of infection is in the gastrointestinal tract of farm animals and birds. Domestic dogs and cats are an additional reservoir. Gastroenteritis due to *Campylobacter jejuni* occurs in people of all ages worldwide and is a common cause of diarrhoea in travellers. Reports of campylobacter have increased recently in England and Wales (see Appendix I, Figure 2).

Transmission to humans is usually by ingestion of contaminated foods, including unpasteurized milk, bird attack on bottled doorstep milk, improperly prepared poultry and contaminated water, or by direct contact with animals (especially cats, puppies and lambs) or on farm visits. Person-to-person spread is uncommon but does occur. Organisms are excreted while patients are symptomatic and excretion may continue for up to 7 weeks after the start of the illness. Treatment with erythromycin rapidly terminates excretion.

Incubation period is usually 3–5 days with a range of 1–10 days.

NATURAL HISTORY AND CLINICAL FEATURES

Clinical features are variable and asymptomatic infections occur. Principal features are those of an acute enteric infection: diarrhoea, fever, malaise, abdominal pain, nausea and vomiting. Diarrhoea may show mucus, blood and pus. The illness may be mild and over in a few days. However, infection may also mimic acute appendicitis and it can also be severe and prolonged, especially in older children and adults. It may be invasive with positive blood cultures. Febrile convulsions can occur. In prolonged cases it may be mistaken for ulcerative colitis. Uncommon manifestations include reactive arthritis and Guillain–Barré syndrome.

Diagnosis Rapid presumptive diagnosis can be achieved by microscopic examination (dark-field or Gram staining) of stool smears. Rapid transfer of stool specimens to the laboratory is essential. Definite diagnosis is by culture of *C. jejuni*. The organism may also be isolated from blood.

MANAGEMENT

Management is symptomatic in most cases (see Chapter 6). Enteric precautions should be applied, though are less crucial than for other, more infectious, gastrointestinal infections. Severely affected children and adults should be given a 5–7 day course of antibiotics (usually erythromycin).

PREVENTION OF FURTHER CASES

When more than one case occurs, the consultant in communicable disease control or the director of public health should be informed in case a common-source outbreak is occurring. Pasteurization of milk, provision of clean water, proper cooking of poultry, care in handling pets and deterring wild birds from drinking 'doorstep' milk will prevent many cases. Children visiting farms need to be supervised to ensure that hand-washing precautions are applied. Enteric precautions need to be applied for managing symptomatic cases; however, if these are well applied to affected hospital workers and infected food handlers they need not be excluded once symptoms have subsided.

35

CANDIDIASIS (Thrush, Moniliasis)

For systemic candidiasis, see Chapter 18.

ORGANISM

Candida albicans, a yeast, is the most common pathogen, but *C. tropicalis* and others can be important in immunocompromised individuals.

EPIDEMIOLOGY

The organism is found worldwide. It colonizes the skin and mucous membranes. Colonization is increased by the use of broad-spectrum antibiotics. Oral and perineal thrush is common in neonates, and vaginitis in women of child-bearing age. In girls and women it can be sexually transmitted. Chronic mucocutaneous candidiasis may be associated with endocrine disorders or immunodeficiency. Systemic candidiasis is very unusual in normal hosts. Premature babies, immunodeficient patients and those with indwelling catheters may develop fungaemia with multiorgan disease or extensive superficial disease.

Transmission is via person-to-person contact and contaminated feeding bottles, etc.

Incubation period is variable, but probably 2–5 days for oral thrush.

NATURAL HISTORY AND CLINICAL FEATURES

Oral thrush presents as white areas on the mucous membranes of the mouth. They may look like milk patches but leave a raw area when scraped off. The mouth may be sore, making it difficult to feed. In the immunocompromised patient there may only be raw areas rather than white patches. In the napkin region there is a clearly demarcated edge to the area of inflammation and satellite lesions are common.

Diagnosis is clinical. The organism is so common on mucous membranes and skin that isolation of the organism from suspect lesions in these sites cannot be taken as diagnostic.

MANAGEMENT

Topical nystatin is first-line therapy. Miconazole can also be used. In perineal disease oral treatment should be given as well as directly to the lesions. Hygiene is also important. Strict disinfection of feeding bottles and dummies is essential, and wet napkins should be changed as soon as possible. Once inadequate hygiene has been excluded, recurrent candidiasis should raise the possibility of an impairment of immunity and the appropriate investigations should be undertaken (see Chapter 16). Systemic treatment with fluconazole may be useful for recurrent or persistent infection.

PREVENTION OF FURTHER CASES

Dummies, feeding bottles and other objects destined for a baby's mouth must not be shared. Where eradication is difficult, then sterilization by boiling may be necessary. Treatment of candida on the breast-feeding mother's nipples may be necessary to prevent reinfection.

CAT-SCRATCH DISEASE 36

ORGANISM

The disease is probably caused by a rickettsial-like organism—*Bartonella henselae*, previously *Rochalimaea henselae*.

EPIDEMIOLOGY

Cat-scratch fever is an uncommon infection, but it occurs worldwide.

Transmission is believed to occur when a cat (usually a kitten) scratches a human. There is no evidence of person-to-person infection.

Incubation period A papule appears 3–10 days after the scratch. Lymphadenopathy follows 2–6 weeks later.

NATURAL HISTORY AND CLINICAL FEATURES

The presenting complaint is lymphadenopathy which may progress to suppuration. Usually there is a history of a cat scratch followed by the appearance of a small papule. Fever and malaise may not occur. A small number of cases with hepatosplenic granulomas have been described. These were seen in children with persistent fever, both with or without an external lymphadenopathy and cat scratch or superficial papule.

Diagnosis is from the history and presence of necrotizing granuloma on lymph node biopsy. Cat-scratch disease may be confused with atypical tuberculosis (Chapter 72). In some cases micro-organisms are identified on the Warthin–Starry silver stain. The bacterium can be cultured on simple medium. Specialist diagnostic services for cat scratch disease and bacillary angiomatous are available on an experimental basis from the A-typical Pneumonia Unit, Central Public Health Laboratory (Tel: 0181 200 4400).

MANAGEMENT

Aspiration of lymph nodes except as a diagnostic procedure is not indicated. Rifampicin has been used in some cases of abdominal granulomas and was probably effective. In most cases of lymphadenitis recovery occurs without treatment.

CHICKENPOX AND HERPES ZOSTER (VARICELLA- ZOSTER) 37

ORGANISM

Varicella-zoster virus (VZV) is also known as human herpesvirus 3 (HHV-3); it is an enveloped DNA virus.

EPIDEMIOLOGY

Humans are the only reservoir of infection. Chickenpox is highly infectious and the majority of individuals become infected in early or middle childhood and remain immune into adulthood. In the UK and the USA in the past 20 years, first infections have increasingly been taking place in older age groups. As the likelihood of severe morbidity and even mortality (estimated at 1 per 4000 cases in adults) increases with age of occurrence, this secular change is of significance. However, more morbidity results from herpes zoster (recrudescence of infection) with a lifetime risk of about 25%. In England and Wales there are estimated to be 3000 admissions to hospital for chickenpox (60% are children) and 6000 admissions for herpes zoster. Though varicella infection in childhood is normally benign it may be severe in the immunosuppressed child, in the newborn infant when infection develops in the mother close to the time of delivery and in those with severe dermatological problems such as Ehrlers Danlos syndrome.

Transmission is by direct contact, droplet infection or recently soiled materials such as handkerchiefs.

Incubation period is from 10 days to 21 days, with the commonest period 14–17 days. The incubation can be prolonged in someone given varicella-zoster immune globulin. The period is somewhat shorter in the neonate infected perinatally, with the usual period between appearance of the rash in the mother and clinical signs in the neonate being 8–16 days; shorter periods have been recorded.

Period of infectivity is from 1–2 days prior to eruption of the rash (when infectivity is maximal) and then until all the lesions are encrusted, usually about 5 days after onset in an immunocompetent individual. In immunocompromised patients the course of the illness (and infectiousness) is prolonged, and patients should be considered infectious as long as new lesions (vesicles) continue to appear on the skin.

NATURAL HISTORY AND CLINICAL FEATURES

Primary infection with VZV results in chickenpox. There may be a short (less than 24 hours) coryzal prodrome followed by fever and an itchy, vesicular rash. Severity varies and asymptomatic infections occur. Crops of vesicles, sparser on the limbs than on the trunk, appear over 3–5 days. The most common complication is staphylococcal infection of the skin. Other complications are unusual in immunocompetent children but are protean, including hepatitis, thrombocytopenia, arthritis, glomerulonephritis, bacterial superinfection (staphylococcal and pneumococcal pneumonias sometimes associated with empyema and pleural effusion), cerebellar ataxia, hemiplegia, post-infective polyneuropathy and encephalitis. Aspirin given during the illness is thought to increase the risk of Reye's syndrome. Recurrences are unusual but have been described in immunocompetent children. Following chickenpox the virus persists as a latent infection in the dorsal root ganglia and may reappear following reactivation of the virus as herpes zoster (shingles), a painful vesicular rash in the dermatome of the affected nerves. Zoster occurs in immunocompetent children but is more common in adults. In adults the acute illness of varicella, fever and constitutional disturbance is more severe and pneumonia is a more common complication than in children. Immunosuppressed children have continued cropping of lesions, generalized zoster, encephalitis, pancreatitis, hepatitis and pneumonia.

Infection during early pregnancy may result in varicella embryopathy, which shows as bone and muscle hypoplasia (normally in one limb) resulting in atrophy, skin and eye lesions or multisystem anomalies (varicella syndrome). This is difficult to diagnose prenatally. Maternal exposure to VZV occurring late in pregnancy in a non-immune mother puts the neonate at risk of severe, overwhelming varicella with a particularly high mortality from varicella pneumonia.

Diagnosis is usually made on clinical features. Virus isolated from vesicle fluid can be identified by electron microscopy, virus culture and specific monoclonal antibodies. Anti-VZV antibodies can be confirmed by enzyme immunoassay, but such tests are usually used to demonstrate immunity in an individual exposed to VZV.

MANAGEMENT

Treatment of infected immunocompetent children Symptomatic treatment only is required in childhood but *aspirin should never be used as an antipyretic*. Children with chickenpox should not be admitted to hospital unless absolutely necessary because of the risk to immunosuppressed patients. Those hospitalized with proved or suspected varicella should be barrier nursed in isolation. Children may gain relief from itching by use of local antipruritics.

Treatment of infected immunocompromised children and infected pregnant women is essentially the same as for the immunocompetent child, but complications are more likely. Varicella-zoster immune globulin (VZIG) is of no help.

PREVENTION OF FURTHER CASES

Exposed immunosuppressed children The immunosuppressed child (see Chapter 16 for definition) should be given VZIG if known to be varicella seronegative and in close contact with a case of chickenpox or shingles. This includes children on systemic steroids and children infected with human immunodeficiency virus. If VZIG is not available, commercial normal intravenous immunoglobulin may be used (see Appendix VII).

Pregnant women (see also Chapter 3)

Exposure in early and mid-pregnancy Risk of varicella syndrome seems highest in the second trimester (2% risk) and lower in the first trimester (under 0.5% risk). It is unclear whether VZIG given following exposure will protect the fetus against varicella syndrome; however if the woman is susceptible (see next paragraph) and in the first 20 weeks of pregnancy VZIG is usually given. Infection during pregnancy is not an indication for termination of pregnancy. Herpes zoster in pregnancy seems to confer little risk to the fetus.

Exposure in late pregnancy Pregnant women exposed to varicella will usually be VZV-immune and there is almost always opportunity to test for anti-VZV before having to give VZIG. If the woman is susceptible and in the first 20 weeks of gestation or near term, then VZIG should be given. Though it may not prevent infection it will usually ameliorate the severity of infection when given up to 10 days after contact.

Exposed neonates Varicella-zoster immune globulin should be given to the newborn if the mother has developed varicella or herpes zoster in the 7 days before or after birth; VZIG should also be given to any exposed premature neonate (prior to 30 weeks or under 1 kg birth-weight) *even if the mother is immune*, because maternal antibody is poorly transferred to the preterm fetus. Intravenous acyclovir is indicated following development of lesions in the newborn and is sometimes used in the mother and in her baby prophylactically where maternal infection occurs just before delivery.

Hospital outbreaks A number of hospital occupational health departments enquire routinely about prior chicken pox in staff and test those without a history for antibody to VZV. Susceptible staff (history and anti-VZV negative) can sometimes then be excluded from contact with vulnerable patients from 8–21 days after exposure and may monitor their own condition for varicella.

Immunization A live attenuated vaccine is available on a named patient basis from Merieux (Pasteur Merieux, Clivemont House, Clivemont Road, Maidenhead, Berks SL6 7BU). The recommended regimen is two doses 3 months apart. It is thought to give at least 6 years of immunity in immunocompetent individuals. No country has yet adopted wide-scale varicella vaccination and at present immunization should only be considered for immunocompromised children and their families. As the vaccine is live, specialist advice should be sought when it is given to immunocompromised children and it may be necessary to stop immunosuppressive therapy for a time.

38

CHLAMYDIA PNEUMONIAE INFECTION

ORGANISM

Chlamydia pneumoniae is an obligate intracellular parasite. It was originally referred to as the TWAR strain and has distinct morphological and serological differences from *C. psittaci* and *C. trachomatis*.

EPIDEMIOLOGY

The disease occurs worldwide. The original isolate was made in Taiwan. Antibodies are uncommon in preschool children, the incidence rising among teenagers so that 50% of those 20–30 years old are positive. Prospective studies in young adults have suggested that up to 20% of lower respiratory tract infections are caused by this organism. Humans are thought to be the only host.

Transmission is by droplet spread from an infected individual. Incubation period is more than 10 days.

NATURAL HISTORY AND CLINICAL FEATURES

The infection is thought to be spread by droplets and the incubation period is more than 10 days. Most infections resemble those caused by *Mycoplasma pneumoniae*, with fever, cough, malaise, headache and pharyngitis. A small number of cases have resulted in respiratory failure and pleural effusion. Auscultation of the chest may identify crackles, and chest X-ray may show a patchy infiltrate restricted to only part of the lungs.

Diagnosis Culture is difficult and diagnosis is usually made on serology. Criteria for diagnosis of infection have been defined and are as follows: a fourfold rise of

IgG titre, or a single IgM titre of 1 in 16 or higher, or a single IgG titre of 1 in 512 or higher.

MANAGEMENT

Because studies have shown that the organism is slow to clear with antibiotics, long courses are recommended: doxycycline 100 mg daily in two doses for the older child for 21 days; or erythromycin for younger children, 50 mg/kg daily in four doses, for the same period.

CHLAMYDIA PSITTACI INFECTION

ORGANISM

Chlamydia psittaci is an obligate intracellular pathogen. It differs from *C. trachomatis*, in lacking glycogen in the inclusions. There are several serovars with preferences for different hosts.

EPIDEMIOLOGY

Chlamydia psittaci infection occurs worldwide. Although most cases occur in adults, children may be affected. Disease occurs among individuals, or in families exposed to infected psittacine birds (parrot family—parrots, cockatiels and budgerigars), turkeys, pigeons and ducks. Usually the birds appear unwell, with anorexia, ruffled feathers and green droppings. Outbreaks have been reported in workers in duck and turkey processing plants. The infection also occurs in some animals. The ewe abortion agent can also infect pregnant women and result in intrauterine death, premature delivery and a septicaemic illness in mother and neonate.

Incubation period is 5–21 days.

NATURAL HISTORY AND CLINICAL FEATURES

The onset of illness is abrupt with fever, cough and often severe headache. Examination of the chest reveals crackles. Chest X-ray usually shows signs of patchy infiltrates and sometimes pleural effusions. Little diagnostic help is obtained from the white blood cell count, but liver function may be abnormal.

Diagnosis A history of contact with psittacine or other birds at risk of infection is invariably a feature. If culture of *Chlamydia psittaci* is not available, the diagnosis can be confirmed by serology. A fourfold rise in complement fixating antibodies is considered diagnostic, however the test is genus-specific so that infection with *C. pneumoniae* may also produce high titres.

MANAGEMENT

Treatment is with oral erythromycin, or tetracycline in the older child. Treatment for 7–10 days is recommended.

PREVENTION OF FURTHER CASES

When pet birds die with suggestive symptoms they should be examined by a veterinary pathologist. If infection is confirmed, exposed individuals should be made aware of the most likely signs of infection (fever and respiratory symptoms). Cages used by the dead bird should be thoroughly disinfected and surveillance maintained of other exposed birds.

40

CHLAMYDIA TRACHOMATIS INFECTION

Chlamydia trachomatis ophthalmia neonatorum is notifiable

ORGANISM

Some serotypes of *Chlamydia trachomatis* (A–C) cause endemic trachoma and others (D–K) sexually transmitted infections. Serotypes L1–L3 cause lymphogranuloma venerium. It is an obligate intracellular pathogen.

EPIDEMIOLOGY

Chlamydia trachomatis is the most common cause of sexually transmitted infection in the UK. Prevalence surveys among sexually active women usually find prevalence of infection of around 4% to 8%. Prevalence tends to be higher among younger women and is usually asymptomatic. Infection is acquired during sexual intercourse or parturition. If the mother is infected, up to 50% of infants develop conjunctivitis after delivery and almost half of untreated infants with conjunctivitis will develop pneumonia. *Chlamydia trachomatis* ophthalmia is more common than that due to the gonococcus and is notifiable. Identification in the genital tract of children means the possibility of sexual abuse must be considered (Chapter 8).

NATURAL HISTORY AND CLINICAL FEATURES

A purulent neonatal conjunctivitis may develop 5–14 days after birth and cannot be distinguished on clinical appearances from gonococcal or other infections. Inadequate treatment may result in recurrence and, rarely, in corneal scarring. Pneumonia may develop 4–6 weeks after birth and is associated with poor feeding, a cough and tachypnoea. The chest X-ray shows hyperinflation and generalized patchy shadowing. Pneumonia, although requiring treatment, is often self-limiting, but the outcome may be more serious in the preterm infant with coexistent chronic lung disease (bronchopulmonary dysplasia). Infection in the adolescent may lead to non-specific or non-gonococcal urethritis (NSU, NGU) and, in the female, salpingitis, pelvic inflammatory disease and possible infertility.

Diagnosis A Gram stain on the exudate should be performed quickly in all cases of purulent conjunctivitis, to exclude gonococcal infection. Because *Chlamydia trachomatis* is an intracellular bacterium the specimen should include cells from the conjunctivae collected by firmly drawing a cotton-wool swab over the everted lower eyelid. Rapid diagnostic tests using monoclonal antibodies have been introduced and allow diagnosis of *C. trachomatis* from a smear on a microscopic slide. An enzyme-linked immunosorbent assay (ELISA) is also available. All these tests, but particularly the ELISA, may yield false positive results and for this reason the definitive tissue culture test should be performed when there is a suspicion of sexually transmitted disease in children, following sexual abuse. The rapid diagnostic tests may be too insensitive to detect organisms in nasopharyngeal or tracheal aspirate for diagnosis of pneumonia, but are recommended for use in conjunctivitis.

MANAGEMENT

A topical eye preparation (e.g. tetracycline) is used in combination with oral erythromycin in treatment of chlamydial ophthalmia. Erythromycin must be given to reduce the risk of recurring conjunctivitis when the topical preparation is discontinued, and to prevent development of pneumonia. Erythromycin is used for treatment of pneumonia (for dose see Appendix III) and there is good evidence that it can be used alone in management of ophthalmia. Children with genital infections should be treated with erythromycin, and adolescents with tetracycline. Parents of infants with neonatal ophthalmia should be investigated and treated in a genitourinary medicine clinic.

PREVENTION OF FURTHER CASES

There is a strong case for screening all women receiving antenatal care for *C. trachomatis* and for screening sexually active adolescent girls. All those testing positive (and their sexual partners) should receive treatment. Prophylactic topical eye treatments given at birth will not reliably prevent development of ophthalmia neonatorum due to *C. trachomatis.*

CHOLERA

Notifiable disease

ORGANISM

Widespread epidemic disease is associated with *Vibrio cholerae* serogroup O1, a Gram-negative, motile, rod-like bacterium. There are two biotypes, *cholerae* and El Tor; the latter dominated the seventh pandemic. These were joined in 1992 by a new and distinct epidemic strain, *V. cholerae* 0139. Other species (for example *V. parahaemolyticus*) may cause severe diarrhoea.

EPIDEMIOLOGY

Humans are a reservoir of infection, as are algae and plankton. Since 1961 the 'seventh pandemic' of cholera spread from south Asia to south-east Asia, Africa, the Middle East, some parts of southern Europe and finally (in 1991) South America. In 1993 a total of 376 845 cases were reported to the World Health Organization from 78 countries, including 6781 deaths with a global case fatality ratio of 1.8%. In the first ten months of 1994 a further 2339 cases were reported in Europe, including 47 deaths. Those cases occurring in western Europe were almost all imported following infection elsewhere. Endemic infection has been reported in parts of Eastern Europe and former USSR. In 1992 an outbreak of cholera due to *V. cholerae* serogroup 0139 appeared in south Asia and spread rapidly. Some authorities are characterizing this as the start of the eighth pandemic. Disease tends to be milder in children and is especially severe in young adult males.

Transmission *Vibrio cholerae* is particularly suited to survival in aquatic environments, and transmission from infected person is through contaminated water and food. Shellfish are important vehicles of transmission and a particular hazard arises from use of waste water or sewage to irrigate vegetables. With modern sanitation, widespread transmission is uncommon in industrialized countries and in areas of developing countries with reasonable sanitation.

Epidemics typically follow natural disasters where there is contamination of food and water and a breakdown of hygiene and sanitation.

Incubation period is usually 1–3 days with a range of a few hours to 5 days. The greater the infective dose ingested, the shorter the incubation period and the more severe the disease.

Period of infectivity is highly variable; a carrier state may last several months or longer. Antibiotics such as co-trimoxazole can shorten the period.

NATURAL HISTORY AND CLINICAL FEATURES

Asymptomatic infection is more common than disease, but cholera is unique among diarrhoeal diseases in its rapidity of onset and its very high mortality rate. Illness is caused by an enterotoxin consisting of two subunits: A (the toxin itself) and B (a carrier). It works on cyclic AMP-dependent secretion and absorption. Its action is characterized by rapid onset of severe diarrhoea followed by vomiting. Profuse, frequent and sometimes painless bowel evacuations accelerate severe dehydration. Shock and collapse may occur, and hypoglycaemia and convulsions are particularly common in children. 'Rice-water diarrhoea' describes the stools, which are typically colourless and contain flecks of mucus. Complications of delayed treatment are hypovolaemic shock, uncompensated metabolic acidosis and renal failure. Untreated, the mortality is up to 50%, but with proper management it should be less than 1%.

Diagnosis In endemic areas, especially during epidemics, there is no difficulty in diagnosis, but sporadic cases will require differentiation from other forms of severe diarrhoea. Diagnosis can be made by microscopic examination of the stool. Culture on bile-salt agar will produce characteristic colonies in 24 hours. The organism can be typed from culture colonies by agglutination with specific antisera. This is rarely done routinely on diarrhoea specimens. Specific antibody titres can also be measured and a rise in titre used for diagnosis.

MANAGEMENT

The most important aspect of treatment is the restoration of plasma volume and electrolyte balance. In most cases this can be achieved using oral rehydration solution (ORS) which promotes absorption via cyclic AMP-independent mechanisms. The introduction of ORS has resulted in a dramatic decrease in mortality in many countries. Antibiotics are used for eradication of *Vibrio cholerae* from the gastrointestinal tract. Co-trimoxazole should be given to children under 9 years of age, and tetracycline to older children. The infected child needs to be barrier nursed during the acute phase, and special care taken with handling of stools (see Table 26.1) until demonstrated to be non-infectious. Stools of close contacts should be cultured and carriers should be given antibiotics (treatment dose). Attempts must be made to identify the source of infection and appropriate control measures taken. Persons with confirmed cholera (and their close contacts) and at higher risk of causing further transmission (Chapter 27) should be excluded from school or work until three consecutive faecal specimens are negative.

PREVENTION OF FURTHER CASES

Prevention is achieved by good standards of hygiene and a clean water supply. The currently available parenteral vaccine confers only limited protection (estimated at 50%) for a few months and has no role in disease control. No country officially requires certification for visitors; however, it may occasionally be demanded by officials at some border crossing-points in developing countries. Oral vaccines are under development. They are based on the non-toxic B subunit of the toxin and have been shown to be safe and efficacious, at least in the short term, in clinical trials.

CONJUNCTIVITIS

Ophthalmia neonatorum is notifiable*

ORGANISMS

Causative organisms are *Chlamydia trachomatis*, serotypes D to K; *Neisseria gonorrhoeae*; other bacteria such as *Haemophilus influenzae* and *Streptococcus pneumoniae* (*Staphylococcus aureus* and *Pseudomonas aeruginosa* in neonates); adenoviruses, especially types 3, 4 and 7; picornaviruses, especially enterovirus 70 and coxsackievirus A24; and herpes simplex virus.

EPIDEMIOLOGY

All these organisms are found worldwide. About 35–50% of neonates will acquire chlamydial eye infection when delivered through an infected cervix. One in 300 people with a genital infection develops eye disease. Chlamydial conjunctivitis can also occur in the sexually inactive. Gonococcal conjunctivitis is also acquired at birth. Other bacterial conjunctivitis most often affects preschool children. It is common especially in warmer climates and may be epidemic. Viral conjunctivitis may be sporadic or occur in epidemics. Enteroviral acute haemorrhagic conjunctivitis (AHC) occurs mainly in the tropics but also in some European countries and in people coming from areas with AHC outbreaks. Adenoviral conjunctivitis often occurs as summer epidemics.

Transmission The spread of non-gonococcal bacterial conjunctivitis is by infected material, either directly or on objects such as make-up, clothing and multiple-dose dispensers of eye-drops or ointment. Viral conjunctivitis is spread by direct or indirect contact with infected material from a discharging eye. Transmission within a household is common. Adenoviral disease has been associated with the use of poorly chlorinated swimming pools.

Incubation period *Chlamydia trachomatis*, 5–12 days; *Neisseria gonorrhoeae*, 1–5 days; other bacterial infections, usually 1–3 days; adenovirus, 4–12 days; picornavirus, 12 hours to 3 days.

NATURAL HISTORY AND CLINICAL FEATURES

For gonococcal and chlamydial conjunctivitis, see Chapters 40 and 50. Non-gonococcal bacterial conjunctivitis presents with irritation and redness of the conjunctiva, followed by oedema of the lids, photophobia and mucopurulent discharge. The severity varies from minor hyperaemia and a slight discharge to

***Ophthalmia neonatorum is defined as a purulent discharge from the eye of an infant within 21 days of birth.**

ecchymoses and infiltration of the cornea. Adenoviral conjunctivitis usually presents with lymphoid follicles and often small subconjunctival haemorrhages. It usually lasts 7–15 days and may be accompanied by upper respiratory illness (pharyngoconjunctival fever). The onset of AHC is sudden with redness, pain and swelling, frequently in both eyes. The inflammation subsides over the next 4–6 days, but petechiae appear on the conjunctivae. These enlarge and coalesce to produce subconjunctival haemorrhages, which resolve over the next week or two. Some outbreaks have been associated with polio-like paralysis starting anything from a few days to a month after the conjunctivitis. Often there is some residual paralysis.

Diagnosis It is important to exclude gonococcal and chlamydial conjunctivitis (see Chapters 40 and 50). Bacterial cultures should be taken before antibiotics are started.

MANAGEMENT

For gonococcal and chlamydial conjunctivitis, see Chapters 40 and 50. If a bacterial aetiology is suspected, topical neomycin or chloramphenicol is first-line treatment. Neomycin is to be preferred in the neonatal period because, unlike chloramphenicol, it will not mask a chlamydial infection. Ointment is often better than drops, especially in young children, as it can be difficult to administer drops reliably. Both eyes should be treated, as the infection, even if initially unilateral, often spreads from one eye to the other. Different dispensers should be used for each eye to prevent cross-infection.

PREVENTION OF FURTHER CASES

Strict attention to hygiene may prevent the transmission of non-gonococcal bacterial conjunctivitis and viral conjunctivitis. Swimming pools should be properly chlorinated.

43 CRYPTOSPORIDIOSIS

ORGANISM

Cryptosporidium parvum is a protozoan parasite. Infected individuals excrete large numbers of thick-walled oocysts which can persist in the environment.

EPIDEMIOLOGY

Cryptosporidia can be found worldwide in a variety of hosts including humans, domestic animals and pets. Prevalence of infection in humans is higher in developing countries. Both children and adults are affected, though cases in children less than 1 year old are unusual. Outbreaks occur in child-care centres, and major outbreaks through contamination of water supplies have been increasingly recognized. Numbers of reports of cryptosporidium have increased in England and Wales since the 1980s (see Appendix I, Figure 2).

Transmission may be faecal–oral, person-to-person or animal-to-person, or through contamination of water supplies. The infective dose is as low as one oocyst.

Incubation period is not clearly known—a likely range is 2–14 days with an average of 7 days.

NATURAL HISTORY AND CLINICAL FEATURES

The parasite invades epithelial cells in the intestine and then produces oocysts which are infectious and excreted. Infection rarely produces a severe illness in immunocompetent children in whom the most common signs are watery diarrhoea, low-grade fever, abdominal pain, anorexia and mild weight loss. Asymptomatic infections occur. Symptoms frequently wax and wane. The infection is usually self-limiting, lasting 10 days on average (maximum 3 weeks). Persistent infection leading to failure to thrive may occur in those with severe immunosuppression such as acquired immune deficiency syndrome.

Diagnosis relies on microscopic examination of stool specimens for oocysts. These are small bodies, and false positive and negative results occur such that repeated specimens and specialist assistance may be required.

MANAGEMENT

Treatment in the immunocompetent child is usually symptomatic, with rehydration therapy as required. In an immunocompromised child (e.g. a child with human immunodeficiency virus infection), specialist opinion should be sought. There is no effective anticryptosporidial agent. Although spiramycin and erythromycin may suppress the symptoms, they are not curative.

PREVENTION OF FURTHER CASES

Enteric precautions should be applied for persons excreting oocysts. Those at higher risk of causing further transmission (Chapter 27) do not need to be excluded from school or work once symptoms have subsided. Water supplies must be well maintained and protected against environmental contamination. Some clinicians suggest immunocompromised patients should only take water-based drinks, using domestic water that has been treated (e.g. by heating to 50 °C for 5 minutes).

CYTOMEGALOVIRUS INFECTION

44

ORGANISM

Cytomegalovirus (CMV), also known as human herpesvirus 5 (HHV-5), is an enveloped DNA virus.

EPIDEMIOLOGY

Serological studies show that approximately 50% of women of child-bearing age are seropositive. Congenital infection occurs in about 3 per 1000 newborn infants in the UK. Most cases result from primary rather than reactivated or secondary infection during pregnancy. Infection in the infant may be acquired later, either at delivery or after birth. Cytomegalovirus is one of the most common causes of congenital hearing loss in the UK, with an estimated 200 cases per year.

Transmission Cytomegalovirus can be cultured or identified in a number of body fluids. Congenital infections are thought to occur via transplacental blood-stream spread at any stage of pregnancy, with acquired infection in the newborn resulting from contamination by cervical secretions. The virus is present in the white blood cells of seropositive individuals and transfusion of CMV-infected blood to preterm infants results in a systemic illness with pneumonia and hepatitis. Transmission may also occur through breast milk. Most transmission in children is thought to be through saliva. Urinary spread may also be a factor, but is less important even in a nursery setting. The agent is transmitted sexually and can be identified in semen and cervical secretions. Organ transplantation is also a source of infection. Immunosuppressed individuals may experience a reactivation of latent CMV infection.

Incubation period is unknown for person-to-person spread. The incubation period for transmission during blood transfusion or transplantation is 1–4 months.

NATURAL HISTORY AND CLINICAL FEATURES

Congenital and acquired infection in the newborn Three to five per cent of infants with congenital infection develop cytomegalic inclusion disease (CID) with features which include petechiae from thrombocytopenia, hepatitis, chorioretinitis, intracranial calcification and microcephaly. Survivors may develop cerebral palsy. Sensorineural deafness alone may occur in up to 10% of infants with congenital infection. Excretion of virus may persist for many years.

Acquired infection in the child Children at risk are those immunosuppressed with symptomatic human immunodeficiency virus (HIV) infection or following bone marrow and organ transplantation. They can develop disseminated disease, with pneumonia, hepatitis and retinitis. Mortality rates of up to 10% have been reported following CMV infection in this group.

Diagnosis is difficult. To make a diagnosis of congenital infection, specimens have to be taken for culture within 3 weeks of birth. Such evidence of infection is supported by a positive IgM anti-CMV antibody. Virus can be isolated in tissue culture from a number of sources, including throat swabs, urine, breast milk, semen, cervical secretion and peripheral blood leucocytes. Although routine tissue culture is usually slow to produce results, neonatal isolates grow quickly and more rapid identification is obtained by a short period of culture following a specific immunofluorescence test. This is particularly useful when treatment is being considered in asymptomatic children with acquired CMV.

MANAGEMENT

There is no evidence that any antiviral agents alter the course of the disease in congenital infection. Ganciclovir, an acyclic nucleoside related to acyclovir, has been shown to eradicate CMV excretion for a short period following treatment of an infant with congenital infection. Case reports describe the successful use of ganciclovir in acquired neonatal infection when used in a dose of 5 mg/kg twice daily for 14 days. Ganciclovir has been used with success in both the prevention and treatment of CMV infection following bone marrow and organ transplantation. The dose used has been 5 mg/kg twice daily, and it is recommended that CMV immune globulin is used at the same time. The main side-effect of ganciclovir is a neutropenia. Foscarnet is the treatment of choice in CMV retinitis and acquired immune deficiency syndrome.

PREVENTION OF FURTHER CASES

Children with congenital CMV infection excrete virus. The importance of hand-washing for staff looking after such children should be stressed. CMV negative blood products should be used in immunocompromised children not previously exposed. A vaccine is unlikely to be available for some time.

DERMATOPHYTOSES: TINEA CAPITIS, CORPORIS, PEDIS AND UNGUIUM

TINEA CAPITIS (scalp ringworm)

ORGANISM

Fungi from the genera *Trichophyton* and *Microsporum* are responsible.

EPIDEMIOLOGY

The disease is found worldwide. It can affect some animal species as well as humans. All ages can be infected. Recently increasing numbers of cases due to *Trichophyton tonsurans* have been seen in the UK.

Transmission Direct contact with infected humans, animals or fomites. Spread may occur via combs, hairbrushes, hats, etc. on which the organism may remain viable for long periods.

Incubation period is 10–14 days.

NATURAL HISTORY AND CLINICAL FEATURES

The lesions often start as small papules which spread outwards leaving scaly areas of hair loss. The remaining hairs are brittle, leaving short stubs when broken. Other presentations are possible—pustules with little scaling or hair loss, or areas of scaling like dandruff with varying degrees of hair loss. The lesions may progress to form a raised, boggy area known as a kerion. Confusion can arise with other conditions such as impetigo, dandruff, seborrhoeic dermatitis, psoriasis, trichotillomania, folliculitis, alopecia areata and, rarely, lupus erythematosus. Reinfection is uncommon.

Diagnosis *Microsporum* spp. will fluoresce under ultraviolet light (Wood's lamp). This is not true for *Trichophyton* spp. and so lack of fluorescence cannot be used to exclude the diagnosis. Scrapings taken from the outer margin of a lesion should be sent to the laboratory on dark paper. There they will be treated with 10% potassium hydroxide and examined for fungal filaments. Culture on Sabouraud's medium provides the definitive diagnosis, and can be important.

MANAGEMENT

Oral griseofulvin (10 mg/kg daily) should be given for 6 weeks; this treatment may fail. An alternative if this occurs is terbinafine 125 mg daily for 2–4 weeks, although specialist opinion should be sought as this drug is not usually recommended for children. Topical antifungal agents have no role.

PREVENTION OF FURTHER CASES

All members of the household, including pets such as cats and dogs, should be examined and treated if infected. Combs, brushes, pillows and hats should not be shared.

TINEA CORPORIS (ringworm of the body)

ORGANISM

Fungi from the genera *Trichophyton* (in particular *T. rubrum* and *T. mentagrophytes*), *Microsporum* (in particular *M. canis*) and *Epidermophyton floccosum*.

EPIDEMIOLOGY

The disease is found worldwide. It can affect some animal species as well as humans. All ages can be infected.

Transmission is by direct contact with infected humans, animals or fomites.

Incubation period is not known for certain, but thought to be 4–10 days.

NATURAL HISTORY AND CLINICAL FEATURES

The typical lesion is found on the hairless parts of the face, trunk and limbs. The groins, hands and feet are spared. The typical lesion is round with a red, scaly border. The border tends to expand slowly outwards leaving a pale centre, often of normal skin. Topical corticosteroid treatment can alter this characteristic appearance. The lesions are usually pruritic.

Diagnosis can often be made clinically but should usually be confirmed microbiologically. Scrapings should be collected for microscopy (see tinea capitis).

MANAGEMENT

Topical preparations alone are often ineffective in the long term. Griseofulvin for 6 weeks should be combined with a topical antifungal agent such as clotrimazole, ketoconazole or miconazole for 2 weeks. When the fungus is resistant to griseofulvin, oral ketoconazole should be used instead.

PREVENTION OF FURTHER CASES

The lesions should be covered. All infected members of the family, and any infected pets, must be treated at the same time.

TINEA PEDIS (athlete's foot)

ORGANISM

Fungi from the genus *Trichophyton* (in particular *T. rubrum* and *T. mentagrophytes*) and *Epidermophyton floccosum*.

EPIDEMIOLOGY

Tinea pedis occurs worldwide, affecting adults more frequently than children and men more commonly than women. It is more common in summer.

Transmission is from infected skin scales, by direct contact with an infected person or from places on which an infected person has shed scales, e.g. changing rooms, swimming pools and bath mats.

Incubation period is unknown.

NATURAL HISTORY AND CLINICAL FEATURES

The typical appearance is of scaling and cracking of the skin of the feet, especially between the toes. It is usually pruritic. Occasionally there may be a hypersensitivity reaction with vesicular lesions on the palms of the hands and sides of the fingers.

Diagnosis is usually on the basis of the appearance of the lesions. The diagnosis can be confirmed by taking skin scrapings (see tinea capitis).

MANAGEMENT

Topical treatment with an antifungal such as clotrimazole, ketoconazole or miconazole for 2 weeks.

PREVENTION OF FURTHER CASES

Good hygiene is necessary in communal places where feet may be uncovered.

TINEA UNGUIUM (nail ringworm)

ORGANISM

Fungi from the genus *Trichophyton*, *Epidermophyton floccosum*, and rarely *Microsporum* spp.

EPIDEMIOLOGY

The fungi are found worldwide, but the only important reservoir is in humans.

Transmission is thought to be predominantly by direct contact with infected skin or nails. It is not very contagious and spread within families is low.

Incubation period is unknown.

NATURAL HISTORY AND CLINICAL FEATURES

The nail becomes thickened, brittle and discoloured. White caseous material may collect under the nail, which in turn may disintegrate.

Diagnosis must be made by examination of scrapings (see tinea capitis).

MANAGEMENT

Oral griseofulvin should be given until the nail has grown out. Topical antifungal agents have no role.

PREVENTION OF FURTHER CASES

No special measures are necessary as the condition is not very contagious.

DIPHTHERIA

Notifiable disease

ORGANISM

Corynebacterium diphtheriae is a Gram-positive bacterium. There are three biotypes (colony types): gravis, mitis and intermedius. Strains may be toxigenic or non-toxigenic depending on the presence of the *tox*+ gene which is thought to be transmitted by a bacteriophage. Toxigenic strains are considered to have some selective advantage in non-immune populations. A diphtheria-like illness is also occasionally caused by toxin-producing *Corynebacterium ulcerans*.

EPIDEMIOLOGY

Humans are the only source of infection of *C. diphtheriae*. *Corynebacterium ulcerans* is a zoonosis associated with cattle and goats, and infections in humans are usually (but not always) associated with the consumption of unpasteurized milk. There are two major sites of infection, the upper respiratory tract and the skin—cutaneous diphtheria. Diphtheria is now rare in most industrialized countries because of routine immunization (see Appendix I, Figure 1). It still causes considerable morbidity and mortality in the developing countries where much of the circulating infection is through cutaneous diphtheria, and an important source of strains in the UK, toxigenic or otherwise, is from the Indian subcontinent. There has recently been a resurgence in what was the USSR and adjoining parts of eastern Europe, seemingly because of breakdown in immunization programmes, large numbers of susceptible adults and increased mixing of populations. In 1994 there were 47802 cases in the Russian Federation and other newly independent states of the former USSR. Imported cases in western Europe and the USA are uncommon but include both throat and cutaneous diphtheria.

Transmission Human beings are the only known reservoir of *Corynebacterium diphtheriae*, which is spread by droplet infection from nose and throat secretions. Cutaneous diphtheria spreads from direct contact through fomites. Untreated patients with pharyngeal diphtheria are considered infectious for 2–3 weeks. Correct antibiotic treatment usually renders the patient non-infectious in 24 hours.

Incubation period is usually 2–5 days but can be longer.

NATURAL HISTORY AND CLINICAL FEATURES

The disease is clinically classified according to the anatomical site of infection: pharyngeal, laryngeal, nasal or cutaneous. In pharyngeal, laryngeal and nasal diphtheria disease usually involves cervical lymphadenopathy and the development of a membranous nasopharyngitis or laryngotracheitis. Onset is often insidious with a low-grade fever for 1–2 days and perhaps a sore throat. The membrane may be classical, grey/white, thick and spreading and firmly adherent to the throat, where it may cause respiratory obstruction (diphtheritic croup). However, it may be more focal on one tonsil or deeper in the larynx causing stridor, while nasal diphtheria will manifest itself as a serous and then serosanguineous nasal discharge. Because of these atypical presentations and the severity of the illness, a high degree of suspicion should be maintained if a patient has travelled to an endemic area or has been in close contact with a case. The bacterium releases a powerful exotoxin that causes local tissue necrosis and attacks the myocardium of the heart and motor nerves—notably of the soft palate, eyes and diaphragm. The course of the illness depends on the severity of the toxaemia and the degree of immunity conferred by previous immunization. Milder infections in the partially immune may lead to uneventful recovery with the membrane sloughing off in 6–7 days. Severe infections occur in the unimmunized, and (untreated) are characterized by increasing toxaemia. Cardiac symptoms appear in the second week and neurological features after 2–6 weeks. These may progress to cardiovascular collapse, stupor, coma and death. Case fatality rates are 5–10%.

Diagnosis Although diphtheria is a rare condition in the UK, cases still occur and the diagnosis must be considered in any membranous condition of the throat, especially in children recently arrived from abroad, or their unimmunized contacts, and in those of doubtful immune status. Cultures should be taken from the nose and throat or from any site which may be contaminated (e.g. weeping skin ulcers). If possible, the swab should be taken from under the membrane. The laboratory should be consulted in advance as special media will be used to accelerate growth and thus identification of the organism. Most isolates of *Corynebacterium* *diphtheriae* from the upper respiratory tract or skin in the UK are non-toxigenic, including those associated with time spent abroad. It is often the case that *C. diphtheria* is isolated but it is unclear whether a toxigenic strain is involved and whether control measures should be employed. The rapid identification of toxigenic strains is possible by the use of methods such as polymerase chain reaction (PCR).* A serum sample should also be obtained for measurement of antibodies to toxin.

MANAGEMENT

Individual management consists of counteracting the effects of the toxin and treating the infection to eliminate the organism and prevent transmission. Patients should be isolated and the antitoxin administered immediately the diagnosis is suspected. The dose is calculated according to the size of the membrane, the degree of toxicity and the duration of illness. A diluted test dose must be given first intradermally. If the test is negative, antitoxin may be given intramuscularly or intravenously depending on the volume required and the severity of illness. If the patient is hypersensitive then expert advice must be sought to discuss the possibility of attempting desensitization. Dosages of antitoxin that have been recommended are as follows:†

- Nasal diphtheria: 10 000–20 000 units IM.
- Tonsillar diphtheria: 15 000–25 000 units IM or IV.
- Pharyngeal or laryngeal diphtheria: 20 000–40 000 units IM or IV.
- Combined or delayed diagnosis: 40 000–60 000 units IV.

Antitoxin is not generally considered useful for cutaneous diphtheria, though wounds should be cleaned with soap and water and antibiotic treatment given. Penicillin (penicillin G, 100 000 to 150 000 U/kg daily in four divided doses for 14 days) is the treatment of choice and should be given intravenously or intramuscularly. An alternative is parenteral erythromycin (40–50 mg/kg to a maximum of 2 g daily for 14 days). Treatment with parenteral therapy should be continued until the child can swallow again, at which point treatment can change to oral medication.

PREVENTION OF FURTHER CASES

Once it is clear that a toxigenic strain is involved (see above) or is very likely, specialist advice is essential and public health measures must be instituted with urgency. The consultant in communicable disease control (or director of public health) and the Communicable Disease Surveillance Centre or the Scottish Centre for Infection and Environmental Health must be contacted. Close contacts (defined as household members, regular household visitors, kissing contacts, classroom contacts and health-care staff exposed to oropharyngeal secretions), whether immunized or not, must have throat swabs (carriage may be up to 25%)

***In England and Wales isolates can be rapidly tested by the Diphtheria Reference Unit at the Central Public Health Laboratory which maintains a 24-hour service (telephone 0181-200-4400).**

†Other dosage regimens are also suggested. In England and Wales diphtheria antitoxin is available from the Immunization Division at the Communicable Disease Surveillance Centre, and in Scotland a small stock is held at the Glasgow Royal Infirmary.

and given a 7-day course of penicillin or oral erythromycin irrespective of the swab result or vaccine history. Carriers should have a second swab to ensure clearance. Patients with cutaneous diphtheria should have the lesion covered and be isolated. Contacts previously immunized should receive a booster dose of monovalent diphtheria vaccine or tetanus/diphtheria (as appropriate for age and previous immunizations) if they have not received a diphtheria-containing vaccine in the previous 12 months. A low dose diphtheria vaccine is available for persons 10 years or older.

IMMUNIZATION

Diphtheria immunization, using a toxoid based vaccine, has been routinely available in the UK for about 50 years. In the UK it is given at 2, 3 and 4 months of age with tetanus and pertussis (the 'triple' vaccine) and before starting school with tetanus (the 'preschool booster'). Since the end of 1994 diphtheria vaccine has also been given with tetanus (Td) before leaving secondary school and may also be given as part of antitetanus prophylaxis for wounds or burns. The strength of this diphtheria toxoid is much less than that given to children below 10 years old as the strength used in young children is reactogenic in older children and adults. A monovalent vaccine is available for children up to age 9 years and a low-dose single antigen diphtheria vaccine for children of 10 years and older and adults. If the latter is not available and it is possible to give one-fifth (0.1 ml) of the monovalent diphtheria vaccine for children (under 10 years) in adults and in children 10 years or older. This must be done on a named patient basis. Contraindications to the vaccine are few and adverse events rare.

FURTHER READING

Begg N (1994) *Diphtheria: Manual for the Management and Control of Diphtheria in the European Region*. The expanded programme on Immunization in the European Region of WHO. Available from the PHLS Communicable Disease Surveillance Centre.

Efstratiou A & Maple PAC (1994) *Diphtherai: Laboratory diagnosis of diphtheria*. The expanded programme on immunization in the European Region of WHO. Available as above.

47

ENTEROVIRUS INFECTION

This chapter excludes poliovirus, which is discussed in Chapter 79.

ORGANISM

Enteroviruses are genera within the family Picornaviridae, which are small, non-enveloped RNA viruses in four major groups:

- Coxsackieviruses—two sub-groups A and B.
- Echoviruses.
- Enteroviruses.
- Heparnaviruses (includes hepatitis A virus, see Chapter 55).

EPIDEMIOLOGY

Enteroviruses are found worldwide with infection rates highest in younger children. Epidemics of particular virus types occur, most notably in the autumn in the northern hemisphere. These are more frequent in institutional settings such as day-care centres for the under-fives and primary schools. Enteroviruses can persist in a watery environment if the temperature remains low, pH is neutral and there is sufficient organic material. Recreational or occupational exposure to contaminated water may result in infection.

Transmission is by the faecal–oral and respiratory routes. Infectivity is high in the acute phase of illness and may be prolonged, since virus may be present in the faeces for up to 2 months.

Incubation period is variable—considered usually to be between 2 hours and 6 days.

NATURAL HISTORY AND CLINICAL FEATURES

Infection is usually asymptomatic (60–70% of echovirus infections and 40–50% of coxsackievirus infections). A range of clinical conditions can result from infection with these viruses. Although certain viruses tend to be associated with particular syndromes there is considerable overlap:

- Viral (aseptic) meningitis and encephalitis: echovirus 3–7; coxsackievirus A9, B1–5; enterovirus 71.
- Conjunctivitis: coxsackievirus A25; enterovirus 70.
- Hand, foot and mouth disease (see Chapter 53): coxsackievirus A5, A16; enterovirus 71.
- Myocarditis, pericarditis: coxsackievirus B1–5.
- Exanthems: echovirus 7, 9, 16; coxsackievirus A4.
- Enanthems: echovirus 3, 6, 9, 16, 17; coxsackievirus A1, A3; B1–5.
- Pleurodynia (Bornholm disease): coxsackievirus B1–6.
- Upper respiratory tract disease: echovirus 1, 3, 4, 20, 22; coxsackievirus B.
- Lower respiratory tract disease: echovirus 9; coxsackievirus B1, B4).
- Neonatal infections: echovirus 9, 11, 14; coxsackievirus B1–5.

Each condition can be caused by a number of viruses, including others outside this group—respiratory conditions are more commonly caused by rhinoviruses, and mumps, polio, herpes and varicella viruses and arboviruses also cause aseptic meningitis. Hence, there is a wide clinical range of signs and symptoms that can result from these viruses. While most infections are self-limiting, some may require substantial supportive therapy.

Diagnosis of one of these viral infections is useful to exclude other causes which may be more serious. Specimens for viral culture should be taken using throat swabs and stools, which are placed in viral culture medium; it must be borne in mind, however, that viral isolation may represent asymptomatic infection, particularly during epidemics. If illness is severe specimens should also be taken from cerebrospinal fluid and blood, if samples are being taken. It is worthwhile setting serum aside and taking a convalescent specimen later to check for a rising titre.

MANAGEMENT

Management is usually supportive. Intravenous immunoglobulin may be of benefit in neonatal outbreaks of echovirus infection.

PREVENTION OF FURTHER CASES

Enteric precautions are obligatory during hospitalization and in institutional outbreaks (Chapters 26 and 27).

48

ESCHERICHIA COLI DIARRHOEA

This chapter deals only with those strains of *Escherichia coli* that cause diarrhoea. Details of meningitis and septicaemia in neonates and of urinary tract infection due to *E. coli* are to be found in Chapters 2 and 7 respectively. There is a separate chapter on the haemolytic uraemic syndrome (Chapter 51).

ORGANISM

Escherichia coli is a Gram-negative, motile bacillus. Strains can be differentiated for epidemiological purposes on the basis of O-antigens (on lipopolysaccharide on the bacterial surface), H antigens (on the flagellae used to propel the bacterium) or K antigens (on the capsule). Although these antigens were used originally to define *E. coli* that caused diarrhoea (all were termed enteropathogenic *E. coli*), serogrouping is not a useful method except when an epidemic occurs. Currently five different mechanisms of pathogenicity have been described. The strains are thus described as enteropathogenic (EPEC), enterotoxigenic (ETEC), enteroinvasive (EIEC), enterohaemorrhagic (EHEC) and enteroaggregative (EAggEC) *E. coli*. (Table 48.1)

EPIDEMIOLOGY AND CLINICAL FEATURES

Enterotoxigenic *E. coli* produces a non-inflammatory (secretory) small bowel diarrhoea. These bacteria produce one or both of heat-labile toxin (LT, similar to cholera toxin) and heat-stable toxin (ST), which have secretory and antiabsorptive effects on the enterocytes. They are a major cause of infantile diarrhoea in developing countries (up to three episodes per child per year) and of travellers' diarrhoea (60–70% of cases). The incubation period is 24–48 hours, followed by anorexia, vomiting, abdominal cramps and voluminous, watery diarrhoea with a frequency of up to ten times per day. The infection is self-limiting and usually resolves in 1–5 days. In malnourished children it may be more prolonged (up to 3 weeks). Dehydration occurs in up to 46% of adults and 16% of children.

Enteroinvasive *E. coli* produces an inflammatory large bowel diarrhoea. The pathogenesis is identical to that of shigellae. These bacteria invade and kill colonic enterocytes. They are responsible for up to 4% of cases of diarrhoeal disease in children in developing countries but are rarely found in babies under 1 year old. They may also be a cause of travellers' diarrhoea. After an incubation period of 2–4 days patients develop fever, abdominal pain and dysentery characterized by frequent but scanty stools with blood and mucus. The illness is less severe than that due to *shigellae*.

Enteropathogenic *E. coli* produces a non-inflammatory (osmotic) small bowel diarrhoea. These bacteria adhere intimately to the enterocyte brush border and cause loss of the microvilli (attaching effacement). This results in a loss of absorptive area and of the brush border disaccharidase enzymes. Enteropathogenic *E. coli* is rarely encountered in developed countries but are a major cause of

Table 48.1 Characteristics of *Escherichia coli* types

Type of *E. coli*	Epidemiology	Mechanism of action	Clinical features	Transmission	Incubation period	Period of infectivity
Enteropathogenic (EPEC)	Acute and chronic endemic and epidemic diarrhoea in infants and neonates	Adherence, effacement	Watery diarrhoea	Contaminated infant formula and weaning foods. Nosocomial infection	9–12 hours in adults	While organism is being excreted. May be prolonged
Enterotoxigenic (ETEC)	Infantile diarrhoea in developing countries and travellers' diarrhoea	Adherence, enterotoxin production	Watery diarrhoea and abdominal pain	Contaminated fo0od, especially weaning foods, and less commonly water	10–12 hours in adults	While organism is being excreted. May be prolonged
Enteroinvasive (EIEC)	Diarrhoea with fever at all ages	Adherence, invasion of mucosa. Similar to *Shigella*	Fever, often bloody diarrhoea, vomiting, abdominal pain and tenesmus	?Contaminated food	About 18 hours	While organism is being excreted
Enterohaemorrhagic (EHEC)	Haemorrhagic colitis and HUS in all ages and thrombocytopenic purpura in adults	Cytotoxin production, adherence, effacement	Non-bloody diarrhoea progressing to bloody diarrhoea and abdominal pain. Fever in one-third.	Contaminated food including hamburgers and milk	12–60 hours	While organism is being excreted; short period
Enteroaggregative (EAggEC)	Incompletely defined	Adherence, ? toxin	Bloody chronic diarrhoea	Food and water	Not known	While organism is being excreted; long period

Key: HUS, haemolytic uraemic syndrome.

infantile and neonatal gastroenteritis in developing countries. The incubation period varies from 8 hours to 60 hours, after which there is a profuse, watery diarrhoea, fever and dehydration. Infection can be prolonged, with relapses over a period of weeks.

Enterohaemorrhagic *E. coli* produces an inflammatory large bowel diarrhoea (haemorrhagic colitis). The bacteria produce attaching effacement on the distal ileum and colon and release one or both of verocytotoxin 1 and 2. These toxins inhibit protein synthesis and kill the enterocytes. In some cases the toxins enter the blood stream and result in haemolytic uraemic syndrome (see Chapter 51). The EHEC (also called verotoxin-producing *E. coli* or VTEC) can be part of the normal intestinal flora of cattle and pigs, and are transmitted via undercooked meat or unpasteurized milk. Outbreaks of infection due to serotypes 0157:H7, 026:H11 and 0111:H8 have been described, for example linked to undercooked beefburgers. After an incubation period of 3–4 days, the patient experiences abdominal cramps and a watery diarrhoea followed rapidly by haemorrhagic diarrhoea containing frank blood. The patient is rarely febrile and diarrhoea lasts for 5–7 days.

Enteroaggregative *E. coli* produces a chronic inflammatory diarrhoea. The bacteria adhere well to colonic mucosa and produce haemorrhagic necrosis of villi. They were responsible for 13% of cases of acute diarrhoea and 30% of cases of chronic diarrhoea in rural Indian children. They have not been described in developed countries. The incubation period is unknown but they produce fever, vomiting and diarrhoea with frank blood in the stool. The mean duration of diarrhoea in one study was 17 days.

Infectivity is for as long as the bacteria are excreted; however, the infective doses for EPEC and EIEC are high (about 10^6 bacteria).

Diagnosis is by culture of stool; however, *E. coli* is part of the normal intestinal flora (see Chapter 24) and commensal *E. coli* must be differentiated from pathogenic strains. Therefore, in symptomatic cases, isolates should be sent to reference laboratories. The majority of EHEC are serogroup 0157 and are sorbitol non-fermenting.

MANAGEMENT

Dehydration and electrolyte imbalance should be corrected (see Chapter 6). Antibiotics should not be used unless diarrhoea is severe, chronic or dysenteric, or systemic spread has occurred, and should be based on antimicrobial susceptibility testing.

PREVENTION OF FURTHER CASES

In babies one of the most potent preventive measures is the promotion of breast-feeding and good household hygiene. In hospitalized cases enteric precautions are obligatory. In outbreaks it is important that consultants in communicable disease control are informed. In England and Wales *E. coli* isolates should be forwarded for typing by microbiologists to the Laboratory of Enteric Pathogens at the Central Public Health Laboratory or, in Scotland, to the Scottish Centre of Infection and Environmental Health. This is particularly important for VTEC and where a food source is suspected. If VTEC are isolated or one or more cases of haemolytic uraemic syndrome occur the possibility of an outbreak must be considered (see Chapter 51).

GIARDIASIS

ORGANISM

Giardia lamblia, also called *G. intestinalis* or *G. duodenalis*, is a primitive, binucleate, flagellate protozoan.

EPIDEMIOLOGY

The life-cycle of *Giardia lamblia* is one of the simplest of those seen in parasites. There are only two stages: the trophozoite, which exists freely in the human small intestine, and the cyst, which passes down the intestine into the environment. The cycle is completed when the cyst is reingested, and excysts in the stomach and duodenum, releasing the trophozoite. The parasite is found worldwide and in animal species including sheep, cattle, cats and dogs, though epidemiologic studies have failed to confirm them as an important source, and cysts from human sources may be more infectious to humans than those from animal sources. Children are infected more frequently than adults, though breast-fed infants may receive protection from breast milk. Prevalence is higher in areas with poor sanitation and in institutions with young children such as day-care centres. The prevalence of stool positivity in different areas may range between 1% and 30%, depending on the community and age surveyed. Water-borne outbreaks occur most often in communities that derive drinking water from streams or rivers without a water filtration system. Giardiasis is prevalent in certain temperate as well as tropical countries, with frequent infection of tourists related to drinking inadequately treated water or eating contaminated food. Reports from laboratories in England and Wales have changed little in recent years (see Appendix I, Figure 2).

Transmission Person-to-person transmission occurs by hand-to-mouth transfer of cysts from the faeces of an infected individual, especially in institutions and day-care centres. Asymptomatic infected individuals (being more common) are probably more responsible for transmission than those with diarrhoea. Localized outbreaks may occur from ingestion of cysts in faecally contaminated water and less often from faecally contaminated food. The cysts are hardy and partially resistant to chlorification. Concentrations of chlorine used in routine water treatment do not kill *Giardia* cysts, especially when the water is cold; unfiltered stream and lake waters that are open to contamination by human and animal faeces are a frequent source of infection.

Incubation period is 5–25 days or longer; the median is 7–10 days.

Infectivity persists through the entire period of infection.

NATURAL HISTORY AND CLINICAL FEATURES

Giardiasis is a protozoan infection principally of the upper small intestine; although usually asymptomatic (asymptomatic carrier rate is high and infection is frequently self-limited), it may occasionally be associated with a variety of intestinal symptoms, such as chronic diarrhoea, steatorrhoea, abdominal cramps, bloating, frequent loose, pale, greasy stools, fatigue and weight loss. Malabsorption of fats or of fat-soluble vitamins may occur. There is usually no extraintestinal invasion, but occasionally trophozoites may migrate into the bile or pancreatic ducts producing inflammatory processes; damage to duodenal and jejunal mucosal cells may occur in severe giardiasis. Chronic or recurrent infection is a particular problem in immunocompromised individuals.

Diagnosis is made by the identification of cysts or trophozoites in faeces. Specimens need to be repeated at least three times over a number of days (because of intermittent release) before being considered negative. An alternative is searching for trophozoites in duodenal fluid (by aspiration or string test) or in mucosa obtained by small intestine biopsy. The latter may be tried when results of stool examination are questionable, but only rarely provides more information than well-conducted stool testing. Because *Giardia* infection is usually asymptomatic, the presence of *G. lamblia* (either in stools or duodenum) does not necessarily indicate that *Giardia* is the cause of an illness. Faecal specimens are examined by microscopy, looking at a fresh specimen for active trophozoites (in liquid stools) or for cysts in preserved specimens and formed stools. Tests for *G. lamblia* antigen in the stool are becoming available. However, since the clinician frequently requires a search for multiple parasites, for example in a child returning from a developing country, such specific tests cannot replace a search for ova and parasites.

MANAGEMENT

Metronidazole is the drug of choice. Tinidazole 50–75 mg/kg as a single dose or quinacrine are alternatives; furazolidone is available in paediatric suspension for young children and infants, but relapses may occur with any medication. When *Gardia lamblia* is found in well-nourished, asymptomatic children it is not always necessary to treat. Considerations should include an assessment of whether other children are being put at risk, for example if the child attends a day-care centre.

PREVENTION OF FURTHER CASES

When a case is found it is worth testing other close household members whether symptomatic or not, supplemented by a search for environmental contamination. If a child is hospitalized enteric precautions should be taken and soiled articles disinfected. In communities with a modern and adequate sewage disposal system, faeces can be discharged directly into sewers without preliminary disinfection. Epidemiologic investigation of clustered cases in an area or institution is needed to determine the source of infection and mode of transmission; a common vehicle, such as water, or association with day-care centre, should be sought; and applicable preventive or control measures should be instituted. Control of person-to-person transmission requires special emphasis on personal cleanliness and sanitary disposal of faeces. Education of families, personnel and inmates of institutions, and especially adult personnel of day-care centres, in personal hygiene and the need for handwashing before eating and after toilet use is of use. As for other enteric pathogens, public water supplies need to be protected against contamination with human and animal faeces. Persons at high risk of causing faecal–oral transmission (Chapter 27) must not be excluded once they are symptom free.

GONOCOCCAL INFECTION

Notifiable as eye infection in the newborn—ophthalmia neonatorum

ORGANISM

Neisseria gonorrhoea B is a Gram-negative diplococcal bacterium.

EPIDEMIOLOGY

Humans are the only reservoir of infection. There are essentially two clinical entities in children.

- Newborn infants: infection usually involves the eye (ophthalmia neonatorum*) though systemic infection can also occur.
- Children and adolescents: infection involves the genital tract and extragenital sites.

Infection in prepubertal children is commonly the result of child sexual abuse (see Chapter 8) and in adolescents through sexual activity. Though the incidence of gonorrhoea has been declining in the UK in recent years, levels of infection are highest in females in the age group 16–19 years among those attending sexually transmitted disease clinics. The incidence of infection in younger adolescents is not well known because of asymptomatic infection (especially common in females) and the reluctance of young people to use clinics or family doctors.

Transmission occurs through close intimate contact. In the newborn this is during the passage through the birth canal from an infected mother; infection at later ages occurs from sexual contact. Casual transmission does not occur.

Incubation period is 36–48 hours for neonatal infection, and 2–7 days for infection in older children.

Period of infectivity Infectivity continues as long as no treatment is given and discharges continue, though infectivity may occur with no or minimal symptoms in females. In adults without treatment, infectivity can continue for 3–6 months.

NATURAL HISTORY AND CLINICAL FEATURES

Newborn infants Acute inflammation and exudate of the conjunctiva of one or both eyes develops within 2 days of birth. Without treatment corneal ulceration, perforation and blindness can occur. Chlamydial ophthalmia usually presents after 48 hours.

Children and adolescents Sites involved are any mucosal membrane that is exposed to sexual contact, i.e. the genital tract, urethra, pharynx and rectum. The genital tract of prepubertal and adolescent girls is considered to be more susceptible to damage than in older women. The clinical spectrum runs from asymptomatic infection through a simple discharge to pelvic inflammatory disease, epididymitis and perihepatitis. Systemic spread is uncommon but septicaemia and meningitis have been described.

***Ophthalmia neonatorum is also caused by other organisms, notably *Chlamydia trachomatis* (see Chapter 40).**

Diagnosis is by microscopic examination and culture of exudate. Culture media which inhibit other organisms should be used when sampling from mucosal surfaces which will be colonized by non-pathogenic organisms.

MANAGEMENT

Newborn infants Treatment of uncomplicated gonococcal ophthalmia neonatorum is with parenteral penicillin with or without chloramphenicol eye-drops. Eye-drops alone are inadequate, though irrigation of the eyes assists in clearing infection. The possibility of chlamydial infection should also be considered (see Chapter 40). Investigation and treatment of the mother is obligatory and should involve a specialist in genitourinary medicine.

Children and adolescents Treatment is with ampicillin and probenecid which can be given at all ages. Spectinomycin (40 mg/kg up to 2g) can be used in penicillin hypersensitive children. Many specialists also give treatment for chlamydial infection because of the likelihood of dual infection and because of difficulties in reliably detecting *Chlamydia trachomatis*. In the prepubertal child treatment is with erythromycin while in those aged over 12 years doxycyline is the drug of choice. Where complications have occurred, such as pelvic inflammatory disease, advice should be sought from specialists in genitourinary medicine who can also assist in tracing and treating the sexual contacts of adolescents through partner notification. The possibility of child sexual abuse should be considered for children at all ages but is obligatory for the prepubertal child (see Chapter 8).

PREVENTION OF FURTHER CASES

Newborn infants Where incidence of gonorrhoea is high, antimicrobial eye-drops are used routinely after birth.

Children and adolescents Children require protection from adults who seek underage sex and sex without consent in older children. Sex education and accessible sexual health services are necessary for adolescents.

51

HAEMOLYTIC URAEMIC SYNDROME

Haemolytic uraemic syndrome (HUS) is a clinical syndrome defined by the presence of microangiopathic haemolytic anaemia, thrombocytopenia and acute renal dysfunction. It is closely related to thrombocytopenic purpura. It comprises a set of heterogeneous conditions but more than 90% of cases are caused by toxin-producing diarrhoeal organisms. There are other rare aetiologies (atypical HUS) which have a worse prognosis, for example some are inherited disorders and patients tend to relapse. The condition has also been reported in association with some drugs (such as antineoplastic agents and cyclosporin) and some other diseases such as systemic lupus erythematosus.

ORGANISMS

Most commonly HUS occurs following an episode of bloody diarrhoea caused by enterohaemorrhagic *Escherichia coli* producing a verotoxin.* These are also called verotoxin-producing *E. coli* (VTEC). Among *E. coli* serotypes the most commonly associated with HUS in the UK is *E. coli* 0157 and the most prevalent exotoxin is VT2. Other organisms have been reported to be associated with HUS and produce a similar toxin to VTEC, such as *Shigella dysenteriae* serotype 1.

EPIDEMIOLOGY

Around 90% of cases of HUS occur in early childhood and most are in children between the ages of 6 months and 5 years. A survey in the UK between 1986 and 1989 through the British Paediatric Surveillance Unit found an incidence of 0.82 per 100 000 child population per annum. The main reservoir of VTEC is considered to be in cattle, though the organism is also found in sheep, pigs and goats as well as humans. Infections with *E. coli* 0157 occur both sporadically and as outbreaks.

Transmission Substantial outbreaks of HUS due to VTEC in the UK, North America and Australia have been associated with consumption of undercooked hamburgers, unpasteurized milk, contaminated water and other food products (such as vegetables) that have been contaminated. Person-to-person spread, presumably faecal–oral, of VTEC is also important.

Incubation period *Escherichia coli* 0157 has a usual incubation period of 3–4 days, though both shorter and longer periods have been observed with the outside limit being 10 days. When HUS follows there is usually a period of about a week between the onset of diarrhoea and the first signs of HUS.

NATURAL HISTORY AND CLINICAL FEATURES

Verotoxin-producing *E. coli* can cause asymptomatic infection, diarrhoea, haemorrhagic colitis or complete or partial HUS. The chance of a child with VTEC-induced diarrhoea progressing to HUS is about 10%. In those who proceed to HUS the diarrhoea is often non-bloody to begin with, but becomes grossly bloody in 75% of cases and is often associated with severe abdominal pain. Intussusception or rectal prolapse may occur, and some signs suggest an intra-abdominal surgical emergency. The acute oliguric renal failure develops abruptly and usually coincides with the onset of anaemia. The abruptness of oliguria is such that it may soon lead to extracellular fluid overload, hyperkalaemia, acidosis and hypertension. Fever occurs in less than 20% of affected children. Broadly speaking, those with the worst colitis have the worst renal damage, but this is not always the case. A helpful adverse prognostic feature is an elevated peripheral blood neutrophil count at presentation. Counts in excess of 20×10^9/l are correlated with poor outcome. Complications in addition to renal failure include cardiomyopathy, diabetes mellitus and central nervous system manifestations (irritability, fits, hemiplegia and coma). The central nervous system involvement is the major cause of death in the acute stage of the illness. Post-diarrhoeal thrombocytopenic purpura can occur as well as, or in addition to, HUS.

Diagnosis of HUS is on the basis of the clinical triad of microangiopathic haemolytic anaemia, thrombocytopenia and acute renal dysfunction, remembering that the thrombocytopenia is often transient. Important differential diagnoses

***Also known as shiga-like toxins or SLTs.**

for non-diarrhoeal HUS include 'atypical' HUS, thrombotic thrombocytopenic purpura, systemic lupus erythematosus and renal vein thrombosis. Diagnosis of infection with VTEC can be on the basis of detection of either the specific verotoxin-producing *E. coli* or the toxin itself. The organism may be isolated from stool specimens though it can be undetectable by the time that HUS develops. Specialist and reference laboratories will be able to detect the toxin from organism-negative stools, and antibody tests for anti-*E. coli* 0157 (IgG and IgM) are becoming available and will be useful in establishing whether a single-source outbreak is occurring.

MANAGEMENT

The child with diarrhoea only (see also Chapter 6) Electrolyte and fluid balance should be corrected and maintained in all children with diarrhoea irrespective of whether HUS develops. Stool specimens for culture should be obtained from all children with diarrhoea; and when the diarrhoea has been bloody the culture should specifically be for VTEC, and the laboratory should be apprised of the likelihood of this diagnosis. If the diarrhoea is severe, or VTEC is found, it will also be wise to establish a baseline blood count and metabolic status. All children with haemorrhagic colitis require parental education and close follow-up to detect the appearance of pallor, oedema or oliguria as early as possible so as to prevent fluid overload. If VTEC is found then observation must be particularly close to allow early detection of HUS. Antibiotic therapy is not thought to reduce the likelihood of HUS developing and antidiarrhoeal agents may be harmful.

The child with haemolytic uraemic syndrome In most cases of VTEC-caused HUS meticulous care will achieve a successful outcome. Specialist advice should be sought early. Fluid balance must be monitored with great care. In the first instance vascular volume must be corrected with isonatraemic fluids. Thereafter fluid prescription should be restricted to the estimated insensible losses plus urine output. Particular attention must be given to the restriction of potassium and the correction of acidosis. Transfusion of packed red blood cells should be undertaken if the haemoglobin level falls below 60 g/l, though transfusion should be slow and cautious to avoid fluid overload. Dialysis is needed in about 50% of cases to support homeostasis. With meticulous attention to care, mortality from acute HUS has declined to under 5%, though HUS due to non-infective causes and atypical HUS (see above) have a worse outlook, as do infective cases where the clinical course has been complicated by central nervous system involvement or rectal prolapse. Chronic renal failure follows HUS in about 10% of cases, but one-third of survivors exhibit renal impairment, proteinuria or hypertension. Some of these abnormalities appear after many years and therefore long-term follow-up of these children is mandatory.

PREVENTION OF FURTHER CASES

General considerations for prevention of gastrointestinal infections apply (see Chapter 6). In any single case of infection-associated HUS it is important that the consultant in communicable disease control is informed at an early stage. Isolates of *E. coli* should be forwarded for typing (in England and Wales) by the Laboratory of Enteric Pathogens at the Central Public Health Laboratory or (in Scotland) by the Scottish Centre of Infection and Environmental Health. This is particularly important for VTEC and where a food source of VTEC is suspected. Serum samples should be retained from affected children to identify serotypes retrospectively where there are outbreaks.

HAEMOPHILUS INFLUENZAE INFECTION

Notifiable disease if resulting in meningitis

Paediatricians also notify all invasive Hib to the BPA Surveillance Unit (1995)

ORGANISM

Haemophilus influenzae is a Gram-negative bacterium. Six serotypes (a to f) are defined by polysaccharide antigens in the capsule. Other isolates are non-encapsulated and hence are classified as non-typeable.

EPIDEMIOLOGY

Humans are the only hosts. *Haemophilus influenzae* type b (Hib) is the most virulent serotype. Before routine vaccination began in the UK, it accounted for more than 90% of invasive *Haemophilus* disease (such as meningitis) in children. The disease rate is maximal in the second half of the first year of life. Day-care attendance and overcrowding are risk factors. Before routine vaccination began, Hib was a principal cause of bacterial meningitis, the predominant cause of epiglottitis and the commonest bacterial pathogen in septic arthritis and cellulitis among children aged less than 5 years. Most serious *Haemophilus* disease in neonates is caused by non-typeable organisms. Later in life, these mainly cause less serious mucosal infections, such as otitis media and bronchitis. However they are becoming relatively more important as causes of invasive disease with the decline in Hib.

Until recent times, the rate of Hib disease in children under 5 years old varied between 1 in 200 and 1 in 600 in the developed world, and was higher in developing countries and in the aboriginal populations of Australia, Canada and the USA. People of Asian and African origin living in the UK may be at increased risk compared with the indigenous European population. Routine immunization with a conjugate vaccine began in the UK in October 1992 and laboratory reports of invasive Hib disease subsequently fell dramatically (see Appendix I, Fig. 3). The few cases of invasive disease now seen are at least as likely to be caused by another serotype or non-typeable *H. influenzae* organisms as by Hib.

Because the organism only infects humans, hope has arisen that disease can be eliminated and perhaps even the organism eradicated. This is supported by studies of the effect of vaccination on Hib throat carriage which have shown a reduced rate of acquisition and transmission within families in which an infant is immunized.

Transmission The respiratory route is most common. Shared handkerchiefs in day-care centres have also been implicated.

Incubation period is uncertain. Although it is suspected that most invasive disease occurs within days of nasopharyngeal acquisition, this has not been proved.

NATURAL HISTORY AND CLINICAL FEATURES

Asymptomatic nasopharyngeal carriage with non-typeable organisms is common. Prior to the introduction of routine vaccination the carriage rate was about 5% for encapsulated strains, and was highest at preschool age. Only a small minority of carriers develop bacteraemia and invasive disease. Meningitis accounts for 70% of invasive Hib disease, epiglottitis about 10%, and cellulitis and bone or joint infections 5% each. Hib pneumonia is more common than diagnoses based on blood culture isolates would suggest, and before vaccination was probably the second most common cause of bacterial pneumonia after pneumococci in children. Cardinal signs of meningitis in the older child include stiff neck and photophobia, but in infants less specific features such as fever, irritability and vomiting may be all that is seen (see Chapter 10).

Diagnosis Accurate diagnosis requires the collection, ideally before antibiotic administration, of samples such as blood, joint fluid or cerebrospinal fluid (CSF) for Gram stain and culture from which serotyping and genotyping can take place. Careful characterization of *Haemophilus* isolates is vital for epidemiologic purposes. Antigen detection by latex agglutination or counter-current immune electrophoresis techniques, where available, are especially useful when antibiotics have been given before samples are obtained. It should, however, be recognized that these tests have a false positive rate which (though low) is especially relevant in the case of a recent recipient of Hib vaccine in whom CSF and urine Hib antigen (polyribosylribitol phosphate, PRP) may be detectable for weeks and perhaps even months. Collection of acute and convalescent sera for antibody to PRP may be helpful if cultures are negative, but do not rule out Hib infection if no rise is seen in an infant less than 2 years old because the immature immune system may not respond to a polysaccharide antigen such as PRP.

Lumbar puncture should be delayed if signs suggesting dangerously raised intracranial pressure are present, such as coma, papillary abnormalities or abnormal posturing. Molecular techniques such as polymerase chain reaction are available in some reference laboratories for typing in cases of diagnostic difficulty.

MANAGEMENT

The treatment of choice for invasive disease such as meningitis is a third-generation cephalosporin such as cefotaxime or ceftriaxone. About 15% of Hib isolates are ampicillin-resistant, as are a similar percentage of non-capsulated isolates. Chloramphenicol resistance in Hib, though rare, is increasing, so its combination with ampicillin is now less justifiable as a first-line treatment. A minimum of 7 days' treatment is required for uncomplicated meningitis. If response to treatment is slow, such as when fever is prolonged, a second lumbar puncture may be helpful by the methods described above. It is reassuring if the CSF is returning to normal, though another source of infection should be sought by the methods described above, and could direct a change in antibiotic treatment if viable organisms, whether resistant or not, are found. Though Hib meningitis has virtually been eliminated it has not been possible to move to penicillin monotherapy as first-line treatment of bacterial meningitis in children aged more than 3 months because of emerging antibiotic resistance, especially in pneumococci.

Hearing tests for sensorineural deafness should be performed in convalescence. Young children, especially those under 2 years old, will often not produce a protective antibody response after invasive Hib disease, whether previously immunized or not, so Hib vaccine should be offered in convalescence if it is not possible to check the serum antibody response. If Hib infection is proved in an adequately immunized child, immunodeficiency—albeit most probably a subtle type, such as IgG_2 deficiency—is a strong possibility and must be investigated (Chapter 16).

In the UK, mucosal infections such as otitis media are usually managed without obtaining an isolate. *Haemophilus influenzae* (usually non-typeable) and *Moraxella catarrhalis*, two of the three most common causes, often produce the enzyme beta-lactamase rendering amoxycillin ineffective. To maximize successful treatment, antibiotics like amoxycillin/clavulanic acid, cefaclor or erythromycin may be required.

PREVENTION OF FURTHER CASES

When a case of Hib disease occurs in a child or an adult the immunization records of all children under 4 years old in the household should be checked and any unimmunized children should be offered vaccine as soon as possible. Elimination of carriage with antibiotic (usually rifampicin) is no longer indicated if *all* contacts aged under 4 years have been fully immunized (three doses for children aged less than 12 months and one dose for those aged 12–48 months). In households where there are one or more children aged under 4 years who are unvaccinated or incompletely vaccinated, then rifampicin should be offered to all home contacts irrespective of age and Hib immunization history. Similar treatment should be offered to all room contacts (teachers and children) when two or more cases of Hib disease have occured in a playgroup, nursery or creche within 120 days. Unimmunized children under 4 years old should also receive vaccine. Cases of Hib disease should be offered both vaccine and antibiotic treatment to eliminate carriage before discharge from hospital as Hib disease occasionally fails to generate immunity, especially in the very young. Rifampicin is the drug of choice for elimination of carriage. The recommended dose is 20 mg/kg (maximum 600 mg) once daily for 4 days. This is longer than the 2-day regimen used for meningococcal infection, which will not always clear Hib. Recipients need to be advised of possible adverse reactions which include interference with the oral contraceptive and red coloration of urine and other body fluids.

IMMUNIZATION

In the UK routine vaccination against Hib in the form of a PRP conjugate is given at 2, 3 and 4 months of age. A booster is not currently offered in the second year of life (unlike in most other western countries). This policy appears to have been successful with the national coverage for three doses approaching 95% (see Appendix I, Fig. 13), estimated vaccine efficacy in the field in those under 2 years old in excess of 95%, and vaccine efficacy is well sustained to the end of the third year of life. The UK's early accelerated schedule ensures that virtually all infants can be protected before reaching the age of susceptibility.

All children under 4 years old should be immunized; however, those at increased risk of invasive infection by encapsulated bacteria such as Hib should be especially targeted for vaccination. These include the premature, children with asplenia and functional asplenia (e.g. children with sickle-cell disease) and children infected with human immunodeficiency virus. There is evidence for adequate, though reduced, immunogenicity in these groups. The widespread use of Hib conjugate vaccines in many western countries has been highly effective in diminishing the incidence of invasive *Haemophilus influenzae* disease. There is no evidence that Hib is being replaced by similarly virulent organisms and neither has the possibility of vaccine escape mutants arisen. However, vigilance will need to be maintained to ensure the continued success of the vaccine programme, and this should include characterization of invasive *Haemophilus* isolates from all children with this infection.

53

HAND, FOOT AND MOUTH DISEASE

See also the chapter on enteroviruses (Chapter 47).

ORGANISM

Causative organisms are coxsackieviruses of a number of types, especially A5 and A16, and less often enterovirus 71. They are small, non-enveloped RNA viruses of the picornavirus family.

EPIDEMIOLOGY

The disease occurs worldwide, sporadically and in epidemics, especially in preschool child-care establishments. It is more common in summer and autumn.

Transmission is by droplets, direct contact with nasal secretions and the rash, and the faecal–oral route.

Incubation period is 3–5 days.

NATURAL HISTORY AND CLINICAL FEATURES

The illness may begin with a mild pyrexia followed 3–5 days later by a rash. In the mouth a vesicular rash 4–8 mm across is present on the tongue and buccal mucosa. Similar lesions occur on the hands and less commonly the feet. They are more common on the dorsal surfaces than on the palms and soles. A rash may be present on the buttocks but it is not usually vesicular. The rash lasts about a week. The disease is usually self-limiting.

Diagnosis Virus can be isolated from the lesions and stools, but this is not necessary as the diagnosis can be made clinically.

MANAGEMENT

Management is symptomatic only.

PREVENTION OF FURTHER CASES

Isolation is of little value as the virus may persist in the stools for several weeks. Strict attention to hygiene may have some effect.

HELICOBACTER PYLORI INFECTION

ORGANISM

Helicobacter pylori is a Gram-negative, spiral organism which grows under microaerophilic conditions.

EPIDEMIOLOGY

In developed countries the prevalence of *Helicobacter pylori* colonization of the gastric mucosa increases with age. Serological studies have shown the prevalence of infection is approximately 10% at 15 years of age and rises to 60% at 60 years of age. However, in developing countries the prevalence of infection is between 90% and 100% by 10 years of age. Recent studies suggest that the marked difference in infection rates between children in different countries is related to living standards. Children who come from families with low incomes are more likely to be infected than children from higher income families. The increase in prevalence of *H. pylori* infection with increasing age noted in developed countries is probably due to a cohort effect. *Helicobacter pylori* is acquired in childhood, and the high prevalence of infection in older people in developed countries probably relates to poor living conditions when they were children.

There is marked clustering of infection within families. In one study, more than 80% of the siblings of children colonized with *H. pylori* had serologic evidence of infection in comparison to 13% of age-matched controls. Clustering of *H. pylori* infection has also been identified within institutions for people with severe learning difficulties.

Transmission The method of transmission of *Helicobacter pylori* is still unknown. Recently *H. pylori* has been cultured from the faeces of some infected individuals. The faecal–oral route of infection is therefore possible. The lack of a serotyping system for the organism is a major problem in conducting studies of transmission.

Incubation period is unknown

NATURAL HISTORY AND CLINICAL FEATURES

Helicobacter pylori colonization of the gastric mucosa is always associated with chronic gastritis in children. The organism is present in all cases of primary or unexplained gastritis. There is a strong correlation between duodenal ulceration and *H. pylori* gastritis in children and adults: almost 100% of primary duodenal ulcers are associated with *H. pylori* gastritis. In adults, duodenal ulcers do not recur if *H. pylori* is cleared from the gastric mucosa. Studies in children have produced similar findings. *Helicobacter pylori* colonization of the gastric mucosa and the associated chronic gastritis may be important factors in the development of gastric cancer. Preliminary studies suggest that infection in childhood may be a critical issue in relation to the ultimate development of gastric cancer. There is no evidence that *H. pylori* gastritis in the absence of duodenal ulcer disease is a cause of abdominal pain in children. Children with *H. pylori* gastritis are often asymptomatic. Large serological studies of healthy children have found *H. pylori* infection in up to 30% of asymptomatic children. Furthermore, it is not possible to differentiate children who are infected with *H. pylori* from uninfected children based on their presenting symptoms. Following eradication of *H. pylori*, symptoms appear to improve consistently only in those children who have an associated duodenal ulcer and not in those who have *H. pylori* gastritis alone.

Diagnosis At endoscopy the presence of *H. pylori* gastritis has usually not been associated with any morphological evidence of inflammation. However, the presence of a nodular appearance of the antral mucosa has been noted in over 50% of children with chronic *H. pylori* antral gastritis.

Culture The ultimate test to confirm the presence of *H. pylori* on the gastric mucosa is to culture the organism from a mucosal biopsy. However, culturing *H. pylori* is slow and expensive and many laboratories have difficulty in consistently culturing the organism. An incubation period of 5–7 days is usually required.

Staining techniques Silver stains are almost 100% sensitive in identifying the presence of *H. pylori* in children. A modified Giemsa stain is also sensitive in identifying the organism and is easier to perform. Gram staining of gastric mucosal material is a practical way of identifying this organism but it has a low sensitivity.

Urease test *Helicobacter pylori* produces large amounts of urease which can be detected by various tests. When a full biopsy specimen is placed in urea medium the sensitivity of this test is close to 100%. It is important to note that using only half a biopsy specimen in such tests significantly lowers the sensitivity in children. This is probably due to a lower number of organisms present in children.

Urea breath test The production of urease by *H. pylori* has also resulted in the development of urea breath tests. The patient ingests urea labelled with carbon-13. The presence of urease in the stomach results in the release of ^{13}C-labelled carbon dioxide in the expired air. These tests are very sensitive in detecting *H. pylori* colonization of the gastric mucosa; however, they have not yet been adequately standardized for use in children in a clinical setting. When the test is properly standardized it may present a very effective non-invasive method of diagnosing active *H. pylori* infection of the gastric mucosa. These tests will be commercially available in the near future.

Serology The *H. pylori*-specific IgG response is both highly specific (99%) and sensitive (96%). The sensitivity and specificity of commercially available enzyme-linked immunosorbent assay (ELISA) tests used in routine clinical laboratories may be significantly less. This is especially true in children. It is important that ELISA tests used to diagnose *H. pylori* colonization in children is standardized by use of children's sera. If the assay is based on adult antibody cut-off levels a significant number of children colonized by *H. pylori* are not detected.

MANAGEMENT

In children, as in adults, eradication of *Helicobacter pylori* from the gastric antrum is associated with a healing of antral gastritis. In children dual therapy combining an antibiotic and a bismuth preparation appears to be successful in eradicating *H. pylori*. Colloidal bismuth subcitrate is the bismuth preparation most extensively studied for use in children. Bismuth subcitrate is prescribed at a dose of 480 mg BiO_3 per 1.73 m^2 of body surface area per day. Bismuth should be given four times a day for a total of 4 weeks and combined with either amoxycillin or metronidazole for two weeks. When combined with amoxycillin 250 mg three times a day for a period of 4 weeks this combination results in clearance of the infection in approximately 70% of children. Bismuth combined with metronidazole administered at a dose of 20 mg/kg per day in three divided doses, with a maximum dose of 600 mg per day, administered for 2 weeks resulted in clearance of *H. pylori* in over 80% of treated children. However, children who fail to clear the organism on a regimen which includes metronidazole will almost always develop resistance to metronidazole, whereas resistance to amoxycillin does not develop despite failure of treatment.

The duration of treatment required to eradicate *H. pylori* in children is not adequately defined at present. Further studies are required to identify the ideal therapy as well as the proper duration of therapy. Concern has been expressed about the use of bismuth in the treatment of *H. pylori* gastritis in children. However, no studies of the use of bismuth preparations to treat *H. pylori* gastritis in children have reported any cases of bismuth toxicity or adverse side-effects. Toxic effects of bismuth have been reported in adults and include encephalopathy which is reversible after withdrawal of the drug and acute renal impairment after ingestion of a large overdose. Children with duodenal ulcer disease who have confirmed *H. pylori* infection of the gastric mucosa should all be treated to eradicate this infection. Eradication of *H. pylori* from the gastric mucosa will result in long-term healing of duodenal ulcers in children as in adults. The question as to whether children with chronic *H. pylori* gastritis who do not have duodenal ulcer disease should be treated remains debatable. As noted above, the evidence suggests that these children do not have symptoms as a result of the chronic *H. pylori* gastritis: there is therefore at this point no definite indication that demands eradication of this infection. However, this situation may change in the next few years if evidence supporting an association between early infection with *H. pylori* and chronic gastritis with the subsequent development of gastric cancer continues to increase.

FURTHER READING

Drumm B (1993) *Helicobacter pylori* in the pediatric patient. *Gastroenterology Clinics of North America* **22**: 69–122.

HEPATITIS A

55

Hepatitis A is a notifiable disease*

ORGANISM

Hepatitis A virus is an RNA enterovirus and has its own genus, heparnavirus, within the picornavirus family. Humans are the only host. The virus can survive for some time outside the body so that water or food contaminated by sewage or faeces constitute environmental reservoirs.

EPIDEMIOLOGY

Hepatitis A virus is the most common cause of childhood jaundice in most countries. In developing countries most individuals are infected in childhood and acquire lifelong immunity. In industrialized countries rates of infection in the

***In the UK the reporting doctor is currently asked to report viral hepatitis and to categorize it as type A, B, non-A, non-B (includes hepatitis C and E) or type not known.**

population are highly variable but lower than in the developing world and many children and adults remain non-immune. In 1994 2543 cases were reported by laboratories in England and Wales to the Public Health Laboratory Service Communicable Disease Surveillance Centre; most occurred in children and young adults. Cases occur either sporadically or as outbreaks. In industrialized countries such as the UK, outbreaks occur within families and in settings where there is close physical contact and the potential for faecal–oral spread is high. Examples would include day-care centres, nurseries and primary schools. In addition, common source outbreaks occur through consumption of food or water contaminated by sewage, consumption of contaminated shellfish (shellfish concentrate the sewage content of seawater) and food contaminated by infectious food handlers. Travel to developing countries places individuals at higher risk of infection, especially if they fail to take precautions against enteric infections and are unimmunized (see 'Prevention of Further Cases' below).

Transmission The virus replicates primarily in the liver and is shed through the biliary tree and bile duct into faeces. Most transmission is via the faecal–oral route. Food and water contaminated by sewage are important vehicles in developing countries. Among adults faecal–oral transmission can take place through sexual intercourse. Transmission from transfusion of blood products can occur but is very rare, and the potential for transmission is far less than for hepatitis B and C because of the short duration and low level of viraemia. Vertical (mother-to-fetus) transmission has been recorded but is exceptionally rare.

Incubation period There is a range of 15–45 days with a median of around 28 days.

Infectivity increases during the latter half of the incubation period and is maximal just before the onset of dark urine and jaundice when the virus is replicating and being shed into the faeces. Infectivity of faeces decreases following the darkening of the urine and there is no risk of transmission 3 weeks after this. There is no chronic infection (carrier) state.

NATURAL HISTORY AND CLINICAL FEATURES

Severity of disease is closely related to age. In childhood many infections are asymptomatic or without jaundice (anicteric), especially in younger children. The most specific sign is the onset of dark urine (due to the presence of urobilinogen) which precedes jaundice. In symptomatic cases common symptoms and signs include fever, headache, anorexia, nausea, vomiting and abdominal pain from a tender, enlarged liver. Splenomegaly occurs in a minority of cases. Once the urine darkens the child often feels better, although return of appetite and full vigour may be delayed for 1–2 weeks. However, convalescence is generally brief in children and full recovery is usual. The return of normal stool colour can be taken as indicative of the end of the disease process. In adolescents and adults symptoms are more often severe and prolonged. The development of fulminating hepatitis due to hepatitis A is rare in children, but does occur.

Diagnosis is often made on the basis of the clinical features and a history of likely exposure to hepatitis A. Urobilinogen can be detected in the urine shortly before the onset of jaundice. Laboratory testing will show a transient rise in serum transaminase (alanine aminotransferase, ALT, and aspartate aminotransferase,

AST) levels for 1–3 weeks with a rise in bilirubin levels around the peak of transaminase disturbance. Serological tests for recent hepatitis A infection, i.e. IgM anti-HAV (antibody to hepatitis A virus), as well as tests for antibodies to hepatitis B and C, are in common use. Hepatitis B, C and E infection should also be considered and appropriate tests undertaken, especially when the course of the illness appears to be more severe or prolonged than expected or there has been a likely exposure to these other infections (see Chapters 56–58). Other infections to exclude are infectious mononucleosis and infection with cytomegalovirus. Salivary and urine tests for anti-HAV are becoming available for use in outbreaks where it is impractical or undesirable to take blood.

MANAGEMENT

There is no specific treatment. Hospital admission is undesirable and rarely necessary. However, if admission is unavoidable, the patient should be nursed in a cubicle and enteric precautions taken. Should the hepatitis be severe and hepatic failure seem imminent it is important to contact a specialist liver unit immediately. Important signs include persisting anorexia, progressively deepening jaundice, reappearance of the initial symptoms or the development of ascites. A late sign is behavioural change prior to encephalopathy. Worrying laboratory signs are prolongation of the prothrombin time, a falling serum albumin concentration or hypoglycaemia. Enteric precautions also apply in the community and it may be desirable or necessary to exclude ill children with hepatitis A from nurseries while infectious though many children will be asymptomatic and undetected (see Chapters 26 and 27). If jaundice appears, these precautions can be discontinued 3 days after its appearance.

PREVENTION OF FURTHER CASES

Cases in the UK The importance of personal hygiene in preventing spread of hepatitis A virus and other enteric pathogens must be emphasized to parents and other carers (see Chapter 27). Particular care must be taken within day-care centres, nurseries and primary schools where the potential for spread is higher. Children with clinical hepatitis should be excluded and managed with precautions applicable to hepatitis A, B and C until a specific diagnosis is made. Blood, faeces and other body fluids and products should be the subject of universal precautions (see Chapter 27). All cases of hepatitis A should be notified by the attending doctor. When two or more cases of hepatitis A occur in association the consultant in communicable disease control or director of public health should be contacted immediately, as well as notification made. This is especially important where food or water contamination is possible or where a number of adults and children may have been exposed, for instance in a day nursery. When children, adults or adolescents have been recently exposed they should be advised to have intramuscular human normal immunoglobulin (HNIG) (there is no specific immunoglobulin); HNIG is considered to prevent infection or at least attenuate disease if given within 2 weeks of exposure. It seems to be more effective in reducing transmission. It is not needed for those with a history of two or more doses of hepatitis A vaccine. Dosage is 250 mg for children up to the age of 9 years, and 500 mg for children of 10 years old and over and adults.* Adults who

***An alternative dosage is 0.06–0.12 ml/kg which applies at all ages. Note these regimens contain dosages higher than those recommended for short-duration travel abroad (see Chapter 20).**

are likely to be exposed to infection are those working in a day-care centre where a case has occurred, household contacts, kissing contacts and those sharing meals with an index case. Testing of exposed individuals for anti-HAV IgG (evidence of preceding infection or active immunization) is not normally recommended because of the low prevalence of prior infection and the delay and expense that this will cause. Most hepatitis A cases occurring in schools in children over 5 years old will be the result of household transmission, and so HNIG for school contacts in this age group is rarely of any use in preventing further cases.†

Travel abroad Travellers to endemic countries (most developing countries) should be advised to take precautions to avoid infection with hepatitis A and other enteric pathogens (see Chapter 20). Effective prophylaxis can be obtained from immunization with HNIG as close to the start of travel as is convenient. The dosage is 0.02–0.04 ml/kg (or 125 mg under age 10 years, 250 mg 10 years and over) for travel of under 2 months, and 0.06–0.12 ml/kg (or 250 mg under age 10 years, 500 mg 10 years and over) for up to 5 months' protection. Active immunization is recommended for frequent and long-stay travellers. An inactivated vaccine (Havrix and Havrix Junior) is available for adults and children, but is mostly used in adults at risk of exposure from frequent travel. The vaccine is given in two doses separated by 2–4 weeks and a booster given 6–12 months following the initial dose. It is not licensed for use in children under 1 year old. Adults only need a single dose followed by a booster 6–12 months later.

56

HEPATITIS B

Acute hepatitis B is a notifiable disease‡

ORGANISM

Hepatitis B virus (HBV) is an enveloped DNA virus of the genus hepadnavirus. The virus is a double-shelled particle with an outer lipoprotein coat containing the surface component hepatitis B surface antigen (HBsAg) and a core containing the core antigen (HBcAg) and the e antigen (HBeAg). Humans are the main host. Hepatitis B virus infects other higher primates but they are not a source of human infection and there are no environmental reservoirs.

EPIDEMIOLOGY

The prevalence of hepatitis B infection in the general population varies between global regions and between groups inside countries. In parts of Africa, east Asia and south-east Asia infection is common, with up to 80% of children being infected by adolescence. In a number of these the infection fails to resolve and a

---

† Exceptions would be when cases occur within a limited time (6 weeks or less) in the same class in children who do not come from the same family or in children attending a boarding school.

‡ In the UK the reporting doctor is currently asked to report acute viral hepatitis and to categorize it as type A, B, non-A, non-B (includes hepatitis C and E) or type not known.

persistent infectious state of carriage develops.* The proportion of acute infections that progress to become carriers seems to vary by area. In Africa the population prevalence of HBsAg positivity in adults is over 7%. Most transmission occurs perinatally as vertical transmission from carrier mothers. Some is also thought to occur horizontally from child to child and perhaps also from adult to child. The Middle East, the Amazon basin in South America, the Pacific Islands and parts of eastern Europe have intermediate prevalence of 2% to 7% HBsAg positivity. Population prevalence is generally low (under 2% HBsAg positivity) in indigenous populations in other countries, including western and northern Europe and the UK, and most new transmissions occur between adults in these countries. Exceptions are aboriginal groups in Australia, New Zealand, and Canada and Alaska who have high prevalences. Groups migrating from high to low prevalence areas retain their prior prevalence rates for some time and consequently variations in prevalence, and rates of perinatal exposure, are found between ethnic groups in low prevalence countries according to their country of origin. Mothers at particular risk of being carriers are those who themselves or their families originate in higher prevalence countries, those who have injected drugs or with other behavioural risks and those in particular patient groups (see Prevention of Further Cases). Children at risk of post-natal acquisition in the UK are those who receive frequent transfusions of blood and blood products such as children on haemodialysis and with severe haemoglobinopathies, all of whom should be protected by active immunization (see below).

Incubation period is usually 45–160 days, the average is 120 days (from exposure to initial disease), but may be as long as 6 months.

Infectivity is greatest in individuals who are both HBsAg and HBeAg positive (see Table 56.1). Carriers who are HBsAg positive but have antibody to e antigen (anti-HBe positive) are of low infectivity. Transmission efficiency for perinatal infection from HBeAg positive (anti-HBe negative) mothers is approximately 80% if vaccine and immunoglobulin are not given. Efficiency of transmission after the perinatal period is thought to be much lower.

Transmission Hepatitis B virus may be transmitted through exposure to the following body fluids (in descending order of viral concentration); blood, wound fluid, semen and cervical secretions and saliva. In infants perinatal transmission occurs to infants born to infectious mothers (see above). The virus does not usually cross the placenta and most vertical (mother-to-child) transmission is thought to occur during or just after birth by infant exposure to maternal blood. Mother-to-child transmission is thought also to take place post-natally but it is unclear whether HBV is transmitted through breast-feeding. In countries where prevalence is high and immunization unavailable, child-to-child and late mother-to-child transmission may take place through accidental sharing of blood and wound fluids, particularly within families. In day-care facilities and schools in the UK the risk of child-to-child transmission is very low and can be minimized by normal infection control procedures (see Chapter 27). In adults parenteral exposure to blood and sexual intercourse are the predominant modes of

***Defined as persons who are HBsAg positive and anti-HBc-IgM negative or HBsAg positive on two occasions more than 6 months apart.**

Table 56.1 Interpretation of serologic markers of hepatitis B virus infection

HBsAg	Anti-HBc IgG	IgM	Anti-HBs	HBeAg	Anti-HBe	Interpretation
+	+	+ or −*	−	+	−	Hepatitis B carrier of high infectivity (chronic hepatitis B)
+	+	+ or −*	−	−	+	Hepatitis B carrier of low infectivity
+	−	−	−	+ or −	−	Very early infection/late incubation period
+	+	+	−	+ or −	+ or −	Acute hepatitis B
−	+	−	+ or −	−	+ or −	Immune due to previous infection
−	−	−	+	−	−	Immune due to immunization

Key: *, usually negative.

transmission, with sharing of equipment by injecting drug users, unprotected sex and frequent partner change having the highest associated risk. Health care workers who are exposed to blood are at risk of infection, which have occurred from and to surgeons, and dentists undertaking 'exposure-prone' procedures. The risk can be minimized by ensuring that all such staff are immunized and have serological evidence of immunity.

NATURAL HISTORY AND CLINICAL FEATURES

In most perinatally exposed children infection is asymptomatic or symptoms are minimal and there is no apparent jaundice. Fulminant neonatal hepatitis has been described but is unusual. The risk of perinatally infected babies becoming carriers is higher (approximately 90%) than for any other group of infected individuals, and those who acquire persistent infection as babies are also more at risk of developing chronic liver disease and hepatocellular carcinoma in later life. Children infected after the birth period are likely to experience either no symptoms or a mild illness with anorexia, nausea and general malaise. A prodrome with arthralgia and a rash may occur but is unusual. Although the serum bilirubin level is usually elevated and serum transaminases are disturbed for a number of weeks, obvious jaundice is unusual and less common than in adolescents and adults. Most children resolve their infection. The probability of developing carrier status is approximately 10%. The most serious sequelae of infection are developing fulminant hepatitis as part of acute hepatitis or becoming a carrier, following which severe chronic hepatitis, cirrhosis and primary hepatocellular carcinoma can develop. Fulminant hepatitis occasionally occurs with onset of hepatic failure within a few weeks after the onset of acute hepatitis. Hepatocellular carcinoma is more common among individuals infected in Africa or Asia and is seen in adults with coexisting liver cirrhosis three or more decades after initial infection.

Diagnosis Clinical signs and symptoms and a history of exposure can give rise to a suspicion of hepatitis B but diagnosis is dependent on serology. Serological testing for antibodies and antigens relating to hepatitis B make the diagnosis and indicate whether an individual is infectious, has natural immunity or immunity relating to vaccination (see Table 56.1). Other infections (and non-infectious aetiologies) should be considered, including hepatitis A, C and E, infectious mononucleosis and infection with cytomegalovirus. Clinical hepatitis developing in a child who is HBsAg positive may represent hepatitis A infection is a child who is a carrier for hepatitis B, and IgM tests should be used for distinguishing between acute and chronic hepatitis B infections.

MANAGEMENT

There is no specific treatment for acute hepatitis B infection at any age. The majority of cases can be cared for at home. Where hospitalization is required, infected children should be nursed with standard universal precautions taken in handling blood and other body fluids (see Chapter 26). Patients with undiagnosed jaundice should be managed with universal precautions applicable to both hepatitis A and B until the aetiology is established.

If a child is seeming to progress to fulminant hepatitis referral to a specialist liver unit is urgently required (guidance on the signs of this are given in Chapter 55). Infants born to HBsAg positive mothers do not need to be isolated but will require immunization within 24 hours of birth with hepatitis B vaccine. If the mother is e antigen positive or not known to be anti-HBe positive, or suffered acute hepatitis B in pregnancy, hepatitis B specific immunoglobulin is also given (see below). Some specialists are now using recombinant interferon α to clear infection in adults with chronic hepatitis and trials are under-way in children. However, the course of treatment is long, there are troublesome (though reversible) side-effects and treatment is not always successful.

PREVENTION OF FURTHER CASES

Immunization

Perinatal exposure In the UK it is becoming standard practice to screen all pregnant women for their hepatitis B status rather than to rely on screening those considered to be at higher risk. All babies born to women known to be HBsAg positive should commence a course of hepatitis B vaccine within 24 hours of birth. Breast-feeding is permissible and should be encouraged as long as immunization is given. Second and third doses of vaccine are given at 1 month and 6 months of age. If the mother is HBsAg positive but also *not* known to be anti-HBe positive, or if she suffered acute hepatitis B in pregnancy, then the baby should also receive 200 iu of hepatitis B specific immunoglobulin (HBIG) intramuscularly within 24 hours of birth and at a contralateral site from the vaccine. Because of the importance of early immunization, preparations to provide immunizations should be made during the pregnancy of the carrier mother. These regimens have an efficacy of over 95% in preventing infection in the infant. There is no clear evidence that giving HBIG to babies of mothers known to be anti-HBe positive has any additional value to giving vaccine alone. Immunized infants should be retested for anti-HBs and HBsAg at 1 year of age. In most cases the child will be anti-HBs positive and HBsAg negative, indicating that immunization was successful and that no further follow-up is needed. In a few cases the child will be HBsAg positive indicating infection has occurred and follow-up is required. Infants that are anti-HBs negative (titre under 10 miu/ml) and HBsAg negative should receive a booster dose and further testing.

Routine immunization In some countries (USA and New Zealand) it is now policy to incorporate hepatitis B immunization in primary immunization courses for children. This is not yet the case in the UK where current policy is to immunize all children and adults at higher risk of infection.

Immunization of individuals at risk Immunization is recommended for those who may have been exposed (see below) and those more likely to be exposed to hepatitis B. Those at higher risk in relation to care of children are:

- Sexual and household contacts of carriers of hepatitis B.
- Health care workers who have direct contact with blood, blood-stained body fluids or patient's tissues.
- Staff and clients of residential accommodation for people with severe learning difficulties (including children).
- Children with chronic renal failure.*
- Haemodialysis patients, haemophilia patients and other children likely to be receiving repeat blood transfusions, and relatives responsible for the administration of such products.

***Response to vaccination is poor in those with advanced disease and HBV vaccine should be given early in the course of the disease.**

Table 56.2 Hepatitis B virus prophylaxis for reported exposure incidents

HBV status of person exposed	Significant exposure*			Non-significant exposure	
	HBsAg positive source	Unknown source	HBsAg negative source	Continued risk	No further risk
One dose HB vaccine or none pre-exposure	Accelerated course of HB vaccine† HBIG × 1	Accelerated course of HB vaccine†	Initiate course of HB vaccine	Initiate course of HB vaccine	No HBV prophylaxis; reassure
Two or more doses HB vaccine pre-exposure (anti-HBs not know)	One dose of HB vaccine followed by second dose 1 month later	One dose of HB vaccine	Finish course of HB vaccine	Finish course of HB vaccine	No HBV prophylaxis; reassure
Known responser to HB vaccine (anti-HBs $\geq$ 10 miu/ml)	Booster dose of HB vaccine	Consider booster dose of HB vaccine	Consider booster dose of HB vaccine	Consider booster dose of HB vaccine	No HBV prophylaxis; reassure
Known non-responder to HB vaccine (anti-HBs < 10 miu/ml 2–4 months post-vaccination)	HBIG × 1 Consider booster dose of HB vaccine	HBIG × 1 Consider booster dose of HB vaccine	No HBIG Consider booster dose of HB vaccine	No HBIG Consider booster dose of HB vaccine	No HBV prophylaxis; reassure

***A significant exposure is one from which HBV transmission may result. It may be (i) percutaneous exposure (needle-stick or other contaminated sharp object injury, a bite which causes bleeding or other visible skin puncture), (ii) mucocutaneous exposure to blood (contamination of non-intact skin, conjunctiva or mucous membrane) or (iii) sexual exposure (unprotected sexual intercourse). Percutaneous exposure is of higher risk than mucocutaneous exposure, and exposure to blood is more serious than exposure to other body fluids. Hepatitis B virus does not cross intact skin. Exposure to vomit, faeces and sterile or uncontaminated sharp objects poses no risk.**

†An accelerated course of vaccine consists of doses spaced at 0, 1 and 2 months. A booster dose is given at 12 months to those at continuing risk of exposure to HBV.

Source: Communicable Disease Review (1992) 2: R97–101.

Details of other persons for whom immunization is recommended are to be found in *Immunisation Against Infectious Disease* (see Further Reading). The routine immunization course is three doses separated by 1 month and 6 months. An alternative accelerated schedule is four doses separated by 1 month, 2 months and 12 months. Immunization is given intramuscularly (not intradermally and not in the buttock). When using the Energix B preparation (Smith, Kline Beecham) the dose is 10 μg (0.5 ml) in those under 13 years of age and in older individuals 20 μg (1.0 ml). For the H-B-Vax II (Merck Sharp and Dohme) the dose for a child is 5 μg (0.5 ml) under 11 years and 10 μg for older individuals. All vaccinated persons require serologic checking (anti-HBs titres) 2–4 months after completing the course. The aim is to achieve antibody levels of over 100 miu/ml. Persons with levels of under 10 miu/ml are given further doses, but if they still show these low titres they are classified as non-responders and will require hepatitis B specific immunoglobulin if exposed to infection (see Table 56.1).

Post-exposure prophylaxis A common occurrence is of a child receiving an injury from a needle found in the community. There is no convincing evidence that transmission has ever taken place in these circumstances, however an immunization course is started but immunoglobulin is not given. It is considered that immunization has to commence within 7 days if it is going to give protection against infection from the needle-stick injury. This and indications for use of HBV vaccine and HBIG following other types of exposure are shown in Table 56.2. When an exposure has occurred a history must be taken which allows an assessment of risk. In the case of a bite from another child, unless the biting child is known to be HBsAg positive, the hepatitis status of the biting child is assumed to be unknown and immunization given (Table 56.2). For further guidance, see PHLS Hepatitis Subcommittee (1992).

HEPATITIS D INFECTION (DELTA HEPATITIS)

Hepatitis D virus (HDV, the delta agent) is a defective transmissible virus which requires the presence of hepatitis B virus for replication. Infection with HDV is therefore acquired either simultaneously with hepatitis B by those susceptible to infection (co-infection), or subsequently by those who are HBsAg positive (superinfection). Hepatitis D virus is mostly found among injecting drug users and in some of the areas where hepatitis B is prevalent such as Africa and southern Europe. Naturally acquired immunity to hepatitis B virus, and hepatitis B vaccine-induced immunity, protect against infection with hepatitis D virus. Chronic infection occurs and most cases are thought to occur from acute superinfection. It is not yet clear if this infection has any additional significance for children.

FURTHER READING

Department of Health (1995/6) *Immunisation Against Infectious Disease 1995/6*. HMSO, London.

Public Health Laboratory Service Hepatitis Subcommittee (1992). Exposure to Hepatitis B virus: guidance on post-exposure prophylaxis. *CDR Review* **2**: R97–101.

HEPATITIS C

Acute hepatitis C is a notifiable disease*

Information specifically relating to hepatitis C in children is limited at the time of writing. Much of this chapter is derived from what is known about the infection in adults. The field is rapidly evolving and the information should be regarded as provisional. The interested reader is advised to consult the review listed under Further Reading.

ORGANISM

An enveloped RNA virus classified as a flavivirus, hepatitis C virus is the major cause of parenterally acquired non-A, non-B hepatitis.

EPIDEMIOLOGY

As tests for antibody to hepatitis C virus (anti-HCV) have become available and more specific, it is becoming clear that hepatitis C is present worldwide. Prevalence is higher in Japan, the southern USA, Africa, the Middle East and European countries bordering on the Mediterranean. In the UK prevalence of confirmed anti-HCV in previously untested blood donors has been around 1 in 2000, with considerable regional variations from 1 in 1000 to 1 in 3000. Most detected HCV-infected adults in the UK are people who have injected drugs, who were born in higher prevalence countries, or who received blood transfusions before screening was introduced (in the UK blood donations have been screened for anti-HCV since late 1991). Many people with haemophilia were infected by plasma products before inactivation with heat or detergent/solvent became standard in 1985.

Transmission Parenteral exposure (blood transfusions), and prenatal and perinatal vertical exposure (mother to child) are the important modes of transmission for children. It is unclear whether or not vertical transmission also takes place through breast-feeding. Transmission from infected blood transfusion is thought to be almost 100% efficient, while the upper limit described in the limited studies of vertically exposed infants is 13%. In adults, parenteral transmission predominates, through injecting drug use and in association with blood donation. Transmission can occur following needle-stick injury with a risk of transmission of between 3% and 10%. Transmission through sexual intercourse is thought to be relatively inefficient.

NATURAL HISTORY AND CLINICAL FEATURES

The natural history of infection acquired at or before birth or in childhood has yet to be described. A few children have seemingly cleared their infections while hepatitis C infection persists in others and a few have developed active hepatitis. In adult transfusion-associated cases the incubation period from infection to appearance of altered transaminase is usually 6–8 weeks (range 2–26 weeks). Infection

***In the UK the reporting doctor is currently asked to report acute viral hepatitis and to categorize it as type A, B, non-A, non-B (includes hepatitis C and E) or type not know. It is likely that in the future doctors will be asked also to categorize acute hepatitis C.**

persists in 80% of cases and although initial disease is mild or asymptomatic it usually leads to chronic persistent or chronic active hepatitis and it is estimated that 20–30% of infected individuals develop cirrhosis. They may also advance to hepatocellular carcinoma. Infection with particular HCV genotypes may be associated with a worse prognosis in adults.

Diagnosis Testing for hepatitis C is an evolving process. Serologic screening enzyme immunoassays (EIAs) for antibodies to hepatitis C (anti-HCV) are in their third generation and improving. Their sensitivity for anti-HCV is close to 100%. However, false positives occur and can contribute a substantial proportion of positives in low-prevalence populations. Seroconversion may not occur in adults for up to 6 months after exposure (the mean period is 12 weeks) so that early tests relying on antibodies may show false negative results following exposure and infection and repeat testing is often required. Anti-HCV seropositivity detected by EIA has to be followed by supplementary testing with recombinant immunoblot assay (RIBA) or synthetic peptide assays. However, there are difficulties in interpretation of results, and tests for the genome are also used to detect HCV viraemia. The most commonly used is the polymerase chain reaction (PCR). If clinical evidence is strong seronegative results should not deter repeat antibody testing and use of antigen (genome) tests. However, these may also show false negatives due to intermittent expression of viral RNA.

MANAGEMENT

There is insufficient experience of disease in children to make any comment. In adults α interferon is considered to be of value in treating hepatitis due to hepatitis C. No vaccine is available.

PREVENTION OF FURTHER CASES

In a number of countries, including the UK, blood donations are screened for anti-HCV and donation by those who have ever injected drugs is actively discouraged. It remains to be determined whether HCV-infected mothers in industrialized countries should be advised to breast-feed. Until the role of breast-feeding in HCV transmission is clarified it would seem wise to advise against it in situations where the risks associated with use of artificial feeds can be minimized.

FURTHER READING

Van der Poel, Cuypers HT & Reesink HW (1994) Hepatitis C virus six years on. *Lancet* **344**: 1475–1479. (This article is mostly concerned with hepatitis C infection in adults.)

58

HEPATITIS E

Acute hepatitis E is a notifiable disease*

ORGANISM

Hepatitis E virus (HEV) is a small, non-enveloped RNA virus similar in morphology to the Calicivirldae.

***In the UK the reporting doctor is currently asked to report viral hepatitis and to categorize it as type A, B, non-A, non-B (includes hepatitis C and E) or type not known.**

EPIDEMIOLOGY

Hepatitis E infection was originally described as enterically transmitted non-A, non-B hepatitis (ET-NANBH). It produces explosive outbreaks of hepatitis in developing countries, on a background of sporadic endemicity. Large epidemics have occurred in Asia (India, Nepal, Kirghizstan, Myanmar, Indonesia, Pakistan, China), Africa and the Middle Eastern crescent (Ethiopia, Sudan, Algeria, Saudi Arabia), North America (Mexico) and eastern Europe (west Ukraine). During epidemics the attack rate is highest in adolescents and young adults. In one survey in Egypt of endemic NANBH in children, 40% of cases were due to HEV. Recent surveys of HEV suggest that is responsible for 50% of cases of non-A, non-B, non-C hepatitis.

Infection has been described in the UK but usually in travellers returning from endemic regions. Blood donor surveys have demonstrated HEV seropositivity rates of 1.7%, 1.1%, 3.4% and 14% from the UK, Netherlands, California and France respectively. However, in most cases those testing seropositive could have acquired the infection outside Europe.

Transmission Direct person-to-person spread via the faecal–oral route can occur but is rare. In most epidemics it occurs indirectly via food or more commonly water.

Incubation period is 2–9 weeks (mean 6 weeks).

NATURAL HISTORY AND CLINICAL FEATURES

The disease is similar clinically to hepatitis A. It has a preicteric phase of 1–10 days with abdominal pain, nausea and vomiting. The icteric phase lasts 12–15 days with complete recovery within 1 month. Chronic infection has not been described. As with hepatitis A, the disease tends to be milder in children. In developing countries mortality rates are higher than for hepatitis A. It has been reported that pregnant women in the developing world are at high risk of death if they acquire hepatitis E infection.

Diagnosis The mainstay of diagnosis is detection of IgM or IgG antibodies by enzyme-linked immunosorbent assay (ELISA) using HEV recombinant antigens. The sensitivity and specificity of the currently available tests are poor (80–85% and 90% respectively). Virus is present in faeces and serum in largest amounts prior to jaundice. Electron microscopy and RIBA-PCR have been used for diagnosis.

MANAGEMENT

There is no specific antiviral chemotherapy, thus treatment is supportive. No vaccine is available.

HERPES INFECTIONS

59

ORGANISM

Human herpes simplex virus type 1 (HHV-1) and human herpes simplex virus type 2 (HHV-2) are enveloped DNA viruses. They grow readily in tissue culture and can be distinguished by differences in cytopathic effect as well as immunologically.

NEONATAL INFECTION

EPIDEMIOLOGY

Most neonatal herpes simplex results from HHV-2 (genital herpes). Data from the British Paediatric Surveillance Unit (BPSU) suggest that in the UK 1 in 50 000 newborn infants have a clinically significant infection . The incidence in the USA is thought to be 1 in 3000 to 1 in 20 000 births.

Transmission

Almost all cases result from transmission of virus from the genital tract of the mother to her infant. Women with a primary herpes simplex virus infection occurring late in pregnancy are at greatest risk of transmitting infection. The risk of transmission in the presence of herpetic lesions where there is an expression of reactivation, is 3–5%. Virus may be shed from the genital tract in the absence of any visible lesions. Most genital lesions are type 2, but a rising proportion are type 1; very rarely neonatal infection may result from transmission of virus from the cold sore of a mother or medical attendant to the baby.

Incubation period is 2–28 days.

NATURAL HISTORY AND CLINICAL FEATURES

Illness takes three main forms:

- A generalized systemic infection with respiratory distress from pneumonia and hepatitis.
- An encephalitic illness, with fits and altered level of consciousness.
- Localized infection of the skin, eyes and mouth (SEM). The typical skin lesion is the vesicle, which may be seen in the mouth also. A conjunctivitis or keratitis may be seen in the eyes, as well as a chorioretinitis. In about one-third of cases, SEM lesions progress to either encephalopathy or systemic infection.

Most cases occur within 1 week of birth, but illness may be delayed for up to a month. There is a high mortality from systemic or neurological disease even when antiviral treatment is used. Severe neurological disability occurs in more than half of survivors of the encephalitis. Those infants who developed SEM are likely to have further local recurrences during childhood.

MANAGEMENT

The high mortality and morbidity may be related to the difficulty in diagnosis, particularly when SEM lesions are not present. Most infections in the newborn follow primary genital infection, which may not be apparent. Treatment of established or suspected infection is with acyclovir intravenously (10 mg/kg per day). Appropriate viral studies should be performed; these include cultures of throat and conjunctival swab, blood and cerebrospinal fluid. Vesicle fluid can be cultured or examined under electron microscopy. A number of rapid diagnostic methods are available but none are in general use.

In infants born vaginally to mothers with active herpetic lesions specimens for viral culture should be collected at 48 hours. If the swabs are positive acyclovir treatment is started if there is a strong likelihood that the mother has a primary infection. In all cases infants should be treated at the earliest sign of symptoms. When there are reactivated lesions then it is appropriate to take specimens at 48 hours and observe the infant in hospital for a week, by which time the risk of infection is very low. Infants with active infection should be isolated.

PREVENTION OF INFECTION

When it is known that a mother has active infection, the infant should be delivered by caesarean section once she goes into labour; this should be performed as soon as possible, preferably within 4 hours. Attendants and mothers with facial sores should be very careful to avoid close contact of the affected area with the infant and wear masks.

CHILDHOOD INFECTION

EPIDEMIOLOGY

Herpes simplex virus type 1 infections are common, and about 50% of adults are seropositive to this virus. Children may develop gingivostomatitis, labial herpes from reactivation, ophthalmic infection and herpetic whitlows on fingers. Herpes tends to be more severe in children with eczema (eczema herpeticum). Very rarely herpes encephalitis may occur *either* as a primary or reactivation of infection. In a child with genital herpes sexual abuse must be considered a likely mode of transmission (see Chapter 8).

Transmission Most oral and skin infections result from person-to-person spread from secretions, either from a lesion or, more often, from the oral secretions of an asymptomatic carrier. Virus is present in particularly high concentrations in vesicles during the first 24 hours.

Incubation period is 2–14 days.

NATURAL HISTORY AND CLINICAL FEATURES

In many children, primary infection is asymptomatic, but reactivation occurs resulting in vesicles on the lips which may be painful or itching. Some children develop a painful gingivostomatitis with lesions on the vermilion borders of the lips, the tongue and mucous membranes in the mouth. They may need hospital admission, because it may be difficult to drink. The symptoms are at their worst for about 2 days. Eye infection may involve the conjunctiva, cornea and skin around the eye. Dendritic ulcers may form on the cornea and can leave permanent scarring. Children with eczema may develop multiple vesicles over the affected areas of skin.

Herpes encephalitis should be considered in any child with an acute encephalopathy. The signs include fever, an altered level of consciousness, and focal fits. There is sometimes a history of previous herpes infection. Cerebrospinal fluid (CSF) may be normal, blood-stained, or show a lymphocytosis or increased protein levels. A computed tomographic scan may show features of temporal lobe ischaemia and inflammation. Although encephalitis does not appear to be any more common in the immunosuppressed, other infection may be more severe and require urgent treatment.

Diagnosis is by electron microscopy of vesicle fluid, and culture of blood, respiratory secretions and vesicle fluid. The virus is rarely found in the CSF. The diagnostic method of choice is PCR of herpes DNA. It has a high sensitivity and specificity. Brain biopsy is rarely indicated.

MANAGEMENT

Management is of particular importance in ophthalmic and encephalitic herpes and in the immunocompromised. The effect of oral acyclovir is only marginal in cases of gingivostomatitis and it should be started very early in the course of infection if it is to be effective. Topical acyclovir is of little benefit for recurrent cold sores. Ophthalmological advice should be sought in the treatment of ocular involvement. In children with herpes encephalitis, acyclovir has been shown to be beneficial. This should be given intravenously in a dose of 500 mg/m^2 three times daily, for at least 14 days otherwise relapse may occur. Similarly high doses should be used in the immunocompromised.

PREVENTION OF INFECTION

People with cold sores on their mouths or face should not kiss children. Medical attendants with herpetic whitlows should wear gloves.

60 INFECTIOUS MONONUCLEOSIS (GLANDULAR FEVER)

ORGANISM

Epstein–Barr virus (EBV) or human herpesvirus-4 is a herpesvirus. Similar clinical illness can occasionally be caused by cytomegalovirus (see Chapter 44) and the protozoan *Toxoplasma gondii* (Chapter 96).

EPIDEMIOLOGY

Epstein–Barr virus only infects the human host. Most people are infected in childhood or adolescence so that serological evidence of past infection is present in up to 90% of individuals by early adulthood. Many seroconversions particularly in early childhood seem to be asymptomatic. Symptomatic infection—infectious mononucleosis or glandular fever—is most common in adolescence.

Like other herpesviruses, EBV exhibits latency and has been shown to reactivate in immunocomprised individuals such as those undergoing renal transplantation. It is associated with lymphoproliferative disease (of B-cell lineage) in such patients which is either polyclonal or true malignant lymphoma. In X-linked lymphoproliferative disorder (Duncan's syndrome), affected boys develop severe illness with EBV, often with a fatal outcome. The virus has been implicated in the oncogenesis of nasopharyngeal carcinoma in SE China and Burkitt's lymphoma in Africa, and may also be involved in the development of other B-cell lymphomas.

Transmission is directly via saliva, by kissing or other close contact, or by droplet transmission. Reactivation disease occurs in the immune suppressed.

Incubation period is 30–50 days.

Period of infectivity is for several months after acute infection and may be lifelong.

NATURAL HISTORY AND CLINICAL FEATURES

The clinical features vary from asymptomatic infection through typical glandular fever to (rarely) severe, prolonged and sometimes fatal illness. Glandular fever is characterized by fever, malaise, pharyngitis (often exudative) and cervical lymphadenopathy. Hepatosplenomegaly and hepatitis (usually anicteric) are relatively common features. Oedema in the throat may occur leading to 'nasal' voice and difficulty in swallowing. A sparse, maculopapular rash is present in 10–15% of cases. Petechiae may be seen on the palate. Most cases develop a florid rash if given ampicillin or amoxycillin. In severe cases central nervous system involvement with meningoencephalitis, transverse myelitis or Guillain–Barré syndrome may develop. Myocarditis, orchitis and blood dyscrasias can also occur. Severe, and usually fatal, disease in X-linked lymphoproliferative syndrome is associated with one or more of the following prolonged and severe infectious mononucleosis, aplastic anaemia, hypogammaglobulinaemia or lymphoma.

Diagnosis is usually based on the typical clinical features. The blood picture shows a lymphocytosis with atypical lymphocytes. A heterophile antibody (agglutinating sheep red blood cells) is produced and is the basis of the slide agglutination tests—Monospot and Paul–Bunnell tests. This antibody does not usually appear until the second week of illness or even later, and in young children may not be produced at all. Specific EBV serology is more reliable. A positive IgM to viral capsid antigen (VCA) is diagnostic early in the disease. Immunoglobulin G anti-VCA indicates past infection but a positive titre with a negative anti-EBNA (antibody to Epstein–Barr nuclei antigen—an antibody produced very late in the illness) is suggestive of recent infection. Antibody response to an 'early' antigen (EA) can also be used in diagnosis.

Differential diagnosis includes other causes of infectious mononucleosis-like illness such as cytomegalovirus infection and acquired toxoplasmosis, as well as other causes of pharyngitis (streptococcus, diphtheria, respiratory viruses) and other hepatitides. The blood picture may be confused with acute leukaemia, necessitating bone marrow examination.

MANAGEMENT

Management is generally symptomatic with analgesics and antipyretics. Corticosteroids help when massive pharyngeal swelling threatens airway obstruction.

PREVENTION OF FURTHER CASES

Isolation is not required and there is no quarantine period. Vaccines against Epstein–Barr virus are not available.

INFLUENZA

ORGANISM

An enveloped helical RNA virus, the influenza virus is a member of the orthomyxoviruses with three antigenic types—A, B and C. The A strains show considerable variability. They are further subclassified by the haemagglutinin (H1, H2 and H3) and neuraminidase (N1 and N2) antigens. Minor changes in antigenic structure are known as antigenic drifts, whereas major changes, e.g. H2 to H3, are known as antigenic shifts.

EPIDEMIOLOGY

Every winter there is an excess of respiratory deaths due to influenza. At intervals, when a sufficiently different strain arises, there are epidemics. The last epidemic in the UK was in 1989–90. When a major antigenic shift in influenza A occurs a pandemic results. There have been four this century, the last being in 1977. The disease is highly infectious and outbreaks in schools and other institutions are common.

Transmission is from person to person by droplet or direct contact. The disease is highly infectious for 24 hours before and 48 hours after symptoms appear.

Incubation period is 1–3 days.

NATURAL HISTORY AND CLINICAL FEATURES

Influenza is predominantly a respiratory illness with a rapid onset of fever, headache, general malaise and generalized aches and pains. Upper respiratory tract symptoms of cough, sore throat and coryza follow soon after but may be absent in young infants where the clinical picture can be non-specific resembling sepsis. A secondary bacterial otitis media is not uncommon. Abdominal pain, nausea, vomiting, conjunctival inflammation, croup and pneumonia may also occur. Especially in debilitated patients, the latter may be due to a secondary *Staphylococcus aureus* or *Klebsiella pneumoniae* infection. Primary influenzal pneumonia also occurs. Influenza B, in particular, has been associated with an acute myositis with calf tenderness and pain on walking. Reye's syndrome may follow influenza, especially influenza B, though this has become less common since many countries have banned the use of aspirin in children. Toxic shock syndrome, myocarditis, encephalitis, Guillain–Barré syndrome and myoglobulinuria have all been reported. There is also some evidence to suggest that meningococcal infection has a higher incidence in the period following influenza.

The mortality in children is low and particularly affects children with pre-existing chronic disorders, including those with neurodevelopmental problems. Influenza has been noted to alter the metabolism of some drugs, in particular theophylline, producing higher blood levels than would otherwise have been expected.

Diagnosis The clinical picture may be similar to that caused by a number of respiratory viruses including parainfluenza viruses types 1, 2 and 3, adenoviruses and coxsackievirus groups A and B. The white cell count may be normal or show a moderate leucopenia. When it is important to make an accurate diagnosis, culture of the virus from nasopharyngeal secretions (aspirate or swab) can be attempted. It takes 2–6 days to grow in tissue culture. Virus isolation is best done in the first 72 hours as virus shedding decreases markedly after this. Antigen detection by immunofluorescence or enzyme-linked immunosorbent assay (ELISA) is also possible. Complement fixation, haemagglutination inhibition and neutralization tests to detect rising levels of antibodies only allow the diagnosis to be made in retrospect.

MANAGEMENT

In the majority of cases management is symptomatic, using antipyretics and analgesics. Prophylactic antibiotics are rarely indicated in children, but suspected bacterial complications should be appropriately investigated and treated. Until the bacterial pathogen has been identified, an antistaphylococcal agent should be included in any 'blind' treatment. Amantadine (5 mg/kg as one or two daily doses) may shorten the course of the primary infection if due to influenza A, but there is no evidence that it prevents secondary infections which are the main cause of serious morbidity and mortality in children. It is rarely used in children. Ribavirin has an effect in vitro against influenza A and B and can be used in severe infection in compromised children, i.e. those who are immunocompromised and those with serious cardiac or respiratory problems.

PREVENTION OF FURTHER CASES

Isolation during the early stages is the only way to prevent the spread of disease. However, even this has only limited effect as the patient is infectious before symptoms appear as well as after.

Chemoprophylaxis Amantidine can prevent infection with influenza A; however, it is rarely used in children and vaccination of high-risk individuals is to be preferred.

Vaccination Vaccination against influenza is recommended for those of all ages with chronic respiratory and cardiac disease; those with chronic renal failure and endocrine disorders; and those who are immunosuppressed. There is also evidence to suggest that it should be given to children with neurodevelopmental disorders, e.g. Down's syndrome and cerebral palsy. It is not usually recommended for healthy individuals. Some would argue that all children in boarding schools should be immunized, because influenza would spread rapidly once introduced.

Because of the antigenic drift, each year the Joint Committee on Vaccinations and Immunizations (JCVI) makes recommendations as to which virus strains should be covered by the vaccine to be used in the forthcoming year. Vaccination should take place in October or early November. Protective levels of antibody take 10–14 days to develop. There is little difference between the vaccines currently available, but not all have a licence for children under 4 years old. Children between 6 months and 12 years old should have two doses of vaccine 4–6 weeks apart, if receiving it for the first time. Subsequently, doses should be given at yearly intervals. No vaccine currently has a licence for children under 6 months old. Current vaccines are prepared in hens' eggs and should not be given to individuals with a history of severe hypersensitivity reactions to egg.

INVASIVE HELMINTHIASIS CAUSING MULTISYSTEM DISEASE (CYSTICERCOSIS, GNATHOSTOMIASIS, HYDATID DISEASE, SCHISTOSOMIASIS, STRONGYLOIDIASIS, TRICHINOSIS)

(See also Chapters 30 (*Ascaris* infection) and 95 (Toxocariasis).

ORGANISMS

This chapter describes conditions caused by a number of organisms: *Clonorchis*, *Echinococcus granulosus*, *E. multilocularis* and *E. vogeli* (causing hydatid disease), *Fasciola hepatica* (fascioliasis or liver fluke disease), *Gnathostoma spinigerum*, *Schistosoma japonicum*, *S. mansoni*, *S. haematobium* (schistosomiasis and Katayama fever), *Strongyloides stercoralis* (strongyloidiasis and *Strongyloides* hyperinfection syndrome), *Taenia solium* (cysticercosis) and *Trichinella spiralis* (trichinosis).

EPIDEMIOLOGY

Gnathostoma spinigerum is mainly confined to south-east Asia and is a parasite of dogs and cats, being accidentally transmitted to humans by the ingestion of undercooked fish or poultry.

Fasciola hepatica, the liver fluke, is a parasite of sheep, cattle and other large animals and occurs worldwide, including the UK. Cysts are ingested in contaminated water plants such as watercress.

Strongyloides stercoralis is a human gut parasite but can also exist as a free-living form in damp soil and occurs throughout the tropics. Infection arises when larvae from stool (including autoinfection) or contaminated soil penetrate the skin or gut wall.

Schistosomiasis (bilharzia) is caused by parasites which are predominantly of human origin and is found in parts of sub-Saharan and northern Africa, the Middle East, south-east Asia, Central and South America and some Caribbean islands. The larvae (cercariae), which have developed in snails, penetrate the skin of anyone swimming or wading in contaminated water.

Cysticercosis occurs following ingestion of food or water contaminated with *Taenia solium* eggs (cf. tapeworm which is due to eating improperly cooked pork containing *T. solium* larvae). The eggs remain viable in soil for many weeks after excretion in human faeces. It is also possible for a patient harbouring an adult worm to autoinfect from anus to mouth via the hands. Cysticercosis is endemic in South and Central America, south-east Asia and parts of Africa. It affects both sexes equally and may become apparent in infancy. The adult tapeworms of *Echinococcus granulosus*, *E. multilocularis* and *E. vogeli* are found in dogs (and other Canidae), foxes (but now also spread to domestic dogs and cats) and Latin American bush dogs, respectively. The larval forms (hydatid cysts) are found normally in herbivores (sheep and cattle) and small rodents (voles, rats and mice) but occur in humans following ingestion of eggs excreted in canine faeces. *Echinococcus granulosus* is the most common cause of human hydatid disease and is found worldwide particularly in association with sheep-raising areas. *Echinococcus multilocularis* is enzootic in subarctic areas and *E. vogeli* in Central America.

Trichinella spiralis has a worldwide distribution in humans and carnivorous animals. The major (but decreasing) reservoir for human infection is the pig. People become infected by ingestion of improperly or incompletely cooked pork containing encysted larvae. In industrialized countries the incidence of infection is decreasing: for example, in the USA autopsy surveys in 1941 and 1970 showed the prevalence had dropped from 16% to 4.7%. This has largely been achieved by banning raw pork scraps from pig feed, deep-freezing meat (which kills cysts) and education on cooking meat.

Incubation period These primary systemic illnesses usually present within 3 months of infection, although *Strongyloides* can be harboured as a symptomless infection for many years until systemic invasion occurs following an event that lowers immunity. For both cysticercosis and hydatid disease the incubation varies according to the site of infection and rate of growth of cysts. For example in cysticercosis, full maturation of cysts takes 3–4 months, when they achieve diameters of 2 mm to 2 cm. Hydatid cysts reach a diameter of 1 cm in 5 months but may continue to grow to a size of 35 cm containing litres of 'hydatid sand'. The incubation of trichinosis is 5–15 days (average 10 days).

NATURAL HISTORY AND CLINICAL FEATURES

Gnathostomiasis may present with recurrent cutaneous swellings, pulmonary and peritoneal effusions. *Strongyloides* hyperinfection syndrome may rarely present with the primary infection, although it is more commonly seen in children who have carried the organism in the gut for many years and then become immunocompromised, for instance following renal transplantation, the onset of leukaemia or human immunodeficiency virus (HIV) infection. This leads to massive tissue invasion by *Strongyloides* larvae. Clinical features include acute onset of severe fever, diarrhoea, pneumonitis and sometimes eosinophilic meningoencephalitis. The blood eosinophil count may not be raised. Gram-negative septicaemia is also a common complication. The mortality is high in the immunocompromised.

Katayama fever is seen 2–6 weeks after infection with schistosome cercariae when the child develops high fever, hepatosplenomegaly and a very high blood eosinophilia. There is always a history of contact with fresh water in an area endemic for schistosomiasis.

Cysticercosis can develop in any organ but the common sites are brain, subcutaneous tissues, muscle and eye. There are usually multiple cysts. The chance of clinical infection is less if infection is light. In muscle, cysts frequently calcify and do not initiate disease, but subcutaneous infection—painless lumps varying in size from that of a rice grain to a pigeon's egg—may become apparent, predominately over the abdomen. Neurocysticercosis usually appears 5–7 years after infection. The most common presentation is of epilepsy but single cysts may present as for a space-occupying lesion, with raised intracranial pressure and focal neurological features. Spinal cord involvement is rare but may present as compression or arachnoiditis. Ocular cysts (often subretinal) may lead to blindness. Death of cysticerci may be accompanied by increased disease manifestation as an intense inflammatory response occurs.

In hydatid disease there is usually a single cyst, but in up to 30% of cases multiple cysts (usually in a single organ) can occur. Cysts have been described in every organ system: favoured sites are liver, lungs, spleen, brain, eye, heart, bone and genitourinary system. Brain hydatid disease is more common in children than in adults and bone cysts are seen in infants. Infection becomes manifest due either to expansion of the cysts or to rupture and release of cyst contents. The signs and symptoms will depend on the site of the cyst; for example, bone cysts give bone pain and pathological fractures; pulmonary cysts give fever, cough, chest pain and haemoptysis (in adults if the cysts rupture into a bronchus the patient may complain about coughing up 'grape-skins'), and brain cysts give raised intracranial pressure and fits but few localizing signs.

Most infections with *Trichinella spiralis* are asymptomatic. When clinically expressed, disease occurs in three phases. The intestinal phase occurs as diarrhoea with abdominal pain due to penetration of the intestinal wall by larvae that have been born to the mature encysted worms. Larvae leave the intestine via lymphatics, enter the blood stream and are distributed to striated muscle throughout the body. In the muscle fibres, they initiate the phase of muscle invasion with fever, eosinophilia, myositis and the classical sign of periorbital oedema. Dyspnoea occurs due to invasions of the respiratory muscles. In moderate infection the convalescent phase begins in the fifth week of disease. Fatalities occur 4–6 weeks after infection owing to cardiac or central nervous system involvement.

Diagnosis The initial diagnosis of each of the individual syndromes is often made on clinical features alone, as specific antibody tests are usually negative at this stage, except in strongyloidiasis. *Strongyloides* larvae can be found in stool or sputum during hyperinfection if examined immediately by an experienced observer. Microscopy of stool or urine may reveal eggs in schistosomiasis. In long-standing cases, the bladder may be calcified. Serology is often difficult to interpret.

The specific diagnosis of cysticercosis generally follows radiological demonstration of calcified cysts in brain or muscle, histological examination of surgically removed subcutaneous nodes or visualization of the cysticercus in the eye. Serological tests—indirect haemagglutination or enzyme immunoassay (EIA)—are available, but false negatives occur regularly in central nervous system disease.

Asymptomatic or symptomatic hydatid cysts are often picked up on radiography where the disease is prevalent. Outlined cysts with fluid levels may be seen. Non-surgical aspiration of cysts is dangerous and should be avoided. Serological tests such as indirect haemagglutination or EIA can be of value but false negatives occur particularly in pulmonary disease and in children. The Casoni skin test is less reliable than serological tests.

The diagnosis of trichinosis is primarily clinical. Muscle biopsy to demonstrate encysted larvae can be of benefit.

Other diagnoses to be considered in a child with acute illness and eosinophilia include haematological malignancies and an acute vasculitic illness.

MANAGEMENT

Strongyloides hyperinfection syndrome requires urgent therapy with thiabendazole 25 mg/kg twice daily for at least 3 days, albendazole 400 mg daily for at least 5 days (by nasogastric tube if necessary). Ivermectin (200 μg/kg as a single dose) is becoming the drug of choice for chronic strongyloidiasis and may soon be the drug of choice for hyperinfection syndrome. Intravenous antibiotics are also required for the septicaemia. This condition carries a high mortality.

The other acute syndromes, especially Katayama fever, may be worsened by anthelmintic therapy in the acute phase, but steroids can be of benefit by dampening the vigorous immune response. Specific anthelmintic therapy, such as praziquantel 20 mg/kg twice daily for 2 days in the case of schistosomiasis, would be introduced after the acute symptoms have resolved and an aetiology has been confirmed.

In cysticercosis many cases are asymptomatic and require no treatment. In some cases surgical removal is needed, but therapy has been revolutionized by praziquantel. For neurocysticercosis, dosage is 50 mg/kg daily in three divided doses for 15 days. Concurrent administration of dexamethasone may be of benefit to suppress inflammation around moribund cysts. Praziquantel should not be used for ocular cysticercosis.

Hydatid disease is often treated by surgical removal (with a 3–5% mortality rate). Albendazole and praziquantel should also be given over the perioperative period. Albendazole can be useful in inoperable or recurrent disease but is of less value in bone disease.

In severe trichinosis corticosteroids should be administered; they can be life-saving.

PREVENTION OF FURTHER CASES

Fasciola hepatica is usually acquired after eating wild watercress or other water plants. Cultivated watercress is safe. *Strongyloides stercoralis* is initially caught by walking barefoot on damp soil in the tropics, and this is prevented by the use of footwear. It is important to screen children from the tropics for this infection prior to the use of immunosuppressives. Schistosomiasis may be avoided by keeping out of rivers, streams and lakes in endemic areas. Prevention of cysticercosis and hydatid disease is by avoiding ingestion of pig and dog tapeworm eggs. Prevention of trichinosis can be achieved by good pig husbandry, storing pork deep-frozen and ensuring that pork (including sausages and 'burgers') is cooked well prior to ingestion.

KAWASAKI DISEASE

Named after the paediatrician who first described it in Japan in 1967, Kawasaki disease is also known as the mucocutaneous lymph node syndrome.

ORGANISM

Unknown. Many features of the illness suggest it has an infectious aetiology but, to date, a causative agent has not been identified.

EPIDEMIOLOGY

The disease is particularly common in Japan, affecting 1 in 1000 children. It is less common in western countries, though probably under-reported. Young children are predominantly affected, with the peak incidence occurring in the second year of life and most cases before the fifth birthday. Asian children show the highest incidence. The male to female ratio is 1.6:1. Second attacks are occasionally seen. Clusters of cases have been described often in the winter months. The epidemiological pattern of the disease as well as the clinical features first led to the suggestion that the disease has an infectious aetiology.

Transmission Direct case-to-case spread has not been demonstrated. The disease is more common in siblings but this may indicate a genetic susceptibility.

Incubation period is unknown.

NATURAL HISTORY AND CLINICAL FEATURES

The illness begins with an abrupt onset of fever which can be up to 40 °C, generally has an unremitting pattern and can last up to 15 days or occasionally longer. The child is usually miserable and may be irritable. Empirical antibiotic therapy has no effect on the fever. The disease induces a vasculitic process and most of the clinical features can be explained on this basis. The characteristic features develop at around the third day of the illness.They include:

- Eyes—non-exudative conjunctivitis.
- Mouth—mucositis with intense erythema; swollen, fissured lips and strawberry tongue.
- Lymph nodes—cervical lymphadenopathy, bilateral or unilateral, with glands more than 1.5 cm in diameter and sometimes much larger.
- Skin—generalized intensely erythematous rash which may be maculopapular or produce a blotchy or confluent erythema.
- Hands and feet—palmar and plantar erythema often with oedema. As the illness subsides in the second to third week, characteristic peeling of fingers and toes occurs.

While classical disease produces at least four of the above features together with fever, atypical cases with fewer features can occur.

Other features of the disease may include diarrhoea, sterile pyuria, arthritis, uveitis and aseptic meningitis. Cardiac involvement is potentially the most serious. In the acute phase a myocarditis or pericarditis may occur leading to heart failure or arrhythmias. Damage to the coronary artery walls by the vasculitic process can lead to aneurysm formation and this usually occurs in the convalescent phase of the illness. This complication has been reported as occurring in up to 20% of untreated cases. Coronary thrombosis may complicate aneurysm formation. In most cases aneurysms resolve over the succeeding 12 months. There is increasing concern, however, that the arteries may not return entirely to normal resulting in a greater risk of coronary artery disease later in life. The acute mortality rate (usually from cardiac involvement) is 0.5–2%.

Diagnosis is based on the clinical features which become more characteristic as the illness progesses. During the acute phase there is usually a neutrophil leucocytosis, raised acute phase reactants and increased sedimentation rate. Thrombocytosis occurs in the convalescent phase and may reach alarming levels ($>1000 \times 10^9$/L). Electrocardiography and echocardiography during the acute phase may show cardiac involvement. However, false reassurance should not be derived from the finding of a negative echocardiogram at this stage since most coronary aneurysms occur later on.

The differential diagnosis of Kawasaki disease is wide. Staphylococcal or streptococcal toxin-mediated diseases such as scarlet fever or toxic shock syndrome have many similar initial features. Since many children will have received empirical antibiotics, drug hypersensitivity reaction may need to be considered. Other differential diagnoses include measles, other viral exanthems, Stevens–Johnson syndrome and systemic onset juvenile chronic arthritis.

MANAGEMENT

Though the disease is self-limiting, early diagnosis is important since treatment with intravenous immunoglobulin (IVIG) at this stage has been shown to reduce the incidence of coronary artery involvement. High-dose IVIG is given either as four daily doses of 400 mg/kg or as a single infusion of 2 g/kg over 12 hours. The latter is marginally more efficacious in shortening the length of the illness. At the same time aspirin therapy (80–100 mg/kg in four divided doses) is commenced and continued until the acute inflammatory phase has subsided. Salicylate levels should be monitored. In the convalescent phase aspirin is continued in low (antithrombotic) doses (3–5 mg/kg as a single daily dose). This is continued for at least 3 months or, if coronary aneurysms have occurred, until these are shown to have resolved on echocardiography. Corticosteroids increase the incidence of coronary disease and are therefore contraindicated. Echocardiographic monitoring is required at approximately 3 weeks and again at 8 weeks after onset of the illness. Follow-up studies beyond this time are only indicated for patients in whom cardiac disease has been detected.

It should be borne in mind that high-dose IVIG may interfere with subsequent immunization with live viral vaccines for several months.

PREVENTION OF FURTHER CASES

Until the identity of the aetiologic agent is established this is not feasible. Increasing awareness of the possibility of this disease in young febrile children and early institution of therapy should help reduce its morbidity and mortality.

LEGIONNAIRES' DISEASE

64

ORGANISM

Legionella spp. (in particular *L. pneumophila*)—a group of Gram-negative bacilli.

EPIDEMIOLOGY

Infection with *Legionella* in normal children is probably uncommon and usually results in a mild and self-limiting illness which would rarely be noticed. However, disease can be severe in immunocompromised children. The effects of *Legionella* species are considerably more common in adults. *Legionella* sp. disease has two manifestations: Pontiac fever, a self-limiting, influenza-like febrile illness, and legionnaires' disease, a severe pulmonary and multisystem infection. It is suggested, but not proved, that Pontiac fever is the result of inhalation of inactive organisms. Legionnaires' disease is frequently fatal (around 15% in reported cases in the UK). The organism can exist long-term in domestic and industrial water systems. It is considered that domestic water systems cause most cases; however, of more community concern are water systems producing aerosols such as incorrectly maintained air-conditioning and water cooling towers—these can lead to outbreaks due to the exposure of numbers of individuals to common sources of infection. Nosocomial infections also occur, especially among debilitated patients.

Transmission is by inhalation of organisms. Person-to-person spread has never been demonstrated.

Incubation period is unknown in children. In adults it is 1–2 days for Pontiac fever and 2–10 days for legionnaires' disease.

NATURAL HISTORY AND CLINICAL FEATURES

In the normal child an infection may be asymptomatic. In the immunocompromised child (e.g. a child on chemotherapy) pneumonia and/or systemic infection can occur. This may include central nervous system, liver, gastrointestinal and renal problems. Pontiac fever is the occurrence of systemic illness without pneumonia and is usually self-limiting.

Diagnosis of legionnaires' disease requires a diagnosis of pneumonia and laboratory evidence of infection with *Legionella* sp. The latter is by direct recovery and culture, or seroconversion or antigen tests on urine or respiratory specimens; DNA probes and monoclonal antibodies are used for further characterization of clinical isolates, which needs to be carried out at a reference centre in order to determine whether a case is sporadic or can be linked to a common source of infection. In England and Wales specialist reference and confirmatory testing is carried out at the Atypical Pneumonia Unit, Central Public Health Laboratory (Tel: 0181 200 4400).

MANAGEMENT

Erythromycin is the drug of choice. In immunocompromised children prompt high-dose intravenous therapy is required, and the addition of another agent such as rifampicin or ciprofloxacin may be beneficial.

PREVENTION OF FURTHER CASES

In all cases of legionnaires' disease, the consultant in communicable disease control or the director of public health should be informed so that epidemiologic and laboratory investigations can be undertaken. Cases in England should be reported to the National Surveillance Scheme for Legionnaires Disease at the Communicable Disease Surveillance Centre (Tel: 0181 200 6868).

Regular maintenance of air-conditioning and hot-water systems in public buildings, especially hospitals, is essential to prevent outbreaks of this infection.

65 LEISHMANIASIS: VISCERAL (KALA-AZAR) AND CUTANEOUS LEISHMANIASIS

ORGANISM

Protozoan species *Leishmania*: visceral leishmaniasis is caused by *Leishmania donovani*; cutaneous leishmaniasis is caused by *Leishmania major* (Old World) or *L. tropica*, *L. brasiliensis* or *L. mexicana* (New World).

EPIDEMIOLOGY

Leishmaniasis is a vector-borne zoonosis. The reservoir is in a variety of warm-blooded animals including dogs and rodents, and the vector to humans is the sandfly. Visceral leishmaniasis is commonly found in rural areas of most tropical and many subtropical countries, including those in Asia, the Middle East, Africa, South and Central America, Russia, the Iberian peninsula and the Mediterranean islands. Cutaneous leishmaniasis is also found in both the Old and New Worlds; the Indian subcontinent, all of Africa (except southern Africa), the Mediterranean, and Central and South America.

Transmission is by the bites of sandflies infected from mammals.

Incubation period

- Visceral leishmaniasis—varies from a few weeks to 6 months after a sandfly bite, though longer periods have been reported.
- Cutaneous leishmaniasis—a few weeks after the sandfly bite.

Period of infectivity Humans are considered an end host and no further transmission has been reported.

NATURAL HISTORY AND CLINICAL FEATURES

Visceral Following penetration of the skin by the sandfly, *Leishmania donovani* move through the reticuloendothelial system and concentrate in the bone marrow, liver and spleen. There is malaise, fever and loss of appetite and weight. Signs include enlargement of lymph nodes, liver and spleen. Reticuloendothelial failure causing anaemia, leucopenia and thrombocytopenia may occur. If infection is untreated, haemorrhage and secondary infections are common and may be fatal.

Cutaneous Local proliferation in the skin results in a red nodule where the bite took place. These are usually on exposed areas, especially the face. The nodule usually later ulcerates. There may be satellite lesion and regional lymphadenopathy.

Diagnosis

- Visceral—By taking samples from affected tissues (e.g. liver biopsy or lymph nodes) and looking for *Leishmania* spp. using Giemsa stain.
- Cutaneous—by taking samples by scraping or a punch biopsy taken from the edge of the lesion and looking for *Leishmania* spp. using Giemsa stain.

Serology and culture may be of value but are only carried out at special centres such as the London and Liverpool Schools of Tropical Medicine.

MANAGEMENT

Specialist advice should be sought. Visceral leishmaniasis is treated by parenteral pentamidine isethionate given as a series of *deep* intramuscular injections; 3–4 mg/kg given on alternate days for up to 15 injections.

In cutaneous leishmaniasis many lesions heal spontaneously, and a conservative approach is recommended if the lesion is not severe and follow-up is possible. If treatment is needed it is the same as for visceral disease.

PREVENTION OF FURTHER CASES

Prevention of the disease is by preventing insect bites.

LISTERIOSIS

66

See also Chapter 2.

ORGANISM

Listeria monocytogenes is a Gram-positive rod with the ability to grow at low temperatures. There are 13 serotypes. Early infection is normally associated with 1/2a and 1/2b, with late disease caused by 4b.

EPIDEMIOLOGY

Listeria monocytogenes is found in cattle, other animals and silage. On occasions it enters the food chain, and food-borne transmission is a frequent source of infection with sporadic cases and common-source outbreaks occurring. *Listeria* has been isolated from unpasteurized soft cheeses, pâté, salads and microwave-ready meals. Outbreaks of infection have been traced to pasteurized soft cheese contaminated during processing, and to silage through occupational exposure. Groups of patients at risk of severe consequences from infection are pregnant women and neonates, immunocompromised patients and the elderly. Mothers can exhibit vaginal, faecal and urine carriage, which can be asymptomatic, and as a consequence neonatal infections occur. There was an increase in neonatal infection during 1988 as a result of contamination of pâté manufactured in Belgium and a major outbreak associated with soft cheese in France in 1993.

Transmission Transplacental transmission can occur to the fetus during acute bacteraemia in the mother. *Listeria monocytogenes* may colonize the genital tract so that the neonate may acquire the organism during delivery and ascending infection can also occur. Transvaginal spread is thought to be unusual. Most late-onset neonatal cases result from hospital cross-infection although they may be acquired from the mother during birth. Nosocomial transmission has been described in day-care centres.

Incubation period For both neonatal and adult food-borne transmission the incubation period is variable from a few days to 10 weeks. Shorter periods, with development of symptoms in the few days after birth are more characteristic of neonatal infection; however, neonates can also develop illness late after birth and longer periods of incubation are more typical in adults.

NATURAL HISTORY AND CLINICAL FEATURES

Congenital infection may result in stillbirth or a septicaemic illness normally within 48 hours of delivery, with meningitis being the most severe complication. Meconium staining of the liquor is said to be associated with infection even in the preterm infant. Infants may develop respiratory distress as a result of pneumonia with a similar presentation to group B streptococcal infection. A characteristic feature of the illness is a red papular rash (roseola) seen on the face, trunk and pharynx. Meningitis may occur. The prognosis is better with later onset infection. In adults (including pregnant mothers) the infection may result in an influenza-like illness with headache, backache, diarrhoea and abdominal pain. Meningitis also occurs in the immunocompromised and elderly patients.

Diagnosis Early-onset infection may be characterized by leucopenia. In meningitis either neutrophils or mononuclear cells predominate in the cerebrospinal fluid (CSF). The organism can be isolated from blood, CSF, meconium, placenta and gastric washings, though it may take several days for the isolate to be confirmed because of the difficulties in distinguishing *Listeria* from other bacilli found in non-sterile sites.

MANAGEMENT

Ampicillin and gentamicin, when combined, have a synergistic effect and are the recommended antibiotics in children. Cephalosporins are ineffective. The organism is intracellular and therefore long courses of treatment should be used, 14 days for septicaemia and 21 days for meningitis. In neonates it is customary to include gentamicin for the first two weeks and then to finish the course with seven days of ampicillin alone.

PREVENTION OF FURTHER CASES

Pregnant women should avoid foodstuffs from which they are at risk of contracting *Listeria* infection. These foods include pâté, unwashed salads, and unpasteurized cheese and other milk products. They should ensure that microwave-ready meals are adequately cooked. Pregnant women should also not work with silage. When cases occur a careful history should be taken so that common-source outbreaks can be detected and the consultant in communicable disease control must be alerted. Isolates of *Listeria* must be referred centrally* to permit the further characterization of organisms and the detection of common-source outbreaks occurring through contamination of the food chain.

Domestic refrigerators should be well maintained to ensure correct temperature control.

LYME DISEASE

ORGANISM

Lyme disease is caused by a spirochaete, *Borrelia burgdorferi*.

EPIDEMIOLOGY

Lyme disease is rare in the UK, but it is endemic in parts of the USA where it is to be found predominantly on the eastern seaboard, and in California and Oregon. In the UK several cases have been reported from the New Forest in Hampshire.

Transmission is through tick vectors (*Ixodes* species). In the UK these are found on deer, and then pass to human beings. It is thought that the ticks need to feed on the human for several hours before the spirochaete is transmitted. Person-to-person transmission does not occur although transplacental spread from mother to child has been described.

Incubation period is 3–32 days.

NATURAL HISTORY AND CLINICAL FEATURES

Infection is usually manifested by a macular or papular skin lesion (erythema migrans or erythema chronicum migrans), red in colour, which expands to become a large, irregular, circular lesion. It is found at the site of a recent tick bite though this may be inapparent, especially in children who have no recollection of a bite. Similar skin lesions may also occur away from the site of the bite. In the early phase there may be many other less specific features including fever, arthralgia, headache and neck stiffness. A secondary phase occurring weeks to months later may manifest as central nervous system (especially seventh cranial nerve palsy and aseptic meningitis), cardiac and joint symptoms. Chronic arthritis is a late manifestation.

***In England and Wales to the Food Hygiene Laboratory, Central Public Health Laboratory, 61 Colindale Avenue, London NW9 5EQ (telephone 0181-200-4400).**

Diagnosis A clinical diagnosis may be possible in the presence of the distinctive skin lesion. Occasionally *Borrelia burgdorferi* can be cultured from a biopsy of the perimeter of the erythema migrans rash or from blood, or from cerebrospinal fluid if there is central nervous system involvement. Serological tests can be performed using an enzyme immunoassay or western blot analysis. Levels of IgM antibodies may not rise until 3–6 weeks after the onset of disease and IgG titres are very slow to rise, hence serology is not always helpful because of the frequent borderline positive results.

MANAGEMENT

Treatment is with doxycycline 100 mg twice daily or amoxycillin 500 mg three times daily for the child over 9 years old. For the younger child penicillin or amoxycillin (25–50 mg/kg daily) is recommended. Erythromycin can be used as an alternative where there is a history of penicillin allergy. A 3-week course is necessary. Some authorities recommend the use of probenecid with the penicillin regimens. Ceftriaxone (75–100 mg/kg as a single daily dose) should be used for later complications.

PREVENTION OF FURTHER CASES

People walking in endemic areas should keep their skin well covered by clothing to avoid tick bites, and inspect themselves for ticks afterwards; any found should be removed as soon as possible.

68

MALARIA

Notifiable disease

ORGANISM

Malaria is caused by four species of *Plasmodium*: *P. falciparum*, *P. vivax*, *P. ovale* and *P. malariae*. This is a protozoan parasite.

EPIDEMIOLOGY

Malaria is endemic throughout most of the tropics below altitudes of 1500 metres and parts of the subtropics. In 1994 there were 1877 cases reported (including 11 fatalities, one in a child), 253 in children under 15 years old. (Figures from the Public Health Laboratory Service Malaria Reference Laboratory of the 1887 cases 1178 were due to falciparum, 501 vivax, 44 malariae, 125 ovale and 39 mixed). Ten of the 11 deaths related to travel in Africa and all were thought to be due to falciparum, the most serious type of malaria. An overall increase in the total number of imported malaria cases had been recorded over the last decade.

The likely species of malaria acquired is related to the country visited. *Plasmodium falciparum* accounts for 85% of malaria seen in travellers to Africa, whereas 95% of patients from south Asia (including the Indian subcontinent) have vivax malaria, although the proportion with *P. falciparum* has increased in recent years. *Plasmodium ovale* is uncommon, causing only 6% of all infections, and almost invariably is related to African travel. *Plasmodium malariae* is rare (1% of all cases).

Transmission is vector-borne through the intermediary of the female *Anopheles* mosquito when it takes a human blood meal. The main reservoir of infection is the chronically infected human.

Incubation period can be as short as 8 days and as long as 5 years or more. Ninety per cent of cases of falciparum malaria present in the first month after travel, with most of the remaining 10% being seen in the following 4 months. A small minority with falciparum malaria (< 1%) present more than 6 months after leaving the endemic area. The picture is different for the benign malarias, with 25% of cases seen in the first month, 30% in the next 4 months, 35% between 6 months and 12 months and 10% presenting more than a year after travel.

NATURAL HISTORY AND CLINICAL FEATURES

Any child with a fever who has visited a malarious area, especially within the preceding year, should be considered to have malaria until proven otherwise. Malaria can present with any one of a number of symptoms or signs. These include myalgia, rigors, headache, cough, diarrhoea and vomiting, abdominal pain and jaundice. Consequently, common misdiagnoses in the child with malaria include influenza, hepatitis or gastroenteritis. Other than fever, there are no consistent clinical signs. Splenomegaly occurs in less than 50% and hepatomegaly is even less common. Periodic fever is also uncommon and is virtually never seen in travellers with falciparum malaria. Only 30–50% of patients with a benign malaria have a discernible pattern to their fever. Ominous signs are loss of consciousness, especially if associated with decerebrate posturing, fits or focal neurological signs (cerebral malaria). Hypoglycaemia is also a common complication and is especially likely in children given intravenous quinine therapy. Other complications include hypotension and diarrhoea with Gram-negative septicaemia (algid malaria), haemolytic anaemia, haemoglobinuria and renal failure (blackwater fever), disseminated intravascular coagulation, pulmonary oedema, acute renal failure and severe anaemia. The mortality from malaria in the UK is approximately 1% and is usually related to delayed diagnosis. Children who are immunocompromised, asplenic or have homozygous sickle-cell disease are especially prone to severe attacks of malaria.

Two chronic malaria syndromes are recognized in children who have lived for prolonged periods in an endemic area. Nephrotic syndrome can complicate *Plasmodium malariae* infection. Tropical splenomegaly syndrome—a combination of splenomegaly which may be massive, pancytopenia, hypergammaglobulinaemia (especially IgM) and a strongly positive malaria antibody test—is related to recurrent exposure to *P. falciparum*.

Diagnosis The disease cannot be ruled out unless three sets of thick and thin blood films, each set taken as the fever rises, have been examined by someone experienced in the recognition of parasites. A fluorescent microscopy technique using an acridine orange stain (QBC system) is also sensitive but non-specific. In rare cases the blood film can be negative, especially if the patient has taken antimalarial drugs in the recent past. It is also important to consider alternative and additional diagnoses such as typhoid and meningococcaemia. Malaria antibodies can be measured to confirm the diagnosis of a chronic malaria syndrome or may be used retrospectively in the rare instances of 'slide-negative' malaria.

MANAGEMENT

All children with confirmed or suspected falciparum malaria should be hospitalized. The drugs used and their route of administration are dictated by the species of malaria, the country where the infection was acquired and, for falciparum malaria, the degree of parasitaemia. Glucose-6-phosphate dehydrogenase (G6PD) deficiency should be sought as its presence may contraindicate some medications.

Infection with *P. vivax*, *P. ovale* or *P. malariae* Oral chloroquine, 10 mg/kg initially, 5 mg/kg after 6–12 hours, then 10 mg/kg daily for 2 more days will eradicate the acute infection. Primaquine 0.25 mg/kg daily for 14–21 days is subsequently given to eradicate the liver forms of ovale and vivax malaria if the child is not G6PD deficient. There are rare reported cases of chloroquine-resistant vivax malaria from New Guinea, in which case mefloquine or possibly halofantrine may be used. Primaquine-tolerant vivax malaria is also described from that region—this responds to 4 weeks primaquine therapy.

Uncomplicated falciparum malaria Providing the parasitaemia is less than 5%, give oral quinine (10 mg/kg every 8–12 hours) for 5 days. This is followed by pyrimethamine and sulfadoxine (Fansidar—0–4 years, $\frac{1}{2}$ tablet; 5–6 years, 1 tablet; 7–9 years, $1\frac{1}{2}$ tablets; 10–14 years, 2 tablets; over 14 years, 3 tablets) which is normally administered as a single dose. If Fansidar is contraindicated (e.g. in G6PD deficiency), the quinine may be given as a single agent for 10–14 days. Otherwise mefloquine (20 mg/kg in two divided doses, 12 hours apart, starting 12 hours after the last quinine dose) or tetracycline (e.g. doxycycline 200 mg day 1, then 100 mg days 2–7 for children over 12 years) may be substituted. Concern has recently been raised about the cardiotoxicity of halofantrine and it should therefore be reserved for use when other drugs are contraindicated. There are insufficient data on the use of artemether in children.

Severe falciparum malaria Intravenous quinine 10 mg/kg, up to 600 mg, in an infusion of 5% dextrose (50–250 ml) over 4 hours and repeated every 8–12 hours should be given if the parasitaemia is 5% or higher and there are complications such as cerebral malaria, or if the patient cannot tolerate oral quinine. This is ideally undertaken in a paediatric intensive care setting. Some authorities recommend an initial loading dose of quinine (20 mg/kg over 4 hours), especially for falciparum malaria acquired in south and east Asia and the Pacific islands. Dose reduction after the first 24 hours may be required if there is hepatic dysfunction, often related to severe malaria, or there are severe side-effects (tinnitus, deafness, nausea and vomiting—cinchonism). It is normal for most patients to have mild cinchonism at therapeutic blood levels of quinine. Close monitoring for hypoglycaemia is very important. The quinine can be given orally at the same dose after 1–2 days to complete 5 days treatment and followed by Fansidar or one of the alternative drug regimens listed above.

Complications such as renal failure, anaemia, Gram-negative septicaemia and disseminated intravascular coagulation are managed conventionally. Some experts recommend exchange transfusion for very high parasitaemias (> 20%), or high parasite counts (> 10%) in the presence of complications, although this practice is not universally accepted. Some also advise fluid restriction to prevent pulmonary oedema.

Table 68.1 Summary of drug regimens recommended for antimalarial prophylaxis

Geographical location	Preferred regimen	Alternative regimen
East, central and southern sub-Saharan Africa*	Mefloquine†	Proguanil and chloroquine
except for: Botswana, South Africa, Namibia, Mauritania, Zimbabwe	Proguanil and chloroquine	Mefloquine
North Africa and Middle East*	Proguanil and chloroquine	Proguanil or chloroquine
Indian subcontinent‡ and South Asia	Proguanil and chloroquine	
except for: Bangladesh	Mefloquine†	Proguanil and chloroquine
South-east Asia (mainly non-tourist areas)* (including Yunnan and Hainan in China)	Mefloquine†	
Papua New Guinea, Solomon Islands* and Vanuatu	Mefloquine†	Pyrimethamine plus dapsone (Maloprim) and chloroquine
Latin America‡ and Caribbean* Amazon basin of Brazil, Bolivia and Venezuela, Guyana, Surinam, French Guiana and Colombia	Mefloquine†	Chloroquine and proguanil
Bolivia, Equador, East Panama, Peru, Venezuela	Chloroquine and proguanil	Mefloquine
Argentina, Belize, Costa Rica, Dominican Republic, El Salvador, Guatemala, Haiti, Honduras, Nicaragua, West Panama, rural Paraguay	Chloroquine	Proguanil

***No chemoprophylaxis is considered necessary, though mosquito bites should be avoided, in Abu Dhabi, Algeria, Bali, Brunei, Brazil outside the Amazon Basin, Cape Verde, China (main tourist areas), Egypt (tourist areas), Hong Kong, Jamaica, Libya, Malaysia (except Sabah), Mauritius, Morocco, Sarawak, Singapore, Thailand (Bangkok and main tourist areas), Trinidad, Tunisia and Turkey (tourist areas).**

†Proguanil and chloroquine for children less than 2 years old.

‡Prophylaxis may not be needed above certain altitudes (see *British Medical Journal* (1995) 310: 709–14).

Table 68.2 Summary of drug regimens recommended for antimalarial prophylaxis

Preparation	Frequency	Age or weight of child	Dose
Mefloquine	Weekly	11 years or > 45 kg	250 mg (adult dose)
		< 2 years	Not licensed
		> 2 years old, < 15 kg	$\frac{1}{4}$ adult dose
		15–30 kg	$\frac{1}{2}$ adult dose
		31–45 kg	$\frac{3}{4}$ adult dose
Chloroquine	Weekly	> 11 years	300 mg (adult dose)
		0–5 weeks	$\frac{1}{8}$ adult dose
		6 weeks–11 months	$\frac{1}{4}$ adult dose
		1–11 years	$\frac{1}{2}$ adult dose
Proguanil	Daily	> 11 years	200 mg (adult dose)
		0–5 weeks	$\frac{1}{8}$ adult dose
		6 weeks–11 months	$\frac{1}{4}$ adult dose
		1–15 years	$\frac{1}{2}$ adult dose
		6–11 years	$\frac{3}{4}$ adult dose
Pyrimethamine plus dapsone (Maloprim)	Weekly	> 11 years	I tablet (dapsone 100 mg, pyrimethamine 12.5 mg)
		< 1 year	Not applicable*
		1–5 years	$\frac{1}{4}$ adult dose
		6–11 years	$\frac{1}{2}$ adult dose

***Formulation is not applicable as it is difficult to give less than $\frac{1}{4}$ of a tablet.**

PREVENTION OF FURTHER CASES

Mosquito bite avoidance Advice to parents should include the use of insect repellents such as diethyltoluamide (deet); long clothing to be worn especially at dawn and dusk; insecticide-containing mosquito coils or vaporizers; mosquito meshing for non-air-conditioned rooms, and the use of bed nets treated with insecticide (permethrin). All these preparations are non-toxic to children as long as manufacturers instructions are followed.

Antimalarial chemoprophylaxis Current recommendations are shown in Table 68.1 and doses in Table 68.2. The regimen may change with emerging patterns of resistance and advice should be sought from an expert source such as the Malaria Reference Laboratory at the London School of Hygiene (telephone 0171-636-8636).

FURTHER READING

Bradley DJ & Warhurst DC (1995) On behalf of a meeting convened by the Malaria Reference Laboratory. Malaria prophylaxis—guidelines for travellers from Britain. *British Medical Journal* **310**: 709–714.

MEASLES

69

Notifiable disease

All paediatricians in the UK and Eire should currently (1995/6)* also notify cases of SSPE to the BPA Surveillance Unit (see p viii)

ORGANISM

The measles virus is the only member of the genus *Morbillivirus* of the Paramyxoviridae family. The single-stranded enveloped RNA virus is sensitive to heat and cold, ultraviolet light, ether and formalin. Only one serotype is known to cause human infection.

EPIDEMIOLOGY

Humans are the only host. Measles is endemic in most large countries and globally it is estimated that one to two million children die from measles annually, mostly in developing countries. To interrupt transmission requires a protection rate from immunization of 95% or greater for the whole population of susceptibles. In the UK a pattern of epidemics every two years was temporarily interrupted following the introduction of measles, mumps and rubella (MMR) vaccine in 1988 (see Appendix I, Fig. 5). Because of poor immunization uptake in children born before then, and the incomplete protection afforded by immunization, numbers of susceptible individuals increased in the 1990s, especially among older children. The proportion of measles notifications from older children increased and school outbreaks began to occur. This suggested that a major outbreak was increasingly

***May be extended.**

liable to occur, and led to the decision to immunize all school-age children with measles and rubella vaccine in the autumn of 1994. It may be necessary to institute a routine second dose of MMR or MR at school entry if the good results of the 1994 campaign (see Appendix I, Fig. 6) are to be sustained.

Owing to the presence of maternal antibodies, the disease is unusual in infants and very uncommon in those under 6 months old. This pattern may change in an era when most mothers have been vaccinated. Antibody levels are lower and persist for a shorter time in the babies of vaccinated mothers. Prior to the introduction of immunization in the UK, over 90% of individuals had the disease by the time they reached their tenth birthday. The disease is more severe in those exposed to large infecting doses and therefore overcrowded housing is a recognized risk factor. The prognosis is worse in very young children and children at secondary school. Second attacks have been described but are rare. Immunosuppressed individuals are particularly susceptible to complications (at least 5 of the 36 people who died from measles in the USA in 1991 were infected with human immunodeficiency virus, HIV).

Subacute sclerosing panencephalitis is one of the most severe sequelae of measles infection. From 1970 to 1989 in England and Wales 290 confirmed cases were reported. The incidence seems to have declined, with only 3 confirmed cases being reported in 1993.

Transmission The disease is highly infectious and transmission is primarily by droplet spread. Contact with fresh nasal or oral secretions may also cause infection. Patients are infectious from 3–5 days prior to the appearance of the rash and until 4 days after its appearance.

Incubation period Family studies have shown that the rash may appear from 7 days to 18 days (average 14 days) after exposure. The rash appears on the fourth day of the illness and the incubation period to first symptoms is therefore about 10 days on average.

NATURAL HISTORY AND CLINICAL FEATURES

Fever, cough, conjunctivitis and coryza are the initial symptoms. In some cases the pathognomonic Koplik's spots (white spots like grains of sand on a red background) appear on the buccal mucosa a day or two later and are followed on the third or fourth day by an erythematous maculopapular rash. The rash begins at the hairline and progresses down the body over the next 3 days. The rash on the upper part of the body tends to become confluent. After 3–4 days, the rash may have a brownish appearance and then begins to fade in the order in which it appeared. The fever usually declines before the rash disappears. While it is present the child tends to be miserable ('measles miseries') with anorexia, coryza, coughing and conjunctivitis. There is often a mild generalized lymphadenopathy.

Complications In developing countries the case fatality rate is around 5–10%. Though this rate is far lower in the industrialized world, complications still develop in 5–10% of recognized cases in the UK and about 1 in 70 affected children are admitted to hospital. Severe complications are more common in older children and adults. The most important complications are listed in Table 69.1. The rates are derived from reported cases in the USA. The data may be subject to under notification or over diagnosis however the relative rates of the various

Table 69.1 Complication rates derived from reported cases in the USA

Complication*	Age group < 5 years (%)	5–19 years (%)	≥20 years (%)	Total (%)
Otitis media	23	5	3	14
Diarrhoea	16	7	13	12
Pneumonia	11	3	11	8
Encephalitis	0.1	0.1	0.4	0.1
Hospitalization	32	11	36	26
Death†	0.37	0.16	0.43	0.32

***Data for 1991.**
†Data for 1990.

complications at different ages provides useful indications of the different risks at different times in childhood.

Otitis media Five to seven per cent of children with measles develop acute otitis media.

Pneumonia is due to the primary virus infection or bacterial superinfection (*Streptococcus pneumoniae*, *S. pyogenes*, *Staphylococcus aureus* and *Haemophilus influenzae*). It is about as common as otitis media.

Croup A mild laryngotracheobronchitis is a normal part of measles. Some children may go on to develop a severe obstruction requiring intubation.

Convulsions and encephalitis Convulsions occur in 0.5% of cases and an acute encephalitis develops in approximately 0.1% of cases usually between the second and sixth days after the development of the rash. Sixty per cent of cases of encephalitis recover completely, 15% die and 25% are left with neurodevelopmental sequelae.

Subacute sclerosing panencephalitis (SSPE) is a rare neurodegenerative condition with an onset many years after measles infection. Occurring in 1 in 250 000 cases, it is invariably fatal. There is a male to female ratio of 2.8 to 1. The median period between measles and onset is about 8 years with a wide range of 3 months to 20 years. It seems somewhat more common in cases where the primary infection has occurred at an early age. Initially there is a deterioration in intellectual function, followed by incoordination and falling. Myoclonic seizures follow, and death may occur within 6 months of onset or the course can be prolonged.

Death In industrialized countries the case fatality rate is of the order of 1 in 1000 overall and 1 in 2500 in older children. In the immunocompromised child, such as those with leukaemia or HIV infection, measles can produce an atypical pneumonia characterized by giant cell formation in the alveoli. In such cases the rash does not appear and there is a high mortality.

Diagnosis is usually on clinical grounds. However, when incidence is low, the clinical diagnosis is frequently erroneous unless based on the presence of Koplik's spots. Immunofluorescence of nasal pharyngeal aspirate can confirm the diagnosis in difficult cases. Isolation of virus is technically difficult and rarely performed. Serum antibodies appear within 1–3 days after the onset of the rash and peak at 2–4 weeks. Neutralizing and haemaglutination inhibition (HI) antibodies may persist for many years. The presence of measles-specific IgM (detectable from 2 days to 5 weeks after the onset of a rash) or a fourfold rise in antibody titres indicates acute infection. Non-invasive salivary tests detecting anti-measles IgG have now become available.* Diagnosis of SSPE is confirmed by the characteristic electroencephalogram and the detection of oligoclonal measles antibody in the cerebrospinal fluid.

MANAGEMENT

There is no antiviral therapy suitable for management of uncomplicated cases. Treatment is symptomatic unless complications develop when these should be managed appropriately. For secondary bacterial infections antibiotics should be given. Intubation may be necessary for the child with severe laryngotracheobronchitis. Steroids have been used with benefit in encephalitis. Ribavirin and interferon alpha have been used in immunocompromised children with giant cell pneumonia, but without great success. In developing countries lack of vitamin A is associated with severe measles and its administration to infected children has reduced morbidity and mortality from this infection. A case for routine use of vitamin A for children exposed in measles in industrialized countries has yet to be established.

PREVENTION OF FURTHER CASES

Isolation of cases is of little value as the period of infectivity includes a significant period before the diagnosis will have been made, though hospitalized children should be nursed with respiratory precautions until 4 days after the onset of the rash. In the community children should also be kept away from nursery or school until they are no longer infectious.

Vaccination following exposure If given within 72 hours of contact, measles vaccination reduces the chances of developing the disease. For those in whom vaccination is contraindicated (immunocompromised children, see Appendix VI for definition) and in whom the disease is likely to be severe (for example children with severe heart or lung disease or who are immunosuppressed) human normal immunoglobulin (HNIG—for dosage see Appendix VII) can be used within 6 days of contact. It may also be of value if given later in severely immunocompromised children.

Routine vaccination A live attenuated vaccine in the form of MMR vaccine is recommended for all children as soon after their first birthday as possible. Immunization is highly effective in giving protection to any individual; however, because vaccine failures occur for a variety of reasons (an estimated 5% of cases),

***In the UK contact the Virus Reference Division, Central Public Health Laboratory, 61 Colindale Avenue, London NW9 5EQ (telephone 0181-200-4400).**

Table 69.2

	Children aged 1–2 years	Children aged 5 years	Teenagers
Fever	1 in 5	1 in 14	1 in 25
Rash	1 in 5	1 in 17	1 in 14
Febrile convulsion	1 in 1000	Nil	Nil

a single-dose schedule inevitably leads to a slow accumulation of susceptibles. A number of countries have introduced a two-dose schedule, with the second dose given at school entry, or later, to interrupt transmission. Conventional contra-indications for a live vaccine apply (see Appendix VI). Following giving of HNIG, for any reason, 3 months should elapse before immunization.

Side-effects of immunization occur; typical frequencies are shown in Table 69.2. Fever generally starts 7–10 days following immunization, is mild and lasts for a day or so. An unusual side-effect is transient thrombocytopenia; reports of encephalitis following immunization are extremely rare (less than 1 per million doses) and are probably coincidental. Arthralgia occurs in approximately 3% of children and arthritis in 11% of adolescents and adult women. Lasting effects are uncommon.

In developing countries much of the morbidity and mortality due to measles takes place in the first year of life when conventional immunization is relatively ineffective. High-titre vaccines have been developed to overcome these problems but have been dogged by association with increased late mortality in recipients, and are not in regular use.

MENINGOCOCCAL DISEASE

70

Meningococcal meningitis and septicaemia are notifiable diseases

ORGANISM

Meningococcal disease is caused by *Neisseria meningitidis* or meningococcus, a Gram-negative diplococcus. Strains are divided into serogroups according to the surface capsular polysaccharide. Groups A, B, C, Y and W135 account for most invasive disease; B and C have been most prevalent in the UK in the last decade.

EPIDEMIOLOGY

Annual incidence is 2–5 per 100 000 population, with wide geographical variation. Attack rates are highest in children aged 1–4 years and half of all cases are in children aged less than 2 years. Infections are much more common in winter. Males outnumber females 3:2. Rises in numbers of cases occur every few years. Since 1985 the annual incidence has risen, peaking in 1991, but has not yet returned to pre-outbreak levels. During recent years about 1400 meningococcal infections have occurred each year in England and Wales. In 1993 there were 954 notifications to the Office of Populations Censuses and Surveys of meningococcal meningitis and 431 of meningococcal septicaemia. In the same year 1154 isolates of *Neisseria meningitidis* were submitted to the Public Health Laboratory Service (PHLS) Meningococcal Reference Unit for England and Wales (provisional total) 70% were group B and 26% group C. Groups at risk include those in poor general health, living in overcrowded conditions, and with sickle-cell disease. There is some evidence that smoking, both active and passive, increases the risk of disease. Specific immunodeficiencies (terminal components of complement, properdin and IgM deficiency) increase susceptibility to infection with unusual serogroups such as X, Y and W135.

Transmission is via close contact with nasopharyngeal droplets or respiratory secretions. Persons living in the household or 'kissing contacts' are most at risk. Nasopharyngeal colonization is found in 4–25% of the population. Its relationship to infection and invasive disease is obscure. Carriers spread the disease, but outbreaks are not directly related to colonization rate. Cases are due to pathogenic strains which are found in 1% of carriers. It is not clear why invasive disease should occur. Host factors include prior respiratory tract or viral infection (e.g. influenza), smoking (including passive), secretor status, and reduced mucosal and systemic immunity. Organism factors include capsulation (protective against host defences), piliation (which aids bacterial adhesion to the nasopharynx) and presence of outer membrane proteins (which influence epithelial penetration).

Incubation period is usually 2–10 days. Carriers retain the organism in their nasopharynx for several weeks, making time of transmission—and hence incubation—difficult to ascertain.

Period of communicability The child with invasive disease may still be a carrier and systemic antibiotics do not necessarily alter that status.

NATURAL HISTORY AND CLINICAL FEATURES

The meningococcus is the most common cause of bacterial meningitis in the UK, but only 15% of those with meningococcal disease present with pure meningitis; 25% have septicaemia with septic shock; the remaining 60% have mixed features of septicaemia and meningitis. During outbreaks cases of septicaemia increase, while cases of pure meningitis stay approximately constant in number. Arthritis, pneumonia, occult bacteraemia, endocarditis, endophthalmitis and chronic meningococcaemia are rare presentations.

Most children present with features of early septicaemia or mixed septicaemia and meningitis. A non-specific prodrome with coryzal symptoms and fever often lasts a few days, but may only be a few hours in children with the severest disease. A rapidly appearing, red, macular rash precedes the typical petechial rash in 38% of cases. An ill child with an erythematous macular rash of large spots should be examined (and reviewed) for evidence of the typical rash elsewhere (see below). The characteristic rash with petechiae and purpura may evolve extremely rapidly. Clusters of petechiae are often localized: purpuric elements may appear at any stage. Vasculitic spots may develop with central areas of necrosis. Other features of this presentation include (in decreasing order of occurrence): vomiting, drowsiness, neck stiffness, unrousability or coma, diarrhoea, muscular aches, irritability, confusion, headache, photophobia, poor feeding, high-pitched cry and fits.

Meningococcal meningitis is clinically indistinguishable from other meningitides. Its features usually develop over several days. Symptoms include fever, vomiting, headache, anorexia, drowsiness, lethargy and high-pitched cry. Photophobia and meningism are present. Patients with severe meningitis may present with convulsions, focal neurological signs and deteriorating level of consciousness, progressing to coma. The petechial rash may not be present.

Septic shock (see Chapter 12) occurs in 30% of meningococcal septicaemia. It may be heralded by signs of impaired peripheral perfusion, including tachycardia, cold peripheries, reduced capillary filling, a wide skin–core temperature difference (best measured with thermistor probes on a toe and in the rectum), tachypnoea, oliguria and low blood pressure.

- Hypotension is a late sign of septic shock in young children who maintain blood pressure by intense vasoconstriction despite severe hypovolaemia.

A rapidly progressive haemorrhagic rash may occur, followed by rigors and prostration, and later coma and death.

Diagnosis A petechial/purpuric rash in a feverish, ill child is virtually pathognomonic of meningococcal disease. Diagnosis is rarely difficult, but may be delayed if a careful search of all skin areas, including palms and soles, is omitted. The petechial nature of a rash may be confirmed by its failure to blanch or fade with local pressure (e.g. beneath a drinking glass). Bacterial infections which very occasionally present with a similar clinical picture include infections with *Haemophilus influenzae* type b, *Streptococcus pneumoniae* and Gram-negative organisms. Other differential diagnoses are Henoch–Schönlein purpura (rash not on trunk, child afebrile and generally well); idiopathic thrombocytopenic purpura (ecchymoses, purpura and petechiae of different ages in a generally well child); acute leukaemia (child usually afebrile and non-toxic with evidence of lymphadenopathy and hepatosplenomegaly); non-accidental injury (child afebrile with suggestive features in history and examination). Other causes are rare. If the diagnosis is in doubt, treat as meningococcal disease until disproved.

Investigations Blood should be taken for the following tests: full blood count and differential white cell count; clotting studies; blood culture; blood group and save serum; urea and electrolytes. Typical findings include a neutrophil leucocytosis and thrombocytopenia. Neutropenia is a poor prognostic sign. Meningococcus can be grown from blood in approximately 50% of all meningococcal disease. Isolation rate is higher in septicaemia, but only 5% if pretreated with antibiotics. The organism may also be grown from aspirates of the skin lesions. All isolates should be sent for typing, in England and Wales to the PHLS Meningococcal Reference Unit* and in Scotland to Meningococcal Reference (Scottish) Laboratory.† Lumbar puncture (LP) should be considered.

- Defer LP if the child is shocked or has predominantly septicaemia features to avoid deterioration during the procedure. If signs of raised intracranial pressure

***Mengococcal Reference Unit, Manchester Public Health Laboratory (telephone 0161-445-2416; out of hours 0161-445-8111).**

†Meningococcal Reference (Scottish) Laboratory (telephone 0141-946-7120).

are present (grossly bulging fontanelle or papilloedema, reduced level of consciousness, focal neurological signs), delay LP until a computed tomographic scan has excluded cerebral abscess or space-occupying lesion.

- Antibiotics should not be delayed by deferment of LP.

Lumbar puncture findings are those of bacterial meningitis (see Chapter 10). Meningococci may be seen within neutrophils and cultured from the cerebrospinal fluid (CSF) in 80–90% of cases. Bacterial antigen detection may confirm diagnosis when prior penicillin treatment renders blood and CSF cultures negative. Group-specific meningococcal antigens may be detected in CSF and blood (and urine) by latex particle agglutination and counterimmunoelectrophoresis. Biopsy (or aspiration) of necrotic skin spots may reveal Gram-negative intracellular diplococci on microscopy.

MANAGEMENT

Emergency antibiotic treatment If meningococcal disease is suspected, give antibiotics urgently. In primary care use penicillin (see Table 70.1), and transfer the child rapidly to hospital. In hospital the first doctor who sees the child should give penicillin urgently. Treatment should not await transfer to a ward area: some children deteriorate despite rapid intervention.

Initial treatment An experienced paediatrician should assess the child as soon as possible. Establish venous access during venepuncture. Give penicillin 300 mg/kg per day in 6 divided doses and/or cefotaxime 200 mg/kg per day IV in 3–4 divided doses to cover other possible pathogens. Ceftriaxone 80 mg/kg IV once daily is an alternative cephalosporin.

Duration of antibiotic treatment Rationalize antibiotic therapy when culture results are available. Nearly all strains are very sensitive to penicillin. Reduce the dose of penicillin after 48 hours to 200 mg/kg per day IV 6-hourly. Short courses of antibiotics are acceptable, but generally continue treatment intravenously for 5 days for uncomplicated septicaemia and 7 days for uncomplicated meningitis. Antibiotic therapy should not be discontinued until the child has been apyrexial for 48 hours. Penicillin has no effect on nasopharyngeal carriage. Give the index case oral rifampicin or an alternative, such as ciprofloxacin, before discharge to remove the possibility of continuing carriage.

Fluid and other management Assessment of fluid balance is extremely difficult because of the severe capillary leak which accompanies septicaemia.

Table 70.1 Dose of benzylpenicillin for initial treatment of meningococcal disease in primary care

Age	Dose	Route
Over 10 years	1200 mg	IV (or IM)
1–10 years	600 mg	IV (or IM)
Under 1 year	300 mg	IV (or IM)

Children who are allergic to penicillin may be given erythromycin 20 mg/kg IV or chloramphenicol 20 mg/kg IV.

Treat shock vigorously. Commence 4.5% albumin 20–40 ml/kg over 10–30 minutes, followed by 20–40 ml/kg 4.5% albumin over the next hour. Follow guidelines for management of septic shock (see Chapter 12).

Commence maintenance intravenous fluids after restoration of the circulating volume. Restrict to half the usual amounts for weight, to mitigate effects of inappropriate antidiuretic hormone secretion, with fluid retention and the risk of cerebral oedema.

Give antipyretics, but avoid sedatives. Corticosteroids should not be used in either pharmacological or physiological dosage in meningococcal disease without careful consideration. There is no evidence of their efficacy in either septicaemia or meningitis. In septicaemia they may be detrimental.

Research into antiendotoxins and anticytokines as treatments for severe meningococcal disease is in progress. No evidence of efficacy of specific targeted therapies has yet been produced in randomized, double-blind clinical trials. These new therapies may have unappreciated side-effects and are often expensive. They should not be given outside trial conditions.

The first 48 hours The initial course of meningococcal disease is unpredictable. Approximately 25% of children with meningococcal disease require admission to a paediatric intensive care unit (PICU). Children who are alert and haemodynamically stable may be nursed in a high-dependency cubicle on a paediatric ward and observed carefully. Non-invasive monitoring of blood pressure, pulse, perfusion (by core–peripheral temperature difference monitoring), and urine output should be undertaken.

Transfer to PICU is needed for children who arrive in shock and fail to respond to initial resuscitation or those who deteriorate despite adequate fluid and antibiotic treatment. Early selection for transfer to PICU is vital. Important predictors of the need for intensive care are refractory hypotension and deteriorating conscious level or coma. Weaker predictors include: extreme age, variations in breathing pattern, a spreading rash of less than 12 hours duration, necrotic skin lesions, absence of meningism, seizures preadmission, white cell count below 10 000 $\times$ 10^9/l, thrombocytopenia (count below 100 000 $\times$ 10^9/l), erythrocyte sedimentation rate below 20 mm/h, disseminated intravascular coagulation (DIC), metabolic acidosis (pH below 7.3), CSF white blood cell count below 100 $\times$ 10^9/l, and antigenaemia.

Several scoring systems aimed at early identification of children with a poor prognosis have been proposed. None is universally accepted. The Glasgow Meningococcal Septicaemia Prognostic Score (Table 70.2) is a validated, clinically based scoring system, which can be repeated at intervals to identify which children with meningococcal disease should be admitted to a PICU. Children scoring 8 or more have 30% mortality risk even with intensive care, and should be transferred to a PICU.

Central nervous system involvement Meningococcal disease may cause cerebral oedema with raised intracranial pressure. Infarction from vasculitis is an unusual, later complication. Intensive care should aim to preserve cerebral perfusion pressure, ie. the difference between blood pressure and intracranial pressure (ICP). Elective ventilation should keep the $Paco_2$ at 30–40 mmHg (4.0–5.2 kPa) to reduce intracranial pressure. Maintain cardiac output by early use of

Table 70.2 The Glasgow Meningococcal Septicaemia Prognostic Score*

1	SYSTOLIC BLOOD PRESSURE†‡ If < 75 mmHg (age < 4 years) or < 85 mmHg age (> 4 years) **score 3 points**
2	SKIN/RECTAL TEMPERATURE DIFFERENCE†‡ If > 3 degrees Celsius **score 3 points**
3	MODIFIED COMA SCALE†‡ If initial score < 8 or deterioration of 3 or more points at any time **score 3 points**
4	DETERIORATION IN LAST HOUR†‡ Ask parents or nurses; if yes then **score 2 points**
5	ABSENCE OF NECK STIFFNESS **Score 2 points**
6	EXTENT OF PURPURA Widespread ecchymoses, or extending lesions on review then **score 1 point**
7	BASE DEFICIT If > minus 8 then **score 1 point** TOTAL

***Differs minimally from original description by Sinclair et al (1987)** *Lancet* **ii**; 38.
†Undertake on arrival and an hour after admission.
‡Notes to Table 70.2:

1 Blood pressure use Doppler or sphygmomanometer; cuff width not less than 2/3 length upper arm.

2 Apply skin temperature probe to toe; axilla or rectal temperatures taken for 2 minutes.

3 Modified Coma Scale

(i)	**Eyes open**	**spontaneously**	**4**
		to speech	**3**
		to pain	**2**
		none	**1**
(ii)	**Best verbal response**	**orientated**	**6**
		words	**4**
		vocal sounds	**3**
		cries	**2**
		none	**1**
(iii)	**Best motor response**	**obeys commands**	**6**
		localize pain	**4**
		moves to pain	**1**
		none	**0**

Add scores (i)+(ii)+(iii) to give result.

4 Unspecified and subjective rating.

volume expanders and inotropes. Use intravenous mannitol and corticosteroids only when ICP monitoring is available in a PICU, because of the risk of rebound ICP rise. Indwelling ICP monitoring carries risks in severe shock or DIC.

Prognosis Overall 10% of children with meningococcal disease die. Most have haemorrhages into internal organs, especially the adrenal glands (Waterhouse–Friderichsen syndrome). Endotoxic shock with DIC is the usual mode of death. Hence, meningococcal septicaemia has a higher mortality rate (around 30%) than meningitis alone (around 2%). Cases of mixed septicaemia and meningitis have an intermediate mortality.

Early intensive care, especially elective assisted ventilation, aggressive management of shock and anticipation of complications may improve the prognosis for children with septicaemia. Survival rates approach 70% in high-risk patients requiring intensive care. Survival is usually accompanied by total recovery. Fewer than 10% of children have sequelae. The most common complication is deafness: refer all children with septicaemia or meningitis to audiology at time of discharge. Areas of necrotic skin may need skin grafting. Necrotic digits or limbs usually autoamputate. Surgical amputation is required occasionally. Neurological disability is uncommon, but subtle developmental and motor problems, learning difficulties and behavioural disorders can occur. With better intensive care morbidity may increase.

PREVENTION OF FURTHER CASES

Prevention currently rests on three principles:

- Primary care services, parents, carers for children and the general public being aware of the early signs of meningococcal disease and the action to take if it is suspected.
- Eradication of carriage of meningococci in close contacts of cases.
- Immunization (only when two or more type A, C, W137 or Y cases occur, or persons are travelling to endemic areas).

Following diagnosis of meningococcal disease (with or without microbiologic confirmation) the appropriate consultant in communicable disease control (CCDC) or his or her deputy must be informed urgently by telephone even if there is only a single case. Cases with features of both septicaemia and meningitis should also be notified officially according to the predominant clinical picture. Approximately 1% of cases are secondary. If a case occurs in a contact within 48 hours of the index case it is considered a co-primary. The risk to household contacts is approximately 800 times higher than that in the general population (but is still a low absolute rate). The CCDC is responsible for ensuring that antibiotic prophylaxis, or immunization if appropriate, is offered to all eligible contacts.

Antibiotic treatment to eradicate carriage Usually the hospital provides treatment for those living in the index household to eliminate carriage with potentially pathogenic organisms. Staff involved in mouth-to-mouth resuscitation should also receive treatment. The CCDC is usually responsible for ensuring that treatment is given to other such contacts, (see Action in Specific Circumstances). The index case should also be given antibiotic treatment during convalescence to

Table 70.3 Dose of rifampicin for treatment of carriage with meningococcal bacteria

Adult	600 mg twice daily for 2 days
Child	10 mg/kg twice daily for 2 days
Neonate	5 mg/kg twice daily for 2 days

eradicate meningococcal carriage. Oral rifampicin is the agent of choice (Table 70.3). Recipients should be warned about unwanted effects including possible interference with oral contraceptives, and orange staining of soft contact lenses. Ciprofloxacin (500 mg as a single dose) is an (unlicensed) alternative while ceftriaxone (250 mg as a single dose) should be used for pregnant women. It should be noted that 'one-off' treatment of a group to eliminate carriage frequently produces only a short-term reduction in carriage rate and that such treatment to eliminate carriage is not effective in treatment of incubating disease.

Nasopharyngeal swabs Swabbing before treatment to reduce carriage is considered unnecessary. There is generally little point to swabbing except on occasion to gather epidemiological information.

ACTION IN SPECIFIC CIRCUMSTANCES

Single cases

Children attending preschool groups Antibiotic treatment for carriage should be offered to all family contacts of the case and vaccination also offered if the organism is type A, C, W137 or Y. Antibiotic use or immunization should not be offered further unless there is evidence of close contact comparable to that in a household as there is little evidence that classmates are at increased risk from a single case. Information about the case and meningococcal disease in general should be given to parents, carers and general practitioners.

Pupils or students attending primary or secondary schools, colleges or universities during term-time Antibiotic treatment for carriage or immunization should not be offered to contacts in the educational setting unless the exposure has been comparable to that experienced in a household (e.g. 'kissing contacts' or those sharing dormitory accommodation). Information about the case and meningococcal disease should be given to teachers, parents and general practitioners, and in secondary and higher education to the students themselves.

Pupils or students attending preschool groups, primary or secondary schools, colleges or universities out of term-time Antibiotic treatment for carriage or immunization should not be offered to contacts in the educational setting. Dissemination of information should be considered when a case occurs within 7 days of the end of term.

Alerting primary care When cases occur and whether or not incidence is high, consideration should always be given to alerting general practitioners and the community child health services, reminding them of the early signs of meningococcal disease and the importance of giving parenteral penicillin to children and adults in whom the infection is suspected while waiting for transport to hospital. This communication is usually done by the CCDC with the Family Health Services Authority (FHSA).

Patient information Family and contacts of the index case must be made aware of the warning symptoms of meningococcal disease and what action to take should they appear.*

Outbreaks (definition: two or more cases closely connected in place and time) Essentially the preventive action is similar to that of single cases. However, wider treatment to reduce carriage or immunization may be indicated, for example if two children are ill in the same primary-school class. In the UK it is important to contact the Communicable Disease Surveillance Centre (CDSC) or the Scottish Centre for Infection and Environmental Health (SCIEH) and to ensure that specimens are sent to the PHLS Meningococcal Reference Unit, Manchester (0161-445-2416) or the Meningococcal Reference (Scottish) Laboratory (0141-946-7120) so that serogroups may be determined.

Patient information Family and contacts of the index case must be made aware of the warning symptoms of meningococcal disease and what action to take should they appear.*

Publicity When two or more cases occur in temporal association there is often interest from the press. Statements to the media may be given or supervised by the CCDC or other authoritative persons; however, it is advisable that there be a single point of communication between the professionals and the press. Meningococcal disease is still thought to be synonymous with meningitis by many members of the public and the medical profession, and publicity should emphasize the petechial rash and septicaemia presentation, summarize features of meningitis separately and explain these clearly. The FHSA should be prewarned of any press notice. The CDSC or SCIEH can advise over its content from their previous experience.

Immunization If two or more cases occur with the same serogroup for which immunization gives protection (usually serogroup C), consideration should be given to offering immunization to the same groups as received treatment to reduce carriage. Vaccines are available against serogroups A, C, Y and W135. Only the group A vaccine is effective in children below the age of 2 years, and a national immunization programme against serogroup B awaits development of a satisfactory vaccine.

TRAVEL ABROAD

Vaccination should be offered to all those travelling to countries where meningococcal infection with serogroups A and C is endemic (see Chapter 20) and asplenic or hyposplenic children (Appendix VII).

FURTHER READING

Cartwright K, ed. (1995) *Meningococcal Disease*. Wiley, London. Particularly relevant chapters are those on treatment of meningococcal disease in childhood, and outbreak control.

***Leaflets for public distribution are available from The National Meningitis Trust, Fern House, Bath Road, Stroud, Gloucestershire GL5 3TJ and The Meningitis Research Appeal, Old Gloucester Road, Alveston, Bristol BS12 2LQ.**

71

MUMPS

ORGANISM

Mumps is caused by a parainfluenza virus (enveloped RNA virus) of the paramyxovirus family. There is one serotype and there is no animal reservoir.

EPIDEMIOLOGY

Prior to the introduction of a vaccine, mumps was mainly a disease of children and young adults with the highest incidence between the ages of 5 years and 10 years. Epidemics were most common in late winter and spring. Both sexes were affected equally. Widespread use of mumps vaccine has been followed by a decrease of approximately 90% in reported cases in the USA. However, as with measles and rubella, there has been a shift in the epidemiology of mumps to an older age group, with several outbreaks in colleges or in the workplace. These outbreaks appear to be mainly in unvaccinated individuals rather than due to poor vaccine efficacy. When mumps has been introduced into a virgin community serious outbreaks have affected adults as well as children. Mumps is uncommon in the first 9–12 months of life presumably due to protective maternal antibody and less exposure to infection at this age.

Transmission is by droplet infection or saliva and possibly urine. Mumps virus can be cultured from saliva, throat washings, blood (in early stages), cerebrospinal fluid, urine and human milk. Patients are infectious from approximately a few days before salivary gland enlargement to up to 3 days after the glands subside. Most children can be regarded as non-infectious 1 week after onset of parotitis.

Incubation period is 12–25 days with a peak at 16–18 days.

NATURAL HISTORY AND CLINICAL FEATURES

Thirty to forty per cent of infections may be subclinical. Parotitis is the most apparent manifestation but involvement of other organs such as the central nervous system (CNS) may occur without, or preceding, parotitis. Onset of symptoms is usually related to pain and swelling of the parotid gland. Apart from fever, there may be headache, malaise, anorexia and abdominal pain. The temperature usually settles within a week and before swelling of the salivary glands subsides. Parotitis is commonly bilateral and one gland usually enlarges 2–3 days before the other. Swelling of the parotid gland is more easily seen than felt, and particularly important in diagnosis is the swelling between the angle of the mandible and sternomastoid muscle extending backwards beneath the auricle. The earlobe is pushed upwards and outwards. The swelling usually subsides within 7–10 days. Involvement of the submaxillary salivary gland is less frequent and can be very difficult to differentiate from cervical lymphadenopathy. Involvement of sublingual glands is uncommon.

Central nervous system involvement is common and was the most important cause of aseptic meningitis before routine vaccination became available. Many patients may have cerebrospinal fluid (CSF) and electroencephalogram changes compatible with meningoencephalitis without clinical manifestations. Headache and mental confusion with meniningism are the usual symptoms and may occur from a week before to 3 weeks following onset of parotitis. In the CSF there is an increased lymphocyte count, normal to slightly raised protein levels and, uncommonly, a reduced glucose level. The virus can be readily isolated. Prognosis of mumps meningoencephalitis is good; however, in the rare post-infectious type of encephalitis, sequelae and even death may occur. Other CNS complications include facial paralysis (in most cases probably due to local pressure on the nerve), deafness, transverse myelitis, cerebellar ataxia, polyneuritis, and hydrocephalus due to aqueductal stenosis or obstruction elsewhere in the ventricular system.

Epididymo-orchitis About 20% or more of post-pubertal males may develop epididymo-orchitis. It has rarely been described in young children. It usually develops within a week of parotitis but may occur prior to or without parotitis. Severe local pain and tenderness often accompanied by systemic symptoms of fever, headache and backache are usual. A degree of atrophy of the testis is common, which is particularly of concern when orchitis is bilateral (20–30%). However, even in bilateral cases sterility is rare and patients should be reassured.

Pancreatitis Mild involvement of the pancreas manifested by upper abdominal pain, tenderness and vomiting is probably common, but severe pancreatitis is rare. Serum amylase levels are usually raised in mumps which may partly originate from the parotid gland; levels bear no relationship to abdominal symptoms.

Other complications include oophoritis, mastitis, thyroiditis, nephritis, arthritis, myocarditis and thrombocytopenic purpura, all of which are usually self-limiting. Mumps during pregnancy may be associated with an increased chance of abortion, but no definite evidence of embryopathy has been confirmed. Neonatal mumps infection may occur when the mother is infected around the time of delivery.

Diagnosis Mumps is usually diagnosed clinically. However, suppurative parotitis, calculus, recurrent parotitis and infection of the parotid glands by influenza and other virus may cause difficulty. Chronic parotid enlargement is a manifestation of human immunodeficiency virus infection.

Mumps virus can be isolated from throat swabs, saliva, CSF and urine. Paired sera for mumps IgG antibody or a single specimen for mumps IgM antibody are reliable methods for diagnosis. Antibodies to soluble (S) antigen which disappear within 6–12 months indicate recent infection, whereas those against viral (V) antigen persist.

MANAGEMENT

Management of parotitis and meningitis is symptomatic. Orchitis can be very painful, requiring analgesics. Gentle support of the scrotum is helpful.

PREVENTION OF FURTHER CASES

Immunization with measles, mumps and rubella (MMR) vaccine is highly effective in controlling mumps. There has been a marked decrease in mumps notifications since MMR was recommended for routine use in the USA in 1977 and in Britain in 1988. Details of the vaccine are given in Chapter 69. Measles and mumps and monovalent mumps vaccines are also available. Hyperimmune mumps immunoglobulin has not been shown to be efficacious in preventing or reducing complications. Administration of MMR to contracts, e.g. non-immune fathers of children with mumps in the hope of reducing the occurrence of orchitis, is not effective in preventing infection or reducing complications.

Reactions to the mumps component of MMR are uncommon. Transient parotitis may develop in the third week and meningoencephalitis 2–3 weeks after vaccination, and rarely deafness. Initially two types of mumps vaccine were available in Britain, containing the Urabe AM9 and Jeryl Lynn strains, respectively. Studies have suggested that the risk of meningoencephalitis was higher with the Urabe strain and only the Jeryl Lynn strain is now used.

72

MYCOBACTERIAL INFECTION (ATYPICAL)

ORGANISM

Unlike *Mycobacterium tuberculosis* and *Mycobacterium bovis*, atypical mycobacteria are widely distributed in soil, water and cold-blooded animals and are usually of low pathogenicity for warm-blooded animals. They generally prefer warm climates and their geographical distribution is very varied. Runyon's classification system is most commonly used and is based on pigmentation, rate of growth and colonial morphology. In children most infections are due to slow-growing, non-pigment-producing organisms which are closely related, namely *Mycobacterium avium*, *M. intracellulare*, *M. marinum* and *M. scrofulaceum*. There is controversy as to whether these are really distinct species and they are sometimes referred to as the *Mycobacterium avium* complex (MAC) or the MAIS organisms (*Mycobacterium avium intracellulare scrofulaceum*).

EPIDEMIOLOGY

The epidemiology of infection due to atypical mycobacteria differs greatly from that of tuberculosis. Unlike tuberculosis, atypical mycobacterial infection is rarely, if ever, transmitted from person to person and almost all cases appear to follow acquisition of the bacilli from the environment. Thus contact tracing and other public health measures are of no benefit whatsoever. Atypical mycobacterial lymphadenitis is almost exclusively a disease of preschool children which may be due to the relatively poor immunity to mycobacteria found in this age group. It is an uncommon condition although it has been suggested that infection is becoming more common in countries where the incidence of tuberculosis is declining.

Transmission Person-to-person spread does not occur.

Incubation period is not known, but is probably weeks to months.

NATURAL HISTORY AND CLINICAL FEATURES

Cervical lymphadenitis is the most common problem caused by these organisms, suggesting that the buccal mucosa may be the usual portal of entry. Typically, children present with firm, painless, unilateral lymphadenopathy, usually high in the neck or close to the mandible but pre- and post-auricular nodes and occasionally inguinal nodes may be involved. The nodes are usually relatively painless and firm at first; they then gradually soften, rupture and drain for many months. The surrounding skin may become inflamed. Despite this the children remain well without any systemic upset or evidence of haematogenous spread. It is commonly mistaken for a cervical abscess, while tuberculosis, cat-scratch disease, mumps, salivary stone or a malignancy are other differential diagnoses. Very occasionally children present with disseminated atypical mycobacterial infection: such patients almost invariably have an underlying, primary or acquired, immunodeficiency.

Diagnosis Commonly atypical mycobacterial disease is not suspected, and a fine needle aspiration or incision biopsy is performed. While this usually excludes malignancy it often results in a sinus with superficial skin infection, rendering later surgery more difficult. Furthermore, if histology reveals caseating granulomas with acid-fast bacilli, this does not distinguish *M. tuberculosis* from atypical mycobacterial disease and if culture is performed the diagnosis will only become apparent after 2–3 months. Differential Mantoux testing with a panel of antigens including tuberculin and antigens from *M. avium*, *M. intracellulare* and *M. malmoense* can be helpful as in many cases the response to *M. tuberculosis* will be very small or absent, while there will be a much larger response to one of the atypical mycobacterial antigens.

MANAGEMENT

Complete surgical excision of the affected lymph node is by far the most effective treatment and is more likely to be performed if the diagnosis has been made on clinical grounds or from the results of differential Mantoux testing. Sometimes this is not possible because the node is too close to a vital structure such as the facial nerve, or because previous surgical intervention has left a sinus and a significant area of infected skin. Treatment with rifampicin, isoniazid and pyrazinamide is usually unhelpful even if in vitro testing suggests that there is sensitivity to these agents. There are some indications that infection with atypical mycobacteria may respond to agents such as aminoglycosides (in particular amikacin), macrolides (erythromycin, azithromycin, clarithromycin) and quinolones (e.g. ciprofloxicin), rifabutin and cotrimoxazole. The efficacy of this approach is unproven particular its value in reducing residual scarring and the need for further extensive surgery requires evaluation. While this is awaited clinicians confronted with a case should seek expert advice before embarking on either lengthy antimicrobial therapy or a surgical approach.

FURTHER READING

Clark JE, Magee JG & Cant AJ (1995) Nontuberalous mycobacterial lymphaclenopathy. Arch. Dis. child **72**: 165–166.

MYCOPLASMA INFECTIONS

73

MYCOPLASMA PNEUMONIAE

ORGANISM

Mycoplasma pneumoniae is a bacterium which lacks a cell wall. Under the electron microscope, the organism is filamentous and has a terminal organelle used for attaching to respiratory epithelial cells.

EPIDEMIOLOGY

Infections occur worldwide; endemic epidemics occur at intervals of 4–7 years. Among children, those of school age and adolescents seem to be the most susceptible. The incubation period is usually 3 weeks with a range of 6–23 days. Humans are the only host, and the disease is spread by droplets.

NATURAL HISTORY AND CLINICAL FEATURES

Mycoplasma pneumoniae infection is known as 'primary atypical pneumonia'. Onset of illness is gradual with headache, fever and sore throat. The cough tends to be paroxysmal and may be associated with sputum production. Substernal or pleuritic chest pain may occur. Several days after onset of illness chest signs may occur, such as widespread crackles. The chest X-ray may show patchy consolidation throughout the lung; features such as consolidation of single lobes, and pleural effusions may be present. Complications of infection sometimes occurring in the absence of chest disease include erythema multiforme, Stevens–Johnson syndrome, encephalitis and transverse myelitis. Illness tends to be particularly severe in children with sickle-cell disease.

Diagnosis Although the organism can be cultured, the procedure is slow, and diagnosis can be established more quickly by serology (IgM detector by ELISA) and identification of cold agglutinins seen in up to 50% of cases. A fourfold rise in complement-fixing antibodies is considered diagnostic.

MANAGEMENT

The response to antibiotics is much less dramatic than that seen in pneumococcal pneumonia. However, erythromycin has been shown to be effective and is recommended. There do not appear to be any microbiological advantages in using the new macrolides, clarithromycin and azithromycin.

THE GENITAL MYCOPLASMAS

ORGANISMS

Ureaplasma urealyticum and *Mycoplasma taceae hominis*, are bacteria which like other members of the *Mycoplasmataceae* family lack a cell wall.

EPIDEMIOLOGY

The genital mycoplasmas are transmitted sexually, and are associated with non-specific urethritis in males and salpingitis in females. Transmitted to the newborn infant at delivery, both organisms may be a cause of infection particularly in those born prematurely.

NATURAL HISTORY AND CLINICAL FEATURES

Mycoplasma hominis is a rare cause of meningitis in the newborn. The clinical signs and cerebrospinal fluid (CSF) findings are little different from the cases caused by other bacteria. Research has suggested that in certain populations *Ureaplasma urealyticum* infection of the respiratory tract is associated with chronic lung disease of prematurity and results in an increased mortality in this group of babies. *Ureaplasma urealyticum* has been isolated from the CSF of premature infants with a history of intraventricular haemorrhage, but there is no evidence that it is a cause of ventriculitis.

Diagnosis is by culture of secretions. This procedure is expensive and available in only few centres. Frustratingly, even when infection is suspected lack of resources rarely allows adequate investigation.

MANAGEMENT

Erythromycin is the treatment of choice for genital mycoplasma infections. Both organisms may be resistant to this antibiotic, in which case doxycycline. 100–200 mg per day in divided doses is recommended.

NITS AND HEAD LICE

ORGANISM

Pediculus humanus capitis is an arthropod. Humans are the only hosts.

EPIDEMIOLOGY

Children are the most commonly infected (60% of cases) some estimates suggest that approximately 9% of school children are affected at any one time. Contrary to popular belief, head lice are more likely to infect clean rather than dirty hair and have no preference for long hair. Infestations are found in all social groups though they are less common in black children as the lice find it harder to hold on to the shaft of their hair.

Transmission Infestation is predominantly spread by head-to-head contact, and less commonly by fomites and sharing of clothing, combs and hats.

Incubation period The eggs take 6–10 days to hatch.

NATURAL HISTORY AND CLINICAL FEATURES

The adult female louse attaches her eggs (nits) to the base of scalp hair. After a week the eggs hatch. The adult louse lives about 2–3 months, feeding on scalp blood, and can survive up to 10 days off the head. Nits can survive for up to 3 weeks. Many infestations are asymptomatic. Pruritus, although rare, is the most common symptom. It is frequently accompanied by enlarged cervical lymph nodes. A maculopapular erythematous eruption, and occasionally urticarial lesions, can occur. Repeated infections are common and many family members may be affected at the same time.

Diagnosis The presence of nits or lice is diagnostic. It is important to examine near the base of hair shafts. Nits should not be confused with dandruff which is easily removed with a comb.

MANAGEMENT

The only effective treatment is the use of a special insecticidal lotion (shampoos are not as effective as lotions). Preparations are available containing malathion, carbaryl and pyrethroids. It is important that the instructions are strictly adhered to and two applications may be necessary in some instances. All the family should be treated. When properly investigated, reports of resistance to treatment are not substantiated. The reason for failure of the treatment to eradicate the lice usually turns out to be incorrect use of the medication or reinfestation from an infested contact. Clothing and bedding can be readily disinfected by machine washing, as hot cycles (over 50 °C) inactivate lice and eggs. Combs and hair-brushes should be soaked in hot water with a pediculicide for 15 minutes.

There is no need for children to be excluded from school once effective treatment has been given as though dead lice and eggs will persist in the hair they are dead and there is no infection risk. It is not necessary to comb out the hair though many parents choose to do so. It has been suggested that, so as to prevent resistance arising, treatment should be 'cycled'—i.e. one treatment used nationally for some time and then another; however, this policy has yet to be adopted uniformly.

PREVENTION OF FURTHER CASES

It has been suggested that a national 'Bug Busting Day' is may be the most effective way to control this pest. Families with children are encouraged to check their hair on the same day throughout the country. Treatment should be given when lice or nits are found.

75

PARVOVIRUS INFECTION: FIFTH DISEASE (ERYTHEMA INFECTIOSUM OR SLAPPED CHEEK DISEASE)

ORGANISM

Parvovirus B19, a small, non-enveloped DNA virus. (The name does not indicate there are other types which infect humans, it is an accident of history.)

EPIDEMIOLOGY

Humans are the only hosts. Any age may be affected and 50% or more of adults have evidence of past infection, i.e. half the adult population is probably immune. Outbreaks occur in schools and health care settings with transmission both to and from susceptible staff.

Transmission In most cases, the virus is found in respiratory secretions in the early part of the illness and this is thought to be the major route of transmission. By the time the rash appears, virus is no longer present in secretions. The exception to this is the patient with an aplastic crisis, in whom viral excretion may continue for a week or more after the onset of symptoms.

Incubation period is usually 4–14 days, but may be as much as 20 days.

NATURAL HISTORY AND CLINICAL FEATURES

About 50% of infections are asymptomatic. The most common disease pattern is of mild systemic upset with fever in 15% to 30% and a characteristic rash. This usually begins as an erythematous appearance to the face, hence the name 'slapped cheek' disease. It is followed by a symmetrical lace rash on the extremities and trunk. For weeks and sometimes months, the rash may fluctuate with temperature or exposure to sunlight. The changes may be relatively rapid, with the rash fading over a matter of hours and reappearing a few days or even hours later. Arthropathy is unusual in children, but common in adults, especially women.

Parvovirus has been proposed as the aetiological agent in some cases of Kawasaki disease. The virus has a predilection for erythroid precursors and switches off erythropiesis for up to 7 days. This is of considerable consequence in patients with red cell disorders characterized by reduced red cell survival and increased turnover. Patients with disorders such as sickle-cell disease and congenital hereditary spherocytosis may develop an aplastic crisis. This is usually temporary, lasting 5–10 days, but may necessitate blood transfusion. Virus clearance is only slightly delayed. Patients who are immunocompromised, such as those with human immunodeficiency virus infection, may develop an chronic relapsing anaemia due to marrow aplasia.

Infection in pregnancy is considered to occur in about one in three fetuses of infected women but rarely has any pathogenic effects. There is a significant increase in hydrops fetalis (due to fetal anaemia and sometimes myocarditis), fetal death and spontaneous abortion in the second and third trimesters. It has been suggested that the excess risk of fetal death following infection in pregnancy is around 9%. However, this risk is difficult to quantify and may vary between subgroups of women, for example it appears highest when the mother is asymptomatic. Congenital infection has been reported to have caused thrombocytopenia in a infant.

Diagnosis is often made clinically. A slight leucopenia and thrombocytopenia may be present. The main differential diagnosis is rubella. Where it is necessary to be certain, e.g. in pregnancy, specific IgM can be detected at 2 weeks after exposure, but because the exact time of infection is difficult to determine it may be important to repeat the test following an initial IgM negative result. When the fetus is affected ultrasonography may detect hydrops fetalis and serum alphafetoprotein levels may be raised. If cordocentesis is undertaken antigen and polymerase chain reaction tests may be applied, and are also sometimes used with post-mortem material. Detection of specific IgG a year after birth can confirm the diagnosis retrospectively.

MANAGEMENT

Management is symptomatic in most cases. Intravenous normal human immunoglobulin may be helpful in immunocompromised patients. When fetal infection is thought to have taken place specialist advice should be sought. Though interventions such as cordocentesis and intrauterine transfusion have been used, these have their own complications. Where pregnant women become aware that they may have been exposed and are anxious as to the consequences, a test for maternal specific IgG may be useful in demonstrating immunity but can lead to difficulties in knowing what to advise should a mother be non-immune.

PREVENTION OF FURTHER CASES

Studies of individual cases and outbreaks frequently reveal that the source of many infections cannot be traced. Because of this and for practical reasons a policy of protecting all pregnant women from exposure to parvovirus B19 is impractical and probably ineffective. However, women particularly at risk, for example pregnant health care staff, should not be exposed to chronically infectious patients such as patients with aplastic crises.

PERTUSSIS (WHOOPING COUGH)

76

Notifiable disease

ORGANISM

Bordetella pertussis and *B. parapertussis* are Gram-negative bacilli.

EPIDEMIOLOGY

Humans are the only hosts. Pertussis is a very important cause of morbidity and early childhood mortality worldwide, though it seems to be more commonly recognized in temperate countries. In the UK there were three major epidemics in the late 1970s and 1980s following a fall in vaccination uptake in the early 1970s, which itself followed concerns over vaccine safety. The concerns were unfounded, however vaccine uptake and incidence only returned to pre-1977 levels in the 1990s following a determined drive to improve the immunization coverage (see Appendix I). Immunization is currently thought to protect against disease rather than infection; however, the role of asymptomatic infection in transmission is unclear. No maternal immunity passes across the placental and young infants are most susceptible to severe disease. Infection can occur at any age, but in adolescents and adults pertussis may not be recognized because of its atypical presentation.

Transmission is by droplet spread. Pertussis is highly infectious with most susceptible household contacts and 50% of school contacts developing the illness. Treatment with erythromycin usually renders a sufferer non-infectious within 5 days.

Incubation period is 7–10 days, but occasionally longer.

NATURAL HISTORY AND CLINICAL FEATURES

Bordetella pertussis and *B. parapertussis* produce similar illnesses except that disease due to the former is usually more severe. The initial symptoms are coryza and a dry cough. The latter worsens over the next 2 weeks until paroxysms start to occur. The severity and frequency of these increase and the characteristic whoop appears at the end of each paroxysm. This may be accompanied by vomiting. In a severe paroxysm, cyanosis may occur and the child may be utterly exhausted. The paroxysms can be precipitated by feeding, crying or even hearing another person cough. In young infants the typical whoop is usually absent, but there may be a period of apnoea at the end of bouts of coughing. The paroxysmal stage continues for 2–6 weeks and may only subside gradually, giving an illness which often lasts 3 months or more. The course of disease is generally more severe in infants. Even in relatively mild cases weight loss occurs and the distress caused to both the child and family is considerable. Subconjunctival haemorrhages are relatively common. The force of the coughing may be sufficient to produce air leaks (surgical emphysema, pneumomediastinum and pneumothorax). Atelectasis is relatively common, but unlike in the pre-antibiotic era, it now rarely leads to bronchiectasis.

Convulsions may accompany severe cases and an encephalopathy occurs in around 1 in 11 000 cases. There is evidence to suggest that when pertussis is prevalent a proportion of cot deaths are due to undiagnosed pertussis. In adolescents and adults the characteristic whoop is often lacking and the sufferer may consider they have a prolonged cold and cough.

Diagnosis There is usually a lymphocytosis at 2–5 weeks which may rise to over 40×10^9/l. This does not occur in *B. parapertussis* infections. For the first 5 weeks of the untreated illness, the organism may be cultured from the nasopharynx, using a pernasal swab plated onto Cephalexine charcoal agar. Culture takes at least 5 days. However, in only 50% of cases can it be recovered, so alternative methods have been employed. The most useful is fluorescent antibody staining of swabs from the nasopharynx but this is still prone to false positives and negatives.

MANAGEMENT

Hospitalization is sometimes unavoidable if the disease is severe especially for young infants who are prone to apnoea. It can also be necessary when the family is reaching exhaustion from nursing a restless coughing infant. Hospitalized cases should be isolated and subject to respiratory precautions (see Chapter 26). Erythromycin should be given on the basis of a presumptive diagnosis to prevent further transmission. Once the paroxysmal stage has been reached the drug is unlikely to change the course of the illness, but it will eradicate the organism in 3–5 days thus preventing further transmission. No medication has been convincingly shown to reduce the frequency or severity of the paroxysms. The child should be disturbed as little as possible. Vomiting may produce significant dehydration if not treated by nasogastric or intravenous therapy. In a sick infant close respiratory monitoring with pulse oximetry is essential as potentially damaging apnoeic episodes may otherwise go unnoticed.

PREVENTION OF FURTHER CASES

Patients can be infectious for 4–5 weeks of their illness if no treatment is given. Once a 5-day course of suitable antibiotic has been completed, there is little danger of transmission. While infectious the person should be isolated from non-immune individuals, especially young children.

Chemoprophylaxis It as been suggested that treating contacts in the presymptomatic or early symptomatic stages with erythromycin may prevent the development of the illness. This is still controversial, but some authorities advocate giving erythromycin to young children, particularly infants, who have been in contact with a case.

Vaccination A highly effective 'whole-cell' vaccine against *Bordetella pertussis* has been in use in the UK for over 50 years. It is available in combination with diphtheria and tetanus as the 'triple' vaccine. Three doses gives about 85–90% protection. If a fully immunized individual develops the disease, it is much less severe than in the unimmunized individuals. However when cases occur vaccination of contacts is of no value in preventing spread of the disease as a number of doses are needed and immunity takes time to develop.

There are very few contraindications to the vaccine and the Department of Health guidelines are now very clear (see Appendix VI). The current vaccine

Table 76.1 Rates of reaction to whole cell vaccine

	First (2 months)	Second (3 months)	Third (4 months)	Combined*
Fever (> 38 °C)	5%	10%	20%	4–11%
Mild malaise	–	–	–	12–18%
Local pain, redness or induration	< 2%	5%	10%	1–5%

***Combining data for immunizations at 2, 3 and 4 months. A range is stated because of variation according to particular vaccine manufacturer.**

contains at least six active components but frequently causes minor local and systemic reactions in recipients. Reaction rates are age-dependent, increasing with age of immunization in infants, and typical rates experienced with the whole cell vaccine are given in Table 76.1. Reactions are more common with the second and third immunizations. It remains unclear whether permanent harm ever results from the whole-cell vaccines currently in use. If permanent harm ever does take place it is extremely rare in occurrence.

'Acellular' (component) vaccines are not yet licensed in the UK. Recent trial data suggest that some acellular vaccines may be as effective as whole-cell vaccines in producing protection. The data also suggest that they produce less of the mild reactions associated with the whole-cell vaccine. But at present no acellular vaccine has yet to be licensed for use in the primary course of immunization in the UK.

77

PLAGUE

Notifiable disease

ORGANISM

Yersinia pestis, the plague bacillus, is a Gram-negative bipolar-staining bacillus.

EPIDEMIOLOGY

Wild rodents are the natural reservoir of plague, with different rodents (not only rats) being the reservoir in different locations. *Yersinia pestis* is probably endemic in animal populations in a large number of countries mainly in sub-Saharan Africa, the Indian subcontinent and south-east Asia, where outbreaks among adults and children have occurred in the past two decades contributing a global figure of reported cases of 200 to 2000 cases annually. Outbreaks are thought to be due to natural occurrences disrupting rodent populations or humans coming into contact with previously isolated rodent populations.

Transmisson There are two forms of plague: *bubonic plague* is transmitted by an infected flea from an animal biting a human, and *pneumonic plague* is thought to be transmissible by coughing and inhalation of aerosols from a person with acute pneumonic plague.

Incubation period is 2–4 days in pneumonic plague, 2–6 days in bubonic plague.

Period of infectivity is unclear. It is thought that fleas may remain infective only for a few days before they themselves die. Pneumonic plague is considered infective through aerosol in the severe phase but is not thought to be infective prior to symptoms.

NATURAL HISTORY AND CLINICAL FEATURES

Bubonic plague is characterized by high temperature, enlarged lymph nodes draining the sites of flea bites (which can enlarge to become 'buboes'), restlessness, generalized malaise and shock. Extension may occur elsewhere causing meningitis, septicaemia or pneumonia (pneumonic plague) which are frequently fatal without treatment.

Pneumonic plague can be overwhelming and result in a severe productive cough and death in a matter of days due to respiratory failure.

Diagnosis Definitive diagnosis is by isolation and identification of *Yersinia pestis* by an experienced reference laboratory. In endemic areas it will be necessary to treat possible cases on the basis of a presumptive diagnosis made on clinical grounds or microbiologic examination of sputum or bubo material. However, before an outbreak is declared, it is important to make the definitive diagnosis. During a confirmed outbreak a presumptive diagnosis can be made by microbiologic examination of sputum or bubo material. Care must be taken as the bacillus is a highly hazardous organism. It should be cultured and some specimens fixed in alcohol and stained for examination by an experienced microbiologist. Serology may be of benefit in demonstrating rising titres but is not as useful as isolation of the organism.

MANAGEMENT

In suspected cases the patient should be isolated and admitted to hospital, preferably to a specialist centre. If used early in the infection, the drugs of choice chloramphenicol, tetracycline and streptomycin are usually effective.

PREVENTION OF FURTHER CASES

Travellers should be advised against visiting areas where new infections and human-to-human spread is occurring. Those who have to travel should wear insect repellent. If exposure is suspected those infected should take a course of tetracycline (250 mg four times daily for 7 days). Children aged between 6 weeks and 12 years may take a week's course of co-trimoxazole and younger babies can have ampicillin (though protection is probably less). In endemic areas control of fleas and rodent populations is important. Currently no effective vaccine is available.

PNEUMOCYSTIS CARINII PNEUMONIA

ORGANISM

Formerly thought to be a protozoan, *Pneumocystis carinii* is now known to be a fungal species.

EPIDEMIOLOGY

Pneumocystis carinii is a ubiquitous organism which can affect many different animals including humans. Serological studies suggest that most children become subclinically infected within the first few years of life. Clinically significant disease only occurs in those who have immunocompromising conditions affecting cell-mediated immunity. This includes children with congenital immune deficiencies, human immunodeficiency virus (HIV) infection and secondary immune deficiencies such as those induced by chemotherapy or malnutrition. It is probable that clinical disease in the first 2 years of life represents primary infection, while disease in older individuals is due to reactivation. The disease has occurred as outbreaks in populations suffering severe malnutrition and occasionally as an opportunist pathogen in extremely premature sick infants.

Transmission The mode of acquisition of this organism is not clear. It is probable that person-to-person transmission does occur.

Incubation period is unknown.

NATURAL HISTORY AND CLINICAL FEATURES

Pneumocystis carinii produces a diffuse pneumonitis (*P. carinii* pneumonia, PCP) usually with an insidious onset. Typically symptoms build up over a period of a few weeks though more acute forms can occur in patients with acquired immunodeficiency syndrome (AIDS). The symptoms include tachypnoea, fever and dry cough, sometimes associated with hoarseness. As the disease progresses there are increasing signs of respiratory distress and of desaturation. There are usually no abnormal auscultatory findings. Chest radiographs may be relatively normal at the onset of symptoms but diffuse pulmonary infiltrates soon appear, most marked in the perihilar regions but spreading extensively to involve both lung fields. As the child progresses into respiratory failure the typical arterial blood gas findings show a reduced oxygen tension with hypocapnia.

Diagnosis While the chest X-ray is highly suggestive of PCP the differential diagnosis is wide and includes viral pneumonitis, atypical bacterial pneumonia and other fungal pneumonias. Confirmation of the diagnosis requires demonstration of the organism in pulmonary secretions or lung tissue. The classical way of confirming the diagnosis is by lung biopsy either obtained by thoracotomy or at bronchoscopy (transbronchial biopsy). The organisms can be demonstrated using methenamine silver stains. Less invasive (though probably less sensitive) techniques are increasingly used. These include examination of bronchial secretions obtained at bronchoscopy by bronchoalveolar lavage or, in older children, examination of induced sputum produced following inhalation of hypertonic saline. Newer methods have also been developed for demonstrating the organism in respiratory secretions using an immunofluorescent technique. Polymerase chain reaction techniques are also becoming available.

MANAGEMENT

Patients will usually require oxygen therapy and in more severe cases ventilatory assistance. High-dose co-trimoxazole (120 mg/kg per day in 4 divided doses) should be started as early as possible. It is normal to start this intravenously but provided the patient does not have significant gastrointestinal disease therapy can be continued by the oral route. For critically ill patients where it is felt that invasive procedures will not be tolerated this treatment can be commenced empirically—improvement occurring over the first 36–48 hours being fairly strong confirmatory evidence of PCP. In severe pneumonitis it has been shown, in adults, that adjuvant therapy with corticosteroids is beneficial.

In those who show intolerance of high-dose co-trimoxazole treatment or fail to respond, pentamidine (4 mg/kg per day) given intravenously or intramuscularly should be used. Treatment should be continued for a minimum of 2 weeks. Thereafter prophylaxis (see below) should be continued indefinitely because of the risk of recurrent disease.

PREVENTION OF FURTHER CASES

Prophylactic treatment has been shown to be effective in preventing PCP in high-risk individuals. The treatment of choice is co-trimoxazole 450 mg/m^2 twice a day (maximum 480 mg twice daily) given on 3 days in a week or 30 mg/kg per day on each day if antibacterial prophylaxis is also required. (see Chapter 19). This treatment should be given to HIV-positive children, children with congenital cell-mediated immune deficiencies and children undergoing chemotherapy, particularly continuous prolonged chemotherapy as in the protocols for acute lymphoblastic leukaemia. Alternative treatments in those intolerant of co-trimoxazole include dapsone 1 mg/kg daily or inhaled pentamidine (300 mg given monthly). The latter is unsuitable for very young children because of the difficulties in administration. In older children, particularly those with an asthmatic tendency, it may induce bronchospasm and pretreatment with nebulized salbutamol is advisable.

Patients with PCP should not be allowed to come into contact with severely immunocomprised children because of the potential risk of person-to-person spread.

POLIOMYELITIS

Notifiable disease

ORGANISM

Poliovirus is an enterovirus of three antigenic types: 1, 2 and 3.

EPIDEMIOLOGY

Poliovirus infection occurs only in humans but the virus can survive in water in favourable conditions for up to 3 months. It is endemic in parts of the developing world, notably Africa and the Indian subcontinent where the annual incidence of paralytic disease may be 10–30 per 100 000 population per annum. Hence there is a potential hazard to travellers to developing countries. Outbreaks also occur in unimmunized groups in industrialized countries. Because of the success of routine immunization transmission of wild virus does not occur in the UK. However, imported infections and vaccine-associated cases (through rare reversion of attenuated forms of the live oral polio vaccine, OPV) still occur in unimmunized or incompletely immunized persons. From 1985 to 1994 in England and Wales 26 confirmed cases were reported: 17 were vaccine-associated and 6 imported, while for 3 the source was unknown. The British Paediatric Surveillance Unit monitored acute flaccid paralysis from July 1991 to June 1994. A total of 108 cases were reported to the scheme from England and Wales, only 4 of these resulted in paralytic polio.

Transmission is by the faecal–oral route; transmission by food or water contamination is rare. Infectivity of wild virus via faeces may be prolonged for several weeks or longer but is highest in the few days around the onset of symptoms. Infectivity of OPV is shorter (rarely more than 2 months).

Incubation period is 7–21 days for paralytic cases due to wild virus. In vaccine-associated cases the period is 7–28 days in recipients and 7–60 days in contacts.

NATURAL HISTORY AND CLINICAL FEATURES

In children most cases are subclinical or simply present as a mild febrile illness. However, in a minority of infections with wild virus or reverted OPV the infection proceeds to invade the nervous system causing either an aseptic meningitis (non-paralytic polio) or more rarely paralytic polio due to the virus attacking the motor cells in the spinal cord. Paralysis is of a lower motor neurone type, usually asymmetrical and may affect only a single muscle group (usually in the limbs) or more extensive groups. If this includes the muscles of respiration and swallowing it can be fatal. Paralysis frequently improves but residual effects are usually permanent. Older children and adults are more at risk of paralytic disease.

Diagnosis Poliovirus can be recovered from the faeces, throat and (rarely) from cerebrospinal fluid by isolation in tissue culture. Two specimens of faeces, taken 7 days apart, should be obtained from all patients with acute paralytic disease (including where Guillain–Barré syndrome is the considered diagnosis) for isolation of the virus. Use of rectal swabs is a relatively insensitive technique. Viral cultures from two specimens collected within the first 15 days of illness remains the diagnostic test of choice. Serologic testing of acute and convalescent sera can be performed in patients suspected of having paralytic poliomyelitis. However, interpretation of serologic tests can be difficult.

Important differential diagnoses include the other causes of aseptic meningitis and acute paralytic disease; Guillain–Barré syndrome, acute polyneuritis (other including viruses and toxins); localized paralysis following specific infections (Epstein–Barr virus and infective mononucleosis) and other enveroviruses (coxsackievirus A7, echovirus 3) causing a poliomyelitis-like illness.

MANAGEMENT

There is no specific treatment for the paralytic form apart from bed rest in the acute phase.

PREVENTION OF FURTHER CASES

Single cases or outbreaks

Informing In the UK, when a case of polio is suspected the consultant in communicable disease control (or director of public health) must be informed immediately along with the Communicable Disease Surveillance Centre, or the Scottish Centre for Infection and Environmental Health or the Department of Health and Social Services in Northern Ireland so they can institute public health measures. The case should also be notified.

Isolation For patients suspected of excreting wild poliovirus, enteric precautions are indicated for the duration of hospitalization or until virus can no longer be recovered from the faeces.

Urgent immunization If laboratory tests indicate a vaccine-derived virus was responsible immunization of further contacts is not required. In cases due to wild virus, if transmission occurred abroad (imported case) then the vaccination of families should be urgently reviewed and immunization given to any unimmunized or underimmunized persons. After a single case of confirmed polio due to transmission of wild virus in the UK a dose of OPV should be given to all cases in the immediate neighbourhood regardless of immunization history. In unimmunized persons the course must be completed.

- **If it is unclear whether this is a wild or vaccine-associated case it should be assumed that it is a wild case and control measures instituted.**

Routine immunization of infants and children Two types of trivalent vaccine are available; live oral poliovirus vaccine (Sabin) and inactivated poliovirus vaccine (Salk)—given parenterally. Both are effective in preventing poliomyelitis in individuals. Oral poliovirus vaccine (OPV) has the additional benefit of often boosting immunization in other family members through ongoing transmission.

Based on consideration of the risks and benefits, OPV is currently the vaccine of choice in the UK because it induces intestinal immunity, is simple to administer, results in immunization of some contacts of vaccinated persons. Its use has eliminated disease caused by wild polioviruses in the UK. Multiple doses of OPV are given to ensure that infection occurs with all three types of poliovirus and induces complete immunity. In the UK, OPV is given at 2, 3 and 4 months with diphtheria, tetanus and pertussis vaccine, at school entry and school leaving. In households with an immunodeficient person, including those known to be HIV-infected, OPV should not be used because it is excreted in the stool by healthy vaccinees and can infect an immunocompromised household member, which may result in paralytic disease. Only inactivated poliovirus vaccine (IPV) should be used in such households—this includes the households of HIV-infected mothers.

POXVIRUS INFECTION (INCLUDING MOLLUSCUM CONTAGIOSUM)

ORGANISM

Poxviruses are large, complex DNA viruses. They are enveloped but the envelope is not necessary for infectivity. The genera infecting children are Orthopoxviridae (smallpox, vaccinia and cowpox), Parapoxviridae (orf and milker's nodes) and molluscipox (molluscum contagiosum). Smallpox has been eradicated and is not considered further.

MOLLUSCUM CONTAGIOSUM

EPIDEMIOLOGY

Humans are the only host and infection is considered to be present worldwide. In Papua New Guinea a prevalence rate of 22% and incidence rate of 6% per year was observed in children under 10 years old. Attack rates in previously unexposed children vary from 12% to 75%.

Transmission is by direct contact, infectivity is low and no exclusion from school is indicated.

Incubation period is highly variable, from 2 weeks to 6 months.

NATURAL HISTORY AND CLINICAL FEATURES

Infection results in a characteristic pearly papule with an obvious central dimple (molluscum body), varying in size from 1 mm to 5 mm. These papules can occur anywhere in children, most commonly in small crops due to direct contact. Infection usually resolves spontaneously without scarring—usually within 6 months to 2 years—and treatment is not indicated.

Diagnosis is primarily clinical. Negative stain electron microscopy of the crushed molluscum body provides specific diagnosis if this is required.

MANAGEMENT

Anti-wart solutions available from pharmacists are ineffective. More drastic local treatments are not justified since the lesions will resolve spontaneously. If they occur in the child's genital or perianal area the possibility of sexual abuse may be considered, but accidental spread can also occur through self-inoculation from a child's hands.

COWPOX

EPIDEMIOLOGY

Despite its name it appears that cattle are not the main reservoir of cowpox. It is probable that cowpox is enzootic in small rodents. Humans have become infected from contact with cats, cattle (rarely) and possibly small rodents. Cowpox is limited to UK and continental Europe. Approximately 40% of reported cases have occurred in children.

Transmission is by direct contact but infectivity is low.

Incubation period is 6–10 days.

NATURAL HISTORY AND CLINICAL FEATURES

Most often infection results in a single lesion predominantly on hands or face. The lesion begins as an inflamed macule which progresses through papular and vesicular stages over 7–12 days. The vesicle becomes pale blue or purple and increasingly haemorrhagic and evolves to a pustule which then ulcerates (2–3 weeks after onset). The lesion then appears as a deep-seated, indurated black eschar which may be mistaken for anthrax. System symptoms are common including pyrexia, malaise and sore throat, which resolve prior to the eschar stage. In the immunocompromised there may be generalized infection which may be fatal. The lesions heal within 6–8 weeks but scarring is common.

Diagnosis Negative stain electron microscopy of material from the lesion provides the definitive diagnosis which can be supplemented by virus culture.

MANAGEMENT

There is no specific treatment and the condition is self-limiting but patients should be counselled on the risks of autoinoculation to other sites.

PARAPOXVIRUS (orf and milker's nodes)

EPIDEMIOLOGY

In general sheep and goats are the source of orf and cattle the source of milker's nodes. The majority of infections occur in adults but in most series just over 10% of cases are in children. Most infections occur from October to December.

Transmission is by direct inoculation from an infected animal into the skin.

Incubation period is 3–7 days.

NATURAL HISTORY AND CLINICAL FEATURES

Most infections are on the fingers. The lesion begins as an inflammatory papule which enlarges to a large, bluish-red granulomatous lesion. The lesion has been mistaken clinically for a malignancy and resulted in amputation of a thumb. It crusts and regresses over a period of several weeks. The lesion is painless. Immunity is poor and repeated infections have been described.

Diagnosis Negative stain electron microscopy of material from the lesion provides definitive diagnosis.

MANAGEMENT

There is no specific treatment and management is supportive.

PRION DISEASE (SPONGIFORM ENCEPHALOPATHIES)

ORGANISM

The spongiform encephalopathies comprise a group of syndromes—Creutzfeldt-Jakob disease (CJD), fatal familial insomnia, Gerstmann–Straussler syndrome (GSS) and kuru—all of which are characterized by vacuolation of neurones and neuropil in brain tissue. This leads to the appearance of numerous small holes (spongiform) in the brain on histological examination. There is no evidence of inflammatory changes (hence 'encephalopathy'). The disease is transmissible and several hypotheses of the nature of the infective agent) have been propounded. The prion (proteinaceous infectious agent) hypothesis has gained widest acceptance. It proposes that the infectious agent is an indigestible self-replicating form of a normal brain protein. Though some experts would maintain that there is associated nucleic acid. The agent co-purifies with a modified host protein (PrP^{SC} in scrapie) and is resistant to conditions that would inactivate conventional viruses (nuclease, 90 °C for 30 minutes, ultraviolet, disinfectants).

EPIDEMIOLOGY

The most common of these syndromes is CJD ($0.5–1/10^6$ population). Kuru, which was endemic in the Fore language group in Papua New Guinea, has been eradicated. In addition to an infective agent there is a genetic predisposition, for example 10% of cases of CJD and up to 80% of cases of fatal familial insomnia occur in close relatives. Most cases of CJD occur in adults but some recent cases (usually associated with human growth hormone administration) have occurred in teenagers.

Transmission The mode of transmission of sporadic CJD is unknown. For iatrogenic CJD modes of transmission are by direct intracerebral inoculation and include neurosurgery tissue transplantation (cornea, dura mater) and injection of tissue extracts (growth hormone and gonadotrophins). Kuru was transmitted by ritual cannibalism. The possibility of transplacental transmission of CJD has recently been raised.

Incubation period For direct inoculation into brain (neurosurgery or transplantation) the incubation period is 18–54 months, and for injection into muscle (growth hormone, gonadotrophins) it is 5–20 years. For kuru the youngest patient was aged 4 years, which sets a minimum known incubation period by ingestion.

NATURAL HISTORY AND CLINICAL FEATURES

The presentation of iatrogenic CJD differs according to the mode of inoculation. In those infected through neurosurgery or tissue transplantation, mental deterioration is the major presenting feature (70% of cases) with 33% showing cerebellar signs and 20% visual and oculomotor signs. In those infected through tissue extracts (growth hormone gonadotrophin) all presented with cerebellar signs and 15% had visual and oculomotor signs, but none had mental deterioration. During the course of disease—which usually lasts 6–18 months—the disease patterns merge with the above features, myoclonus and pyramidal and extrapyramidal signs. There are none of the usual signs associated with infection and disease progresses inexorably to death.

Diagnosis The definitive diagnosis is by histological and electron microscopic examination of brain biopsy. Characteristic electroencephalographic changes (periodicity) are present in a minority of those with iatrogenic CJD.

MANAGEMENT

There is no specific therapy and supportive treatment does little to alter the course of the disease. Care must be taken to prevent transmission of disease to others (at post-mortem, etc.).

82 RABIES

Notifiable disease

ORGANISM

Rabies virus is a rhabdovirus of the family *Lyssaviridae*.

EPIDEMIOLOGY

Rabies is a zoonosis with reservoirs of infection in a variety of warm-blooded animals, usually wild. Important species include foxes in Europe, racoons and bats in the USA and dogs and foxes in south Asia. A limited number of industrialized countries are rabies-free, including those of Australasia, parts of Europe (the UK, Eire, Greece, Norway, Portugal, Sweden and most of Spain) and a number of islands (including Japan, Singapore, Taiwan and much but not all of the West Indies). Worldwide the most important mode of infection is by bites from domestic dogs that themselves have been infected by wild animals or by other dogs. Human infections from cats and other animals are unusual. Residents of the UK are only at risk when in countries where rabies is endemic, usually from domestic animals. Since 1902 there have been 21 cases of rabies in humans in the UK following exposure abroad (five cases since 1980). All had a fatal outcome. Most of those recently reported have been due to dog bites taking place in South Asia.

Transmission is most commonly from a bite. As the virus is present in saliva licking of injured skin or open mucous membrane also poses a small risk.

Incubation period is highly variable in humans, from a few days to over a year following exposure (one case in the UK was more than 14 months). The virus is neurotropic and travels up nerves to affect the brain. Consequently, the closer the site of infection to the brain the more rapid the appearance of symptoms, with bites on the face, head and neck resulting in the quickest appearance.

Period of infectivity Person-to-person spread is not recorded except in a very unusual example of tissue transfer of infection when rabies infection has taken place through transplantation of corneas following an undiagnosed rabies death. Once a dog or cat is infected it almost always develops symptoms within 10 days.

NATURAL HISTORY AND CLINICAL FEATURES

An affected patient presents with a fever and a deteriorating neurological condition including confusion and convulsions. There will usually be a history of exposure to a rabid animal.

Diagnosis Preliminary diagnosis in humans is by history of exposure and then appearance of symptoms. Pre-mortem diagnosis is very difficult but may be possible by specialist laboratories through detection of virus in saliva or cerebrospinal fluid (CSF). Definitive diagnosis in an animal is by demonstration of the virus in brain tissue. In the UK, the Public Health Laboratory Service unit with special expertise in diagnosis of rabies in humans is the Virus Reference Division, Central Public Health Laboratory (Tel: 0181 200 4400). It also issues prophylactic treatment, both rabies vaccine and specific immunoglobulin. Advice on the need for pre- and post-exposure prophylaxis is also available from CDSC (Tel: 0181 200 6868) or the PHLS Virus Reference Division (Tel: 0181 200 4400) and the Scottish Centre for Infection and Environmental Health (Tel: 0141 946 7120).

MANAGEMENT

Treatment, once symptoms have developed, is supportive but it is very unusual for the patient to survive (the best treatment is prevention). Isolation is recommended.

PREVENTION OF FURTHER CASES

Pre-exposure immunization Some people require pre-exposure immunization because of the risk of exposure through their work. These include the following:

- Laboratory workers handling the virus.
- Persons whose work is expected to bring them into contact with imported animals, e.g. zoo workers and quarantine kennel workers.
- Persons going to work in endemic countries who may be in contact with animals (e.g. veterinary officers).

Pre-exposure immunization consists of three immunizations with the inactivated vaccine at intervals of 7 and 21 days. Immunization is by the deep intramuscular or subcutaneous route (intradermal immunization is not recommended). In addition, some people travelling to, and spending time in, endemic areas where risk is high and post-exposure immunization unavailable choose to have pre-exposure vaccination.

Post-exposure prophylaxis Because of the relatively slow time-course of rabies in which the organism slowly tracks up nerves to affect the central nervous system, there is usually time to successfully apply post-exposure prophylaxis (immunization and sometimes also rabies-specific immunoglobulin).

Hospital exposure Following a case of proven exposure, hospital and laboratory staff need immunization, and also immunoglobulin if their mucous membranes or an open wound have been exposed to saliva, CSF or brain tissue from a rabid animal or a patient with rabies (e.g. performing mouth to mouth resuscitation.

Community exposure—animal bite Any animal bite in any country should be flushed immediately with water or any available clean fluid (bottled drinks will do in the first instance), then the wound should be cleaned with soapy water.* Good drainage is important and stitching should be avoided or delayed unless there are good cosmetic reasons. Exposure is classified according to the level of risk of the area where it took place.

- *No-risk areas*: UK, Eire, Denmark, Norway, Greece, Portugal, Spain (except central areas), Japan, Singapore, Taiwan, Australasia, Malta, Cyprus, Jamaica and Bermuda.
- *Low-risk areas*: Countries where rabies is present in wild animals but very rare in domestic animals and where dogs are routinely immunized. These are USA, Canada and western Europe (except those countries in the 'no risk' category).
- *High-risk areas*: Countries where rabies is widespread in both wild and domestic animals. These are most countries in Africa including North Africa, South and Central America, and most of the Middle East (including Turkey) and Asia.

It is difficult to make completely firm rules as to who should receive post-exposure immunization or immunoglobulin. A good history will always help in making a rational decision covering the following points:

- *The exposure*: which country (level of risk as above)? When? Where on the body? Was the skin broken? Was there a pre-existing wound? Were the mucous membranes exposed? Was local management applied (i.e. was washing undertaken)? Had pre-exposure immunization been received—when, and was it a complete course?
- *The animal*: what species (the risk is predominantly from dogs)? Name and contact details of the owner. Was the animal provoked, or was it behaving oddly? What happened to the animal subsequently? **If a dog is known to be alive and well 10–14 days after the exposure rabies can be ruled out** and a telephone call or fax to a reliable owner may obviate the need for continuing post-exposure prophylaxis.
- Local information that there is no risk because all dogs are immunized should not be regarded as a reason for not giving post-exposure prophylaxis in high risk areas.

If the history reveals any significant exposure, specialist advice must be taken (see diagnosis above).

Even if exposure was months in the past it can be life-saving to give post-exposure prophylaxis which consists of the following:

- *Previously unimmunized individuals*: six doses of vaccine one given on each of days 3, 7, 14, 30 and 90, counting the day of the first vaccine as day zero. It may also be considered necessary to give specific immunoglobulin (20 iu/kg; half infiltrated into the wound or exposure site and half given elsewhere by parenteral injection).
- *Previously immunized individual*: two doses of vaccine at an interval of 3–7 days without immunoglobulin.

***Infections from animal bites are unusual. In addition to rabies they include cat-scratch disease and pasteurellosis (cats).**

RESPIRATORY SYNCYTIAL VIRUS INFECTION

ORGANISM

Respiratory syncytial virus (RSV) is an enveloped RNA paramyxovirus of the genus pneumovirus.

EPIDEMIOLOGY

There is a worldwide distribution with annual epidemics during the autumn, winter and early spring. Infections occur predominantly in infants and young children. The infection is particularly severe in infants with congenital heart disease and those with a history of chronic lung disease following respiratory distress syndrome of prematurity. Passive smoking is a risk factor for infection.

Transmission Humans are the only source of infection, and transmission is mainly person-to-person by droplets from the respiratory tract. The virus is known to be viable for up to 6 hours in secretions outside the body. Infection is communicable for up to 1 week after onset of symptoms. More prolonged sheddng of virus may occur in young infants.

Incubation period is 2–8 days.

NATURAL HISTORY AND CLINICAL FEATURES

Infection with RSV is the usual cause of bronchiolitis in infancy. In the preterm infant infection may result in apnoea, lethargy or non-specific signs of sepsis. In the term infant signs are more localized to the chest, with tachypnoea and subcostal recession. Auscultation may reveal crackles and wheezes. In the majority of children recovery occurs within 5–7 days, but in the high-risk groups described above, respiratory failure ensues which if not recognized quickly may lead to respiratory arrest.

Diagnosis is by immunofluorescence on cells from the nasopharynx. Such tests have 80–90% sensitivity during the first few days of the illness. This investigation should be available in all paediatric units treating high-risk infants, eligible for ribavirin.

MANAGEMENT

Treatment is generally supportive; fluids are given by nasogastric tube or intravenously in sick, hospitalized babies. In severely affected infants, the antiviral drug ribavirin can be used. It is administered by a small particle aerosol generator over 12 hours for 2–4 days, either into a head box or ventilator tubing. Infants likely to require and benefit from treatment include those with congenital heart disease, bronchopulmonary dysplasia and cystic fibrosis; infants with deteriorating respiratory function (an oxygen saturation of less than 90% and rising carbon dioxide levels); and infants requiring mechanical ventilation for RSV infection. Ribavirin has been found to be teratogenic in rodents. There is no evidence of teratogenicity in human beings, but as a precaution, it should not be administered by pregnant attendants.

PREVENTION OF FURTHER CASES

Infants with RSV infection should be isolated. Attendants should pay particular attention to hand-washing. There is some evidence that cohort nursing reduces the risk of cross-infection, but this is usually difficult to organize.

84 ROSEOLA INFANTUM, EXANTHEMA SUBITUM OR SIXTH DISEASE (HUMAN HERPESVIRUS 6/7 INFECTION)

ORGANISM

Human herpesviruses 6 and 7 (HHV-6 and HHV-7) are enveloped DNA viruses.

EPIDEMIOLOGY

Humans are the only hosts and the infection is thought to occur worldwide as a disease of infancy and early childhood (ages 3 months to 4 years) following protection in early infancy from maternal antibody. It is considered that nearly every child acquires infection in that period. There is no seasonal pattern to infection.

Transmission is by respiratory secretion and occurs while the child has a fever, though asymptomatic infections may be important in transmission and are considered to be important for sustaining cycles of infection.

Incubation period is probably 8–10 days.

NATURAL HISTORY AND CLINICAL FEATURES

The child has a sudden onset of pyrexia with irritability. This lasts 3–6 days with the fever climbing to 40–41 °C, following which the fever suddenly falls and a widespread red maculopapular rash appears, which can last anything from a few hours to 2–3 days. Complications are rare, though febrile convulsions may occur. The virus may persist and the disease can reactivate in immunosuppressed individuals, though even in these infection is rarely serious.

Diagnosis is usually clinical. Some laboratories can isolate the virus on a research basis though this is only of value in excluding other causes.

MANAGEMENT

It is important to rule out more serious illnesses: see Chapter 14. Otherwise treatment is symptomatic.

85 ROTAVIRUS AND OTHER VIRAL ENTEROPATHOGENS

ROTAVIRUS

ORGANISM

Rotavirus is a medium-sized, non-enveloped RNA virus with a characteristic double-shelled capsid which gives the characteristic wheel shape (L. rota, wheel). It is a genus within the family Reoviridae and its genome consists of 11 segments of double-stranded RNA. Rotavirus is divided into seven serogroups (A–G). Most infections in children are due to serogroup A although serogroups B and C have been responsible for major epidemics. For epidemiological purposes rotaviruses are further divided into serotypes (1–14) and on the migration pattern of the 11 ds RNA segment on polyacrylamide gel electrophoresis (electropherotypes). Most human infections are due to serotypes 1–4 and antibodies to these epitopes neutralize infectivity.

EPIDEMIOLOGY

Rotavirus is the most important cause of gastroenteritis and dehydration in children throughout the world. In hospital-based surveys rotavirus is responsible for 20–60% of cases of gastroenteritis in infants and children. In community-based surveys the proportion of cases due to rotavirus is lower, ranging from 6% to 35%. Estimated hospitalization rates for rotavirus gastroenteritis in developed countries range from 2.2 to 8.5 per 1000 children. Reports of virus from laboratories in England and Wales have increased slowly since 1980 (Appendix 1, Fig. 2). In developing countries rotavirus is responsible for 125 million cases of gastroenteritis per year; 18 million of these are severe, leading to almost 1 million deaths each year. The peak incidence of rotavirus infection is in children aged 3–15 months. Repeated rotavirus infections are frequent but are usually mild or asymptomatic unless due to serogroup B or C virus. In temperate countries such as the UK rotavirus infection occurs predominantly in the cooler winter months although infections do occur throughout the year. Although most mammalian species are infected by rotavirus, animal strains rarely cross the species barrier to infect humans. Most rotavirus infections are community-acquired, but sporadic and epidemic nosocomial spread has been described.

Transmission Person-to-person spread occurs predominantly by the faecal-oral route. However, because the spread is so efficient in both developed and developing countries it has been suggested that transmission might also occur by the respiratory route. During acute infection a child can excrete up to 10^{11} rotavirus particles per gram of faeces. The infective dose is estimated to be as low as 10^2 particles. Infection can be transmitted from symptomatic or asymptomatically infected children and all four major serotypes (1–4) circulate at a given time, although one serotype tends to predominate.

Incubation period is 1–3 days.

NATURAL HISTORY AND CLINICAL FEATURES

Ingested virus first replicates in the proximal small intestine and spreads distally to the terminal ileum. Rotavirus does not infect the stomach or colon. Virus infects mature villous enterocytes but not the crypt enterocytes. The villous enterocytes are killed leading to blunted villi. This results in loss of absorption and decreased disaccharidase activity and thus to an osmotic diarrhoea.

Rotavirus gastroenteritis can vary in severity from mild, watery diarrhoea lasting 24 hours to overwhelming, dehydrating and occasionally fatal gastroenteritis. It is not possible to distinguish rotavirus gastroenteritis from other causes of small intestinal diarrhoea. Vomiting is a frequent occurrence often preceding diarrhoea. The illness lasts on average 5–7 days in hospitalized children. Virtually all children are febrile and a large proportion have upper respiratory tract symptoms, although the latter assocation may be coincidental. Infection in neonates is frequently asymptomatic and in outbreaks in neonatal intensive care units only 10–20% of those infected are symptomatic. Extraintestinal infections with rotavirus have been rarely described and include hepatic abscess, myositis, meningitis and encephalitis. Immunocompetent children continue to excrete rotavirus for 5–8 days following cessation of diarrhoea. Immunodeficient children may excrete virus for much longer.

Diagnosis It is not possible diagnose rotavirus gastroenteritis on clinical features. Although it is possible to grow rotavirus in tissue culture this is not a useful diagnostic procedure.

Electron microscopy During acute infection sufficient virus is excreted for it to be detected by negative stain electron microscopy (a minimum of 10^6 particles/ml faeces is needed). This has good sensitivity and high specificity which can be enhanced by addition of specific antisera to clump virus particles (immuno-electron microscopy). Electron microscopy will detect most other viral enteropathogens and is thus a 'catch-all' technique. The remaining techniques are all pathogen-specific.

Antigen detection There is a variety of commercially available methods for detection of rotavirus antigen in faeces including enzyme immunoassay (EIA), radioimmunoassay and latex particle agglutination. The sensitivity and specificity of such tests are high; in general EIA tests perform best although all may not detect group B or C rotaviruses.

Genome detection So much virus is excreted during acute infection that it is possible to extract rotavirus RNA directly from faeces, separate its 11 ds RNA segments by polyacrylamide gel electrophoresis (RNA-PAGE) and visualize them by silver staining. This is a sensitive, specific and inexpensive diagnostic test which also provides epidemiological information. Recently reverse transcriptase polymerase chain amplification has been used for diagnosis and to provide information of rotavirus serotypes.

Antibody detection is of little value for diagnosis of infection.

MANAGEMENT

There is no specific therapy available. Management principally involves assessment of dehydration and replacement of fluid and electrolytes orally or intravenously. Therapy with immune colostrum or gammaglobulin has been tried with mixed results and such therapies remain experimental. Breast-feeding may provide pretection by providing both specific IgA antirotavirus and trypsin inhibitor.

PREVENTION OF FURTHER CASES

A variety of live attenuated human, simian, bovine and reassortant vaccines are being developed. Immunization using 'neonatal' strains of rotavirus is a possibility.

ADENOVIRUS

ORGANISM

Adenovirus is a medium-sized, non-enveloped DNA virus with eicosahedral symmetry. It has a double-stranded linear DNA genome. Of the 46 serotypes only adenovirus 40 and 41 are associated with diarrhoeal disease. In comparison to other serotypes they do not grow easily in tissue culture ('fastidious adenoviruses').

EPIDEMIOLOGY

Adenovirus serotypes 40 and 41 are the second or third most common cause of diarrhoeal disease in children under 5 years old. They are found to be responsible for 4–10% of cases of diarrhoea in children in community and hospital-based surveys. Unlike rotavirus there is no seasonality of endemic infection. Most infections occur in those under 2 years old.

Transmission Infection is transmitted person-to-person by the faecal-oral route. Most infection is community-acquired but nosocomial outbreaks occur.

Incubation period is 8–10 days.

NATURAL HISTORY AND CLINICAL FEATURES

Little is known of the pathogenesis of adenovirus gastroenteritis but it is presumed to be similar to that of rotavirus. The clinical features are similar to those of rotavirus. The most prominent feature is a watery diarrhoea which lasts 5–12 days. Vomiting usually occurs after the onset of diarrhoea. The severity is usually less than rotavirus diarrhoea. Virus tends to be excreted in stool for some time (up to 14 days) after cessation of diarrhoea.

Diagnosis is by detection of virus, its antigens or genome using immuno-electron microscopy, EIA or DNA hybridization.

MANAGEMENT

Management is symptomatic. There is no vaccine available for prevention nor is there information available on determinants of immunity.

ASTROVIRUS

ORGANISM

Astrovirus is a small, round, non-enveloped RNA virus with a characteristic six-pointed star on its surface. Astrovirus is difficult to grow in tissue culture.

EPIDEMIOLOGY

There are five serotypes but serotype 1 accounts for 80% of cases in Europe and the USA. Astrovirus is responsible for 5–12% of cases of diarrhoeal disease in children under 5 years old. The majority of infections occur in children under 2 years old, and anti-astrovirus antibodies are detectable in 70% of UK children by the age of 4 years. Astrovirus has a similar seasonal distribution to rotavirus with peaks of infection occurring in winter 2–4 weeks prior to the rotavirus peak.

Transmission is person-to-person by the faecal-oral route.

Incubation period is 1–2 days.

NATURAL HISTORY AND CLINICAL FEATURES

Illness commences with 5–7 days of watery diarrhoea. Vomiting is also a prominent feature. Astrovirus diarrhoea tends to be less severe than that due to rotavirus.

Diagnosis Specific diagnosis is by negative stain electron microscopy, EIA or polymerase chain reaction (PCR) amplification of viral RNA. The latter will also provide information on the serotype.

MANAGEMENT

The management is as for rotavirus diarrhoea. There is no vaccine available for prevention of infection.

CALICIVIRUS

ORGANISM

Calicivirus is a small, round, non-enveloped RNA virus with cup-shaped indentations (*calyx*, cup) that may lead to the appearance of a 'star of David' on electron microscopy.

EPIDEMIOLOGY

Calicivirus is responsible for 2–4% of cases of gastroenteritis in children, and may affect older children and adults. There is no apparent seasonality of infection. Outbreaks of infection occur in schools, orphanages and hospitals.

Transmission is by the faeco-oral route either directly or indirectly (water-borne outbreaks have been described).

Incubation period is 1–3 days.

NATURAL HISTORY AND CLINICAL FEATURES

The illness is clinically indistinguishable from mild rotavirus gastroenteritis. Diarrhoea persists for 4–6 days on average.

Diagnosis is by negative stain electron microscopy, EIA or PCR amplification of viral genome.

MANAGEMENT

The management is as for rotavirus diarrhoea

NORWALK VIRUS

ORGANISM

Norwalk virus is a small, round, non-enveloped RNA virus, closely related to calicivirus.

EPIDEMIOLOGY

Norwalk virus is responsible for up to 40% of outbreaks of gastroenteritis in recreational camps, cruise ships, communities, schools, nursing homes or hospitals. Infections tend to be more common in older children and adults. The seroprevalence to anti-Norwalk virus is low in childhood and rises through adolescence to adulthood where 60% are seropositive. In developing countries infection occurs earlier. There is no seasonality of infection.

Transmission From person-to-person occurs via the faeco-oral route, although air-borne transmission has been suggested since this is consistent with the explosive secondary transmission seen in outbreaks. Indirect spread via drinking or recreational water and food (poorly cooked shellfish, salads and cake icing) is a common occurrence in outbreaks.

Incubation period is 12–48 hours.

NATURAL HISTORY AND CLINICAL FEATURES

The virus replicates in the mucosa of the proximal small intestine. Gastric emptying is delayed which probably accounts for the frequent occurrence of nausea and vomiting. Diarrhoea lasts from 3–6 days.

Diagnosis Virus is excreted in vomitus and faeces in large numbers only in the first few days of illness and negative stain electron microscopy is useful only during that period. Antigen detection by EIA provides the most useful diagnostic test.

MANAGEMENT

The management is as for rotavirus disrrhoea. There is no vaccine available.

OTHER VIRAL ENTEROPATHOGENS

A variety of other viruses have been associated with gastroenteritis, including small, round, structureless viruses (possibly parvovirus), coronavirus, torovirus (e.g. Breda), pestiviruses and picobirnaviruses. However, the evidence linking them to diarrhoeal disease is not strong and they are responsible for a minority of cases, if any. Small round structural viruses are responsible for sporadic cases (see Table 6.1) and outbreaks of diarrhoeal disease.

PREVENTION OF FURTHER CASES

Routine enteric precautions should apply (see Chapter 27). Children with presumed or confirmed viral infection may return to school or day care once symptoms have terminated.

RUBELLA

Notifiable disease

All children in the UK and Eire with congenital rubella should currently (1995–6)* be reported to the BPA Surveillance Unit

ORGANISM

Rubivirus is an RNA enveloped virus in the togavirus family.

EPIDEMIOLOGY

Humans are the only host and the disease is endemic worldwide. It occurs in epidemics about every 6–9 years where rubella vaccine is not in use. In the UK and western Europe infection is more common in late winter and early spring. A downward trend in the incidence of rubella in England and Wales was reversed in 1993 when there were local outbreaks particularly affecting young adult males.

Transmission is by direct contact or droplet spread. The patient is infectious from 7 days before and for 2 weeks after the appearance of the rash. Congenital rubella (see below) is contracted by the fetus when the mother is infected at or after the time of conception or in early pregnancy. Infants with congenital rubella may continue to excrete virus for 6 months or longer after birth.

Incubation period is from 14 to 21 days.

NATURAL HISTORY AND CLINICAL FEATURES

Between 25% and 50% of cases are totally asymptomatic and in the remainder the disease is rarely serious. In children there is usually little if any prodrome. In adolescents and adults a prodrome of low-grade fever, malaise, headache, conjunctivitis, coryza, sore throat and cough may precede the rash by 1–5 days. At all ages there is a generalized lymphadenopathy, the suboccipital, post-auricular and cervical nodes being most affected. This may precede the rash by up to 7 days. An enanthem consisting of small red spots may be present during

*** May be extended.**

the prodrome or on the first day of the exanthem. The exanthem itself consists of discrete pink-red maculopapules, appearing first on the face. These spread rapidly so that after 24 hours the entire body may be covered. On the second day the rash disappears from the face and may coalesce on the trunk. By the end of the third day the rash has usually gone entirely. The lymphadenopathy may take longer to resolve. The rash may appear similar to that caused by measles, scarlet fever or parvovirus B19. Rubella can be distinguished from measles where the general upset is greater and the evolution of the rash slower than in rubella, while in scarlet fever the rash spares the area around the mouth (circumoral pallor).

Complications are unusual. Adults and adolescents are more likely to develop an arthritis than are children and women are more commonly affected than men. This is often a polyarthritis with a predilection for the small joints of the hands. There is rarely any residuum. In approximately 1 in 6000 cases an encephalitis may occur. Fatalities are rare and the survivors are usually undamaged. Purpura (with normal or low platelet counts) rarely occurs and may be accompanied by serious bleeding, e.g. into the intestinal tract or cerebral substance. It is usually self-limiting and resolves within 2 weeks. Idiopathic thrombocytopenic purpura may follow an attack of rubella.

Diagnosis is usually made clinically in children. In acute infection either a single test for rubella IgM or paired tests with a 10-day interval for rising rubella IgG levels are diagnostic. The virus can also be recovered from the nasopharynx and the urine in the acute phase. Because of the uncertainties in clinical diagnosis a history of rubella should never be accepted where it is important to be certain, i.e. when a pregnant woman is involved, without serologic confirmation. The presence of IgG specific for rubella indicates immunity due to prior infection or immunization.

MANAGEMENT

Management is symptomatic.

PREVENTION OF FURTHER CASES

Unless a child is likely to come into contact with a pregnant woman, isolation is not appropriate. The main strategy to prevent further cases, especially of congenital rubella, is twofold:

- Ensuring high herd immunity in children of both sexes through rubella immunization within measles, mumps and rubella (MMR) or MR vaccination.
- Ensuring all women entering pregnancy are sero-immune.

Vaccination A live attenuated vaccine has been available for many years. In the UK it was previously given to 13-year-old girls and women of child-bearing age who were found to be susceptible. Since October 1988, it has also been given as part of the MMR vaccine to all children at 13 months of age. In November 1994 a mass campaign to immunize with MR all schoolchildren aged 5–16 years took place. Since then, rubella vaccine is no longer given to schoolgirls. In most people the vaccine is thought to provide lifelong protection. However, there is a small proportion of people where there is a primary or secondary failure of the vaccine to protect. Congenital rubella has occurred in the babies of mothers known to have been immune in the past. Exactly the same situation applies to protection after the disease. The same contraindications apply as for any live vaccine (see Appendix VI). The vaccine should not knowingly be given to a pregnant woman, however, there is a large body of evidence that while it may infect the fetus it does no harm. Inadvertent vaccination in pregnancy is not a reason for termination.

CONGENITAL RUBELLA

The risk of congenital rubella is maximal in non-immune pregnant women acquiring infection in the first 8–10 weeks of pregnancy. At that stage the probability of some degree of damage, frequently severe, is considered to be 90%. Beyond 13 weeks' gestation the risk of any abnormality apart from deafness is extremely low and by 16 weeks of pregnancy the risk has fallen to 10–20%. Infection beyond 16 weeks' gestation is not thought to cause deafness. Between January 1991 and June 1994 in the UK 14 infants were notified to the National Congenital Rubella Surveillance Programme, including one set of triplets. Nine of the 12 mothers were immigrants, indicating the importance of these groups being immunized after their arrival. Severe clinical manifestations that have been described include fetal death and stillbirth, growth retardation, cardiac anomalies (septal defects, patent ductus and pulmonary artery stenosis), eye involvement (cataract, blindness, microophthalmia), neurologic damage (nerve deafness, meningoencephalitis, microcephaly), thrombocytopenia and jaundice. However, milder cases do occur and congenital rubella is worth considering as a differential diagnosis in any growth-retarded newborn or child with idiopathic nerve deafness.

Notification of cases of congenital rubella Cases of suspected congenital rubella detected in the UK must be notified to the National Congenital Rubella Surveillance Programme.* Paediatricians may do this by ticking the box on the British Paediatric Association Surveillance Unit (BPASU) 'orange card'. Reporting by laboratories, audiologists, etc. also reveals significant numbers of cases.

PREGNANCY AND RUBELLA

Pregnant women exposed to rubella should all be investigated serologically irrespective of a history of immunization, clinical rubella or previous positive rubella serology. As soon as possible after exposure maternal blood should be tested for anti-rubella IgG or IgM. There should be close consultation between the clinician managing the woman and the virologist to ensure prompt taking of further samples and correct interpretation of results. A high likelihood of congenital rubella infection having occurred is an indication for offering the woman termination of pregnancy.

Screening pregnant women and women contemplating pregnancy All pregnant women should be screened for anti-rubella IgG in *every pregnancy* and on request when pregnancy is contemplated irrespective of a previous positive serology. Serologic testing of non-pregnant women should be performed whenever possible before immunization, but need not be undertaken where this might interfere with the acceptance or delivery of vaccine.

Recent migrants Girls and women migrating to the UK from countries where rubella vaccination is not routine are at particular risk of being non-immune and should be tested for anti-rubella IgG or given MMR or MR (which ever is available).

***National Congenital Rubella Surveillance Programme, Department of Epidemiology and Biostatistics, Institute of Child Health, 30 Guilford St, London WC1E 7HT (tel: 0171-242-9789).**

Women found to be seronegative on antenatal screening should not be immunized during the pregnancy but should receive immunization after delivery *before discharge from the maternity unit*. If anti-D immunoglobulin is required the two may be given at the same time at different sites.

HEALTH CARE STAFF

All health care staff, both male and female, should be screened and those who are seronegative should be immunized (some occupational health departments may choose to immunize without prior serology).

87

SALMONELLOSIS*

Food poisoning through whatever cause is a notifiable condition

ORGANISM

Salmonellae are Gram-negative bacilli with a number of species and many serotypes (more than 2200). Important species include *Salmonella enteritidis* and *S. typhimurium*. These two are responsible for most of the cases of salmonellosis in the UK.

EPIDEMIOLOGY

Salmonellae are present worldwide with animals and poultry considered to be the reservoir of infection for non-typhoidal salmonellae. The species seemingly the source of most infections in humans are poultry and cattle and the major vehicles are meat, and eggs. Circulation of infection may occur through spreading of human waste on farmland. Occasional infections in children have occurred though spread from turtles and terrapins kept as pets. Poultry eggs are a potent source of human infection because they are often used uncooked, for example in mayonnaise. Cases occur at all ages and outbreaks occur in families through contamination of food in day-care facilities and schools. Reports of salmonella infections from laboratories in England and Wales have increased fourfold since the start of the 1980s (see Appendix I, Fig. 2). The infection is more apparent in children and the elderly because they experience the highest attack rates. Invasive infections occur with typhoid and paratyphoid infection and in children with certain chronic conditions: notably sickle-cell disease and other haemoglobinopathies, human immunodeficiency virus infection, constitutional immunodeficiencies and malignancies (see Chapter 97). *Salmonella* species occasionally cause meningitis (see Chapter 2).

Transmission is mostly through food products, water and faecal-oral spread.

Incubation period is 6 hours to 3 days (usually 12–36 hours) depending on the infecting dose.

***See also typhoid and paratyphoid (Chapter 97).**

Period of infectivity is during symptoms and up to several weeks after , although the risk of transmission decreases considerably as the diarrhoea subsides. Asymptomatic infection occurs and rarely carriers are found who remain infectious for months. Antibiotic treatment is usually ineffective in rendering carriers uninfectious .

NATURAL HISTORY AND CLINICAL FEATURES

Salmonella infections cause a number of clinical syndromes including asymptomatic infection, gastroenteritis, focal infections, bacteraemia and enteric fever, though the most common are asymptomatic infection and gastroenteritis, and the severe manifestations are more often seen in infection with *Salmonella typhi* and *S. paratyphi* (see Chapter 97). Constitutional illness and bacteraemia may occur without any apparent gastrointestinal illness. Systemic signs can include headache and general malaise; fever is uncommon. Alternatively there may only be diarrhoea and vomiting with abdominal cramps. Diarrhoea rarely contains pus (dysentery) and may be watery; it rarely contains blood. Focal signs can be caused by invasive disease in immunocompromised patients.

Diagnosis is usually by culture of stool or urine. Culture of blood or material from foci of infection will be useful during fever.

MANAGEMENT

Normal management procedures for a child with an infective diarrhoeal disease apply (see Chapter 6). Treatment with antibiotics is not recommended unless there is severe systemic illness or the child is under 6 months or otherwise immunocompromised. It will not shorten the duration of disease or excretion of infective organisms. Ampicillin, trimethoprim, cefotaxime or ceftriaxone and ciprofloxacin are the drugs of choice when there is invasive disease, but should be guided by bacterial drug sensitivity (see Chapter 97).

PREVENTION OF FURTHER CASES

Important measures include good hygiene and proper methods for food production, preparation and cooking. Uncooked eggs should not be used in food without heating or cooking and all poultry should be well cooked. Infected children should be excluded from day-care facilities until the risk of infection is minimal. In schools the provision of well-maintained and provisioned toilet facilities is essential. Antimicrobial therapy is generally not given to asymptomatic infected persons, apart from those persons with typhoid or paratyphoid (see chapter 97). Food handlers and those at a higher risk of causing transmission may return to work when they are asymptomatic and have normal stools for 48 hours (see chapter 27). A prolonged course of ciprofloxacin does eliminate carriage in adults but data is not available for children. Referral of positive isolates to the central reference laboratory is important for detecting common-source outbreaks and contamination. of food products*

***The Public Health Laboratory Service special diagnostic service in England and Wales for *Salmonella* and other food-borne infections is the Laboratory for Enteric Pathogens, Central Public Health Laboratory, Colindale (Tel: 0181-200-4400). In Scotland consult the Scottish Centre for Infection and Environmental Health (Tel: 0141-946-7120).**

88

SCABIES

ORGANISM

Scabies is caused by the mite, *Sarcoptes scabiei*

EPIDEMIOLOGY

Occurs throughout the world, and is no respecter of persons.

Transmission is by prolonged skin-to-skin contact. Scabies is also a sexually transmitted disease.

Incubation period In the first infestation this may be several weeks. It is shorter in subsequent infections.

NATURAL HISTORY AND CLINICAL FEATURES

After mating, the female mite burrows into the skin and lays one to three eggs daily along a linear track. She dies after 4–5 weeks in the burrow. After 3–5 days the eggs hatch into larvae which grow and become nymphs on the surface. They reach maturity in 2–3 weeks, mate and repeat the cycle. Outside infancy the areas most affected tend to be the interdigital spaces, wrists, elbows, ankles, buttocks, groins, genitalia and areola. The rash consists of vesicles, weals, papules, the burrows themselves and a superimposed dermatitis. In infancy the palms, soles, head and neck are often infected. Bullae and pustules may be present while there may be no burrows. Because the pruritus is so extreme, the skin changes resulting from scratching may obscure the underlying lesions.

Diagnosis The presence of burrows is almost diagnostic. Mites and ova can be seen in scrapings from burrows, eczematous lesions and fresh papules. In immunosuppressed patients, there may be a generalized dermatitis with scaling and even vesiculation and crusting ('Norwegian scabies').

MANAGEMENT

Malathion or lindane should be applied to the whole body apart from the head and neck and left for a day without rinsing. A second application is necessary after 3 days. Lindane should not be used in infants.

PREVENTION OF FURTHER CASES

Careful laundering of clothes and bedding is important. Treatment of family members and sexual contacts is recommended.

89

SHIGELLOSIS

Dysentery (diarrhoea with pus) is a notifiable condition

ORGANISM

Shigella species Gram-negative bacilli in the family Enterobacteriaceae include *S. sonnei*, *S. flexneri*, *S. dysenteriae* and *S. boydii*. (*S. sonnei* and *S. flexneri* cause most of the cases in the UK).

EPIDEMIOLOGY

Shigella spp. are present worldwide with humans as the reservoir of infection. Most cases are in children, including neonates and young infants. In the early 1990s there were increases in numbers of cases in England and Wales (see Appendix I, Fig. 2). As is typical, outbreaks occurred particularly in families, day-care facilities and primary schools. Children and adults with severe learning difficulties are at particular risk of involvement in transmission because of the difficulties in maintaining hygiene. Cases also occur in adults where hygiene is poor.

Transmission Faeces are the source of infection through faecal-oral transmission. Occasionally transmission occurs through food or drink when they are faecally contaminated. *Shigellae* spp. are highly infectious and only a few organisms are necessary for transmission.

Incubation period is 1–3 days (longer for some species)

Period of infectivity is during symptoms and up to 4 weeks in the untreated patient, though risk of transmission decreases considerably as the diarrhoea subsides. Asymptomatic infection occurs and rarely carriers are found who seem to remain infectious for months. However, if they are asymptomatic and able to apply simple hygiene precautions they can be regarded as non-infectious. Appropriate antibiotic treatment (see below) renders the patient uninfectious in 5 days.

NATURAL HISTORY AND CLINICAL FEATURES

The infection may be mild with only gastrointestinal symptoms or it may extend to constitutional involvement. Consequently there may only be diarrhoea, perhaps with abdominal cramps (vomiting is unusual) or abdominal tenderness. Diarrhoea may contain pus (dysentery) or it may be watery or contain blood. Constitutional signs include fever, headache and general malaise. Fever may cause febrile convulsions. Unusual complications include gut perforation, and with *S. flexneri*, Reiter's syndrome.

Diagnosis Stool specimens or rectal swabs will normally be sufficient for culture diagnosis. However, routine laboratory methods are relatively insensitive and may miss a significant proportion of asymptomatic cases. The Public Health Laboratory Service special diagnostic service for *Shigella* is at the Laboratory for Enteric Pathogens, Central Public Health Laboratory, Colindale (telephone 0181-200-4400).

MANAGEMENT

Normal management procedures for a child with an infective diarrhoeal disease apply (see Chapter 6). Treatment with antibiotics is recommended if there is marked systemic illness and may be of some use in shortening the length of the illness and making the patient non-infectious to others. A 5-day course of oral ampicillin is usually sufficient, though ampicillin resistance occurs and co-trimoxazole is an alternative. Hospitalization should be avoided, but if children have to go into hospital they should be isolated and enteric precautions applied.*

***See Chapter 26.**

PREVENTION OF FURTHER CASES†

Good hygiene is essential, with hand-washing an important feature. The most important control features are the provision of toilet facilities in schools (including toilet paper) and thorough hand-washing after use of toilets and before meals, using soap and warm water. Where practical children should be excluded from day-care facilities until the risk of infection is minimal. In schools the provision of well-maintained and provisioned toilet facilities are essential (shigellosis is one of the few infections that can be acquired from toilet seats). Persons at higher risk of causing transmission especially food handlers (Chapter 27) and with proven *Shigella flexneri*, *dysenteriae* or *boydii* require exclusion until three stools are negative: in cases of *S. sonnei* it is not necessary to demonstrate negative stools but stool habit should have returned to normal. Very occasionally in families where hygiene cannot be guaranteed it is necessary to issue antibiotic therapy to all members to break cycles of reinfection, but this should be a last resort.

90 STAPHYLOCOCCAL INFECTIONS

ORGANISMS

Staphylococci are Gram-positive bacteria. *Staphylococcus aureus* produces a coagulase enzyme (coagulase-positive staphylococcus). Coagulase-negative staphylococci include a number of species including *S. epidermidis*. Methicillin-resistant *S. aureus* (MRSA) poses problems of nosocomial infection.

EPIDEMIOLOGY

Staphylococci are common surface colonizers of humans: *S. aureus* is found in the nares and on the skin in up to 50% of individuals; *S. epidermidis* is part of the normal 'resident' skin flora in all individuals and is also found on mucosal surfaces. Compromised defences either local or generalized lead to infection with these organisms; MRSA particularly affects surgical patients and the elderly. Coagulase-negative staphylococci are the most common cause of infections associated with implanted foreign materials—central intravenous lines, cerebrospinal fluid shunts, orthopaedic or cardiac protheses. Outbreaks of *S. aureus* infections may be caused by particularly virulent strains such as those producing toxins, as in toxic epidermolysis of infants (scalded skin syndrome).

Transmission Many staphylococcal infections are caused by the body's own endogenous bacteria. Transmission between individuals can occur by close contact via the hands.

Incubation period is 1–10 days for scalded skin syndrome and impetigo.

NATURAL HISTORY AND CLINICAL FEATURES

Staphylococcus aureus most commonly causes superficial infection in the form of boils, paronychia, impetigo or wound infections. Skin disorders such as eczema predispose to such infections. Invasion beyond the skin may result in suppurative localized lymphadenitis and further invasion leads to deep infection such as septicaemia, pneumonia, osteomyelitis, septic arthritis, endocarditis or deep

† **See also Chapter 27.**

organ abscess. Staphylococcal pneumonia produces characteristic cavitating lesions and empyema. Toxin-producing *S. aureus* may result in scalded skin syndrome (Ritter's disease) due to an epidermolysin which produces general effects, though the initiating infection may be very localized and minor. Other toxin-producing *S. aureus* strains can lead to toxic shock syndrome (see Chapter 13). Staphylococcal food poisoning results from the ingestion of food contaminated with preformed enterotoxins elaborated by toxigenic strains of *S. aureus*.

Coagulase-negative staphylococci are of relatively low pathogenicity. However, in those with implanted foreign materials (prostheses, central lines, etc.) they may cause deep infections including septicaemia and endocarditis. Slime-producing species result in indolent infections which are extremely difficult to eliminate with antibiotic therapy and can only be cured by the removal of the foreign body. Coagulase-negative staphylococci are the most common cause of sepsis in premature newborns and in immunocompromised individuals. *Staphylococcus saprophyticus* can cause urinary tract infections mainly in those with urological problems.

Diagnosis Gram stain and culture are the standard diagnostic tests. Cultured staphylococci are then further identified by the coagulase test. Antistaphylococcal antibody tests for both *S.aureus* and coagulase-negative staphylococci are available but have relatively low sensitivity in children even in the presence of invasive disease. Phage typing and toxin identification are sometimes useful in suspected toxic shock or scalded skin syndrome.

MANAGEMENT

Localized *S.aureus* infection often requires surgical drainage of the abscess. In systemic infection antibiotic therapy is required. Many *S. aureus* strains are beta-lactamase producers and therefore penicillin-resistant. Flucloxacillin is the treatment of choice but other useful agents include fucidin, gentamicin, clindamycin and the glycopeptides vancomycin and teicoplanin. In deep-seated infection prolonged (several weeks) courses are required. The glycopeptides are the treatment of choice for MRSA. Coagulase-negative staphylococcal infections require intravenous antibiotic therapies with or without removal of any infected foreign body. Multiple antibiotic resistance is common and so glycopeptides should be used as first-line treatment.

PREVENTION OF FURTHER CASES

Strict hand-washing procedures in newborn nurseries and in the care of surgical patients should be routine. In outbreaks of staphylococcal disease, for instance of scalded skin syndrome, isolation and cohorting is necessary. Screening for MRSA carriage is advisable on transferring patients between hospitals. Those identified as positive, particularly if they have desquamative skin disease or discharging wounds, should be isolated. Elimination of MRSA carriage may be attempted in selected patients and staff members using topical antistaphylococcal agents such as mupirocin. Patients with recurrent furunculosis can be treated with topical anti-staphylococcal agents such as chlorhexidine soap and shampoo and chlorhexidine (Naseptin) or mupirocin nasal carrier cream. Meticulous attention to aseptic technique during insertion and subsequent handling of central venous lines and during surgical implant procedures reduces coagulase-negative staphylococcal infection. Short courses of prophylactic glycopeptides to cover insertion of foreign bodies is potentially useful but generally unproven. In the future, impregnation of implants with combinations of antimicrobials at the time of manufacture is a likely development, and may reduce the incidence of colonization and infection.

91 STREPTOCOCCAL INFECTIONS

ORGANISM

Streptococcus pyogenes is a Gram-positive coccus and is beta-haemolytic. There are about 80 different types characterized by different M proteins in the cell wall. Certain types are associated with rheumatic fever (1, 3, 5, 6 and 18) and another with acute glomerulonephritis (12).

EPIDEMIOLOGY

Infections occur worldwide, although impetigo is more common in tropical countries and in the northern hemisphere. Streptococcal pharyngitis and scarlet fever are more common in the autumn and winter months. During outbreaks of streptococcal pharyngitis asymptomatic carriage may occur in up to 50% of children. Toxic shock syndrome (see Chapter 13) may be a result of streptococcal infection.

Transmission Pharyngitis and scarlet fever result from contact with a person who has active streptococcal pharyngitis. Carriers do not appear to transmit infection. There is no evidence that fomites are a source of infection. Occasionally, food-borne spread can occur. Impetigo results from skin-to-skin transmission of streptococci.

Incubation period is 3–5 days for streptococcal pharyngitis and 7–10 days for impetigo.

Communicability for untreated disease is 7–21 days. With antibiotics this is less (1–2 days) but some children have pharyngeal colonization for weeks or months and may be contagious for much of this time.

NATURAL HISTORY AND CLINICAL FEATURES

The most common manifestation is a purulent tonsillitis or pharyngitis. Complications of this include suppurative cervical lymphadenopathy. In children under 3 years old, infection may result in a low-grade fever with anorexia and cervical lymphadenopathy. In the older child scarlet fever may develop with pharyngitis and a characteristic rash produced by an erythogenic toxin. The rash develops during the first day of fever, is dark red in colour and quickly becomes generalized. Lesions are punctate, the size of pinheads, and give the skin a sandpaper-like texture. There is a generalized erythema of the face and forehead, but the area around the mouth is spared (circumoral pallor). Fever peaks on the second day and in untreated infection persists for another 3–4 days. The tonsils are enlarged and covered with exudate (if present). There are characteristic changes to the tongue: for 1–2 days the dorsum is covered in a white fur; the papillae become red and thickened, protruding through the coat to produce the white 'strawberry tongue'. By the fourth or fifth day, the white coat disappears leaving a red strawberry tongue. Petechiae can be seen on the palate during the illness.

Impetigo is seen in children with eczema. Streptococcal cellulitis characterized by a dark-red induration of the skin is seen following varicella infections in children. In children who develop rheumatic fever, which is very rare, there is usually a history of tonsillitis or pharyngitis in the previous few weeks. Glomerulonephritis may follow skin sepsis—cellulitis or impetigo. This may present with haematuria, oliguria, oedema and hypertension. In most children this resolves spontaneously.

Diagnosis A throat swab culture is the most useful indicator of streptococcal infection in tonsillitis and suspected scarlet fever. Streptococcal throat infections cannot be distinguished from viral infections on clinical grounds. An important disease to be considered in the differential diagnosis of scarlet fever is Kawasaki disease. Skin culture may be indicated for impetigo. Antigen detection tests are available but many are of high sensitivity and low specificity. Antistreptococcal antibody tests may be useful in the diagnosis of possible post-streptococcal glomerulonephritis.

MANAGEMENT

Penicillin V or amoxycillin is the treatment of choice for children with streptococcal infection. Erythromycin or a cephalosporin are acceptable in the presence of penicillin allergy. Research in the 1950s showed that the risk of rheumatic fever was reduced if penicillin treatment was given for 14 days, but shorter courses were not evaluated, and a 10-day course may well be sufficient. Although it is recommended that streptococcal tonsillitis is treated with antibiotics, the need for this in areas where rheumatic fever does not occur is questionable. Treatment of streptococcal impetigo and cellulitis is with penicillin; long intravenous courses (up to 14 days) may be needed in cases of cellulitis. Treatment of acute glomerulonephritis includes penicillin during the illness, with symptomatic treatment—fluid restriction, bed rest and antihypertensive drugs if necessary.

SYPHILIS (CONGENITAL AND ACQUIRED) AND NON-VENEREAL TREPONEMATOSES

92

All children with congenital syphilis or born to mother with syphilis in the UK or Eire should currently (1995/96) be reported to the BPA surveillance unit

SYPHILIS

ORGANISM

Treponema pallidum subsp. *pallidum* is a spirochaetal bacterium.

EPIDEMIOLOGY

Treponema pallidum infections occur only in humans. Syphilis is endemic in many developing countries. Serological studies in Africa suggest infection in 2–20% of pregnant women. A resurgence of adult and congenital infection in the USA began in the 1980s, particularly in blacks in large cities and more recently in rural areas in the south-eastern USA. The risk factor for adult infection was drug use. The major reason for congenital infections is lack of screening of the mother during antenatal care (syphilis screening), usually because of failure of the mother to receive any antenatal care. Levels of infection in the UK are considered to be low for adult infection (300–400 cases per annum) and very low for congenital infection.

Transmission Vertical transmission occurs in later pregnancy from mothers with untreated or inadequately treated syphilis. Infection in children is otherwise very unusual until they become sexually active. Vertical transmission rate varies with the stage of maternal infection. If the mother is untreated, it is 40–50% in primary, secondary or early latent syphilis and 10% in late latent syphilis. Acquired syphilis occurs through sexual intercourse and transmission can take place through blood transfusions.

Incubation period is unknown. Congenital disease often commences *in utero*.

NATURAL HISTORY AND CLINICAL FEATURES

If the mother's infection is untreated, there is a 12–25% probability of any pregnancy resulting in a miscarriage or stillbirth and the infant death rate is doubled. The clinical features are many (Table 92.1) such that a serological test is appropriate for a variety of presentations.

Diagnosis The definitive positive test is dark-field microscopy of exudate showing treponemes. However, usually the first test will be a specific serological test such as a *Treponema pallidum* haemagglutination (TPHA) test, an IgG or IgM enzyme immunoassay or a fluorescent treponemal antigen (FTA) test. Though no laboratory test will distinguish syphilis from the non-verenal treponematoses (see below).

MANAGEMENT

Treponemes remain sensitive to parenteral penicillin. For infants procaine penicillin is recommended—30 mg/mg as a single daily dose or benzyl penicillin 60 mg/kg per day in two divided doses intramuscularly. It is important that a full 10 day course is completed. Mothers with primary, secondary or early latent syphilis should receive 4g of benzathine (long-acting) penicillin. Interpretation of test data in adults is complex and advice should be taken from specialists in genitourinary medicine (STDs).

PREVENTION OF FURTHER CASES

Routine antenatal syphilis screening of each pregnancy is required.

NON-VENEREAL TREPONEMATOSES: Yaws, Bejel and Pinta

Non-venereal treponemal infections are endemic among rural populations in tropical countries (the Amazon Basin, west and central Africa, south-east Asia and Indonesia). These infections are much less prevalent than in the past due to mass treatment campaigns that took place in the 1960s and 1970s and the widespread use of antibiotics in the tropics. The causative organism is indistinguishable from *Treponema pallidum* causing syphilis. Transmission is primarily thought to be by direct physical contact between children. Characteristically yaws and pinta initially show papillomatous skin lesions while with bejel the first lesions are in the mouth. Yaws and bejel can occasionally proceed to destructive gummas of the bones and skin.

Table 92.1 Clinical consequences of congenital syphilis

Prenatal
Increased fetal wastage Late miscarriage and fetal death Still birth Preterm delivery Intrauterine growth retardation
Early congenital syphilis
Lymphadenopathy (50% of cases)* Hepatosplenomegaly (50–90%) Anaemia Leucocytosis or leucopenia Thrombocytopenia Mucocutaneous lesions (30–60%): Rhinitis or 'snuffles' (less frequently seen in recent series) Rash[†] Bullous eruption (palms and soles) Condylomata lata (perioral and perianal) Mucous patches on lips, palate and angles of mouth Bony involvement of long bones (70–80%): Osteochondritis Periostitis Osteitis Neurosyphilis (40–60%) Nephrotic syndrome Pneumonia Myocarditis
Late congenital syphilis
Dental stigmata (Hutchison's teeth and mulberry molar) Frontal bossing of the skull Anterior bowing of tibia (sabre shins) Saddle nose Linear scars from body orifices (rhagades) Nerve deafness Interstial keratitis leading to blindness.

***Percentages are derived from clinical series and may overestimate the percentage of affected children showing a feature.**
[†]Rash can have any distribution, initially red and maculopapular, turning coppery brown and scaling.

93

TETANUS

Notifiable disease

ORGANISM

Clostridium tetani a spore-forming, anaerobic Gram-positive bacillus. In its spore form it is found ubiquitously in soil. It produces a potent exotoxin which acts on the nervous system.

EPIDEMIOLOGY

Neonatal tetanus is a relatively important cause of infant mortality in less developed countries, because of unhygienic birth practices and inadequate care of the umbilical cord stump. In 1993 an estimated 515 000 neonatal deaths were caused by tetanus worldwide, a mortality rate of 4.1 per 1000 live births. In the UK almost all women of child-bearing age are immune, so that antitoxin antibodies are transmitted to the fetus by the transplacental route, but this is not the case in many developing countries where tetanus immunization is not performed. The World Health Organization's global goal (adopted in 1993) is to reduce the incidence of neonatal tetanus to less than one death per 1000 births. Neonatal tetanus has been eliminated from the UK. In the decade 1983 to 1992 there were 117 cases of tetanus reported in England and Wales. most of which were in older persons who would not have been immunized.

Transmission is by the direct transfer of spores of *Clostridium tetani*, which can be found in soil, and the excreta of animals and humans.

Incubation period Varies from 4 days to 3 weeks depending on the infecting dose and the severity of the injury.

NATURAL HISTORY AND CLINICAL FEATURES

Following contamination of traumatized tissue, burns or the umbilical stump, spores multiply in anaerobic conditions and produce tetanus toxin which causes powerful muscle contractions, extreme irritability and death. Case fatality rates in neonates are high.

Diagnosis is on clinical grounds. Though infection is more possible in extensive wounds, the wound or site of entry may be trivial. Bacterial culture is positive only in a small proportion of cases.

MANAGEMENT

Exposed patient If a wound is minor and clean, and a full immunization course for the age has been given (see below) no further action is needed. If the wound is more serious and tetanus-prone (contaminated with dirt, a puncture wound, containing substantial amounts of dead tissue, or with evidence of sepsis) a tetanus toxoid booster should be given even if the last immunization was within 10 years. The wound will also require surgical attention and antibiotic treatment if there is sepsis. Human tetanus immune globulin (HTIG) is given if the wound is tetanus-prone (see above) and it is known that an exposed patient is unimmunized, underimmunized (last tetanus toxoid more than 10 years previously) or of uncertain immunization status,* The HTIG is given in the contralateral limb to the toxoid. Patients known to be suffering from impaired immunity are also given a dose of HTIG.

Patient with tetanus If a diagnosis of tetanus is made, specialist help should be sought. Treatment includes tetanus immune globulin (150 iu/kg given in multiple sites), benzylpenicillin (60 mg/kg per day for 10–14 days), surgical wound debridement where indicated, and supportive medical management. Diazepam has proved beneficial in treating neonatal tetanus.

PREVENTION OF FURTHER CASES

Prevention is achieved by ensuring adequate tetanus immunity through immunization. By the age of 6 months, every child should have had three doses of toxoid within diphtheria, tetanus and pertussis vaccine. A booster of diphtheria and tetanus vaccine is given at or around school entry (age 4 years) and a reinforcing booster of tetanus toxoid (T) or tetanus and adult dose diphtheria (Td) before leaving school. This is considered to give life long immunity unless there is specific exposure.

THREADWORMS

ORGANISM

Enterobius vermicularis, also called pinworm, is a small (circumference 1 mm), white worm.

EPIDEMIOLOGY

Threadworms affect all ages throughout the world, especially preschool children. Infection is common in the UK.

Transmission is predominantly faecal–oral. Eggs may be carried under fingernails and on clothing, bedding or house dust.

Icubation period The life cycle is 2–6 weeks.

NATURAL HISTORY AND CLINICAL FEATURES

Ingested ova hatch in the stomach and the larvae migrate to the caecum where they mature. The gravid female adult worms lay their eggs at night in the perianal area. This gives rise to the most common symptom, namely perianal itching, especially at night. Scratching can result in the transfer of eggs to the mouth and hence a cycle of autoinfection. Vulvovaginitis may occur in young girls giving rise to a vaginal discharge. Tissue invasion does not occur.

Diagnosis Occasionally the worms may be seen around the anus. The diagnosis is best made by pressing a piece of adhesive over the anus and then examining it with a magnifying glass for the presence of eggs. This test may be negative in the presence of highly suggestive symptoms—in this case treatment should be given.

***A guide for older patients is that since immunization began routinely in 1961 patients born before that date are unlikely to have been immunized as infants.**

MANAGEMENT

Treatment consists of a single dose of mebendazole (not to be given to children under 2 years old), or two doses of piperazine 2 weeks apart. Preparations often contain a laxative such as senna, to aid the expulsion of the adult worms. There is a high incidence of reinfection. This can be reduced by keeping fingernails short and wearing close-fitting pants at night to prevent scratching.

PREVENTION OF FURTHER CASES

Strict attention to hygiene will prevent infection. Chemoprophylaxis is also necessary for all family members of the index case; although asymptomatic, they may be infected.

95 TOXOCARIASIS

ORGANISMS

Toxocara canis and *T. cati* are nematode worms.

EPIDEMIOLOGY

Toxocara canis and *T. cati* are common gut parasites of dogs and cats respectively and occur worldwide. The parasite can be transmitted transplacentally in dogs and therefore puppies as young as 3 weeks old can be infectious. Soil from parks has been shown to contain *Toxocara* eggs in up to 25% of samples. Human disease is predominantly caused by *T. canis* and affects children mainly in the age group 1–6 years old. The prevalence of symptomatic infection is unknown but sero-epidemiological studies suggest that 3% or more of children have been exposed to the parasite.

Transmission Disease is caused by tissue invasion with parasite larvae after ingestion of *Toxocara* eggs. The eggs may be swallowed when a child eats soil (pica) contaminated with infective dog or cat faeces. Other potential sources include play-pit sand and unwashed vegetables contaminated with faeces. The eggs require an incubation period of 1–3 weeks before becoming infective and the infection therefore cannot be transmitted by eating faeces that are fresh.

Incubation period The acute illness (visceral larva migrans) can occur within a matter of a few weeks or as long as several months after exposure. The form presenting with an ocular granuloma may take up to 10 years to develop.

NATURAL HISTORY AND CLINICAL FEATURES

There are two relatively distinct forms of disease and it is rare for children to progress from one to the other.

Visceral larva migrans is a syndrome of fever, hepatomegaly, pulmonary symptoms (wheezing) and signs, and eosinophilia, which is often very marked, caused by migrating helminth larvae and the ensuing immune response they provoke. A minority of children also develop splenomegaly and lymphadenopathy. This form is most common in children aged 1–3 years old and symptoms can persist for up to a year.

Eye infection (ocular larva migrans) is detected in older children: most commonly about the ages of 6–8 years when the child's optic fundus is examined because of strabismus or problems with visual acuity. The dead larva causes a granulomatous reaction in the retina which is most damaging when close to the macula but is fortunately unilateral in most cases.

Diagnosis Visceral larva migrans (VLM) is diagnosed clinically on the basis of a multisystem disease accompanied by an eosinophilia, especially in a child who has not been out of northern Europe, although other parasites such as *Fasciola hepatica*, *Gnathostoma spinigerum*, *Ascaris lumbricoides* and *Clonorchis* sp. should also be considered after foreign travel (see Chapter 62). Serum *Toxocara* antibodies may be detected, although not reliably so in the acute infection. Occasionally *Toxocara* larvae may be found if a liver biopsy is performed. Ocular toxocariasis is diagnosed clinically from the appearance of the inflammatory mass in the retina, although it may be difficult to distinguish from other retinal problems. Serum antibodies are not always detected in this form of the disease.

MANAGEMENT

Toxocariasis presenting with VLM can be treated with diethylcarbamazine or thiabendazole, although with limited success, and in mild cases it is probably best to treat the child symptomatically only. There may be some benefit in giving steroids to children with severe disease. Antihelminthic drugs are not effective in the ocular form of disease, but local or systemic steroids may be of benefit.

PREVENTION OF FURTHER CASES

Toxocara infection could be largely prevented if pet owners regularly dewormed cats and dogs and prevented them from defaecating in public places. Sand-pits should be covered after use to prevent cats defaecating in them. There is no advantage in prophylactic antibiotics if a child has ingested dog or cat faeces.

TOXOPLASMOSIS

ORGANISM

Toxoplasma gondii is a protozoan.

EPIDEMIOLOGY

Toxoplasmosis is a common infection, and about half the population of Britain have antibody by middle age. When the first infection occurs in pregnancy transplacental transmission occurs in 30–40% of cases. The incidence of toxoplasmosis during pregnancy in the West of England and South Wales is about 2 per 1000, but the incidence of congenital infection is unknown, because diagnosis is difficult and because most cases present with choroiditis which may not become apparent until late childhood. Some of these cases may have resulted from post-natal infection. Every year 100–300 cases of choroidoretinitis are reported in British patients with *Toxoplasma* antibodies; it is not clear how many of these are caused by *Toxoplasma* infection, and at what stage. A total of 423 reports of toxoplasmosis in pregnancy were received by the Public Health Laboratory Service between 1981 and 1992. The annual rate of toxoplasmosis reported in pregnancy rose in the late 1980s but it is thought that this is due to increased professional awareness rather than increased incidence and the rate of congenital toxoplasmosis changed little over this period. It is estimated that up to 50% of mothers infected during pregnancy pass the infection to the fetus, and a

British Paediatric Surveillance Unit survey during this period found 15 babies per year with a clinical diagnosis of toxoplasmosis.

Transmission Toxoplasmosis is a zoonosis. The organism is found worldwide in many mammals. The cat is the definitive host, acquiring the organism from infected prey such as mice. The parasite replicates in the cat intestine and for 2–4 weeks after a primary infection oocysts are excreted in the stool. They then mature for 24–48 hours outside the cat before becoming infective by the oral route. Infected animals develop tissue cysts in muscle and brain which remain viable for long periods. Humans become infected from ingestion of poorly cooked meat or milk containing tissue cysts or from sporulated oocysts excreted by cats. Transmission through organ transplantation has been reported but otherwise human-to-human transmission does not occur.

Incubation period is 7–21 days.

NATURAL HISTORY AND CLINICAL FEATURES

Congenital toxoplasmosis The classic triad of congenital toxoplasmosis comprises choroidoretinitis, hydrocephalus from aqueduct stenosis and intracranial calcification. Symptomatic infection is most likely when infection occurs in the first trimester. It is unusual for the components of the triad to be present together. Other features include rashes, generalized lymphadenopathy, hepatomegaly, splenomegaly, jaundice and thrombocytopenia. There is a high mortality in the most severely affected infants, but those surviving may develop epilepsy and mental retardation. Children with choroidoretinitis may not develop visual impairment until later in childhood, or early adulthood.

Acquired toxoplasmosis may be asymptomatic, although non-specific symptoms such as fever, sore throat, lymphadenopathy and myalgia may occur. Cervical lymphadenopathy may be a feature of infection. The most serious outcome is in the immunocompromised. In children with AIDS reactivation of infection may result in cerebral toxoplasmosis.

Diagnosis

Infection in pregnancy is diagnosed is by serology. A number of specific enzyme-linked immunoassays for IgM are available which when positive indicate infection over the previous 6 months. The *Toxoplasma* dye test and a number of other IgG tests are in use, but are of less value. When there is serological evidence of maternal infection, fetal blood sampling is recommended for both serology and culture of *T. gondii*. Although it has been suggested that pregnant women should be screened for toxoplasmosis, a Royal College of Obstetricians and Gynaecologists committee concluded in 1992 that this was not appropriate.

Congenital infection can be detected by serology on blood from the infant. If there is strong suspicion of maternal infection, then serology should be performed for the first year at 3-monthly intervals as antibodies may be slow to rise. When infection is suspected, then cerebral ultrasonography should be performed to exclude hydrocephalus and intracranial calcification, and an ophthalmological examination performed. Detection of specific nucleic acid sequences by PCR is also available in specialist centres.

MANAGEMENT

Infection in pregnancy Three antibiotics are used in management: spiramycin, pyrimethamine and sulphadiazine. When a diagnosis of maternal infection in pregnancy is made, spiramycin should be given, which reduces the risk of transmission of infection to the fetus. Fetal blood sampling may be performed and if this confirms infection, then pyrimethamine, sulphadiazine and folinic acid should be given daily for 3 weeks and then alternated with spiramycin, also for 3 weeks, until delivery. Because infection during the first trimester carries the highest risk of fetal morbidity, termination following fetal infection is a reasonable option in this situation.

Treatment of the newborn Following maternal infection during pregnancy, if there is no evidence of infection in the infant either clinically or on serological grounds, spiramycin should be given for 6 months providing serology remains negative. If the newborn infant is infected then alternating courses of pyrimethamine plus sulphadiazine and spiramycin should be given until the age of 1 year.

PREVENTION OF FURTHER CASES

Pregnant women should avoid or exercise caution in contact with cats. By changing cat litter daily, the risk of infection is reduced. Meat should be cooked thoroughly.

TUBERCULOSIS

Notifiable disease

ORGANISM

Tuberculosis is caused by *Mycobacterium tuberculosis* and occasionally by *M. bovis* (the latter has virtually disappeared from the UK following eradication of disease in cattle and pasteurization of milk). These pleomorphic, weakly Gram-positive bacilli are acid-fast and grow slowly in vitro and in vivo. They form stabile complexes with dyes even when rinsed with 95% ethanol and hydrochloric acid so that microscopically bacilli show a characteristic acid-fast red colour when stained with Ziehl–Neelsen stain.

EPIDEMIOLOGY

M. tuberculosis and *M. bovis* are only found in the appropriate mammalian host, unlike the atypical mycobacteria which are commonly found in soil and water. Up to 35% of the world's population are infected, 95% of whom live in developing countries. It has been estimated that in 1990 about 7.5 million people developed tuberculosis and 2.5 million people died from the disease. There is no evidence that the burden has diminished since and it is estimated that, unless control improves, 90 million new cases and 30 million deaths will occur between 1990 and the end of 1999. In 1993 the National Survey of Tuberculosis in England and Wales reported 2422 new notifications of previously untreated cases over a 6-month period (adults and children combined), a rise of 12% from 1988; however, when population changes are taken into account the notification rates fell between

1988 and 1993 in the white, Asian and West Indian ethnic groups while they have risen in people of other ethnic groups including persons of black African origin. The incidence varies considerably from one ethnic group to another among children as it does in adults. Numbers of notified tuberculosis cases in children over aged two years has risen since 1990 (see Appendix I, Figure 12). In the 1988 National Survey 294 children with previously untreated tuberculosis were notified in England and Wales, a rate of $3.1/10^5$; however, incidence rates ranged from $1.5/10^5$ amongst white children to $29/10^5$ amongst children whose families originated in the Indian subcontinent (India, Pakistan or Bangladesh), while West Indian and other children showed an intermediate incidence of between $6/10^5$ and $13/10^5$. The highest rate of $53/10^5$ was in children born in the Indian subcontinent. Ethnic minority children born in the UK generally seem to be at a lower risk than those born in their country of origin. Tuberculosis remains associated with poverty as well as with country of origin. The decline in incidence in the UK in the twentieth century has been attributed largely to rising living standards. It has been suggested that current declining living standards in certain sections of the population may be leading to an increased incidence. The human immunodeficiency virus (HIV) epidemic has contributed to the rising number of cases of tuberculosis in sub-Saharan Africa and the USA, but it remains to be seen whether this will be the case in the UK.

Transmission The tubercle bacillus is usually inhaled in small droplets, and experimental data suggest that a single tubercule bacillus can initiate infection. Children with the disease are almost always non-infectious. Communicability is highest from untreated pulmonary tuberculosis; however, prolonged close contact with an infected adult (most often in the household) is usually necessary for transmission. Such adults will almost always have 'open' tuberculosis (i.e. they are expectorating large numbers of tubercle bacilli from a cavity in the lung). These cases are usually smear positive.

Incubation period The time from exposure to development of the primary complex is 1–3 months. However, because of dormancy and reactivation the period from initial infection to appearance of significant disease can be far longer.

NATURAL HISTORY AND CLINICAL FEATURES

Natural history The progress of tuberculosis and disease depends on the balance between bacterial multiplication and host immune response. On entering the respiratory tract the bacilli settle in peripheral alveoli and are ingested by pulmonary macrophages. Host macrophages may completely eliminate the mycobacteria with no sign of infection or immune response. In other cases multiplication within macrophages occurs both in the distal site (primary or Ghon focus) and the regional lymph nodes. The T lymphocytes are activated and surround the infected macrophages releasing cytokines that should enable the macrophages to kill the organisms in both the primary focus and the regional lymph node—a reaction which may be associated with the development of fever and tuberculin hypersensitivity. A chest X-ray taken at this stage may show a peripheral lung lesion together with hilar lymphadenopathy, the primary complex. In most cases resolution now occurs, sometimes leaving calcification at the Ghon focus and the regional lymph nodes, although viable organisms may lie dormant ready to reactivate many years later. Alternatively, there is sufficient immunity to prevent distant infection but the disease progresses in the lung with clinical sequelae resulting from destructive immune responses to the organism. Pulmonary disease is most common, accounting for 66% of cases in children of whom about half will have parenchymal lung lesions (with or without enlarged intrathoracic nodes). There may be progressive hilar lymphadenopathy which can obstruct bronchi leading to collapse and consolidation of the affected lobe or lobes. Sometimes this obstruction is incomplete and air can enter the affected segment more easily than it can leave, causing a hyperinflated segment (the ball valve effect). Lymph nodes may rupture causing a segmental pneumonia or pericarditis. In other children there may be progressive primary tuberculosis resulting in bronchopneumonia from extension of the pulmonary focus, while in others the disease progresses around a peripheral focus leading to the development of a large pleural effusion. The disease may spread only in the lymphoid system leading to cervical, supraclavicular or axillary node involvement. During this initial phase of infection haematogenous spread probably occurs in many cases but usually does not lead to disease at a distant site. However, in 0.5% to 3% of cases haematogenous spread leads to multiple foci of infection usually within 3–6 months accounting for miliary shadowing seen on chest X-ray or for tuberculous meningitis. For these reasons young children at risk of tuberculosis need to be investigated carefully and early prophylaxis given to prevent such catastrophic consequences. It is important to remember that tuberculosis can infect virtually any part of the body. Dissemination can also cause metastatic lesions in bones or joints in 5–10% of affected children, although these do not usually become apparent until at least a year after infection and their clinical sequelae often have a subacute onset. Renal disease may not be apparent until 5 years or even 20 years after the initial infection.

Clinical features The spectrum of immunopathological responses to tuberculous infection accounts for its protean clinical manifestations. The slow growth of the organism leads to an insidious onset of symptoms and these features together with the relative low incidence means that diagnosis is often delayed. Tuberculosis is still surrounded by considerable social stigma and so a positive family or contact history is rarely volunteered. Thus a high index of suspicion and direct questions concerning contact with tuberculosis are imperative. Pulmonary tuberculosis takes many forms but the child with a fever and weight loss who has unilateral hilar lymphadenopathy with or without segmental lung changes or overinflation of a segment should always be investigated with tuberculosis in mind. Phlyctenular conjunctivitis or erythema nodosum may be seen and other causes are uncommon in children. Pleural effusions in children should be considered to be tuberculous until proved otherwise. Twenty per cent of affected children suffer from extrapulmonary lymphadenitis, 5% from tuberculous meningitis and 5% from bone or joint infection. Small children with miliary tuberculosis present with non-specific features such as weight loss, apathy and poor feeding. They may have hepatosplenomegaly and a chest X-ray will show miliary shadowing. Alternative diagnoses such as Langerhans' cell histiocytosis or atypical pneumonia are usually considered first. The signs and symptoms of tuberculous meningitis evolve over several weeks with a history of a low-grade fever, headache, vomiting and increasing drowsiness. The chest X-ray may be normal and all too often the diagnosis is not made until there are frank neurological signs which are unfortunately associated with a very poor long-term outlook. Choroidal tubercles are a very helpful diagnostic sign in both tuberculous meningitis and miliary tuberculosis, and so careful fundoscopy is essential. The cerebrospinal fluid in tuberculosis meningitis is usually clear containing 50–410 white blood cells $\times 10^6$/l, most of which are lymphocytes. The protein content is raised and the glucose concentration low. Computerized axial tomography often shows a degree of hydrocephalus with contrast enhancement of the brain stem. Bone and joint tuberculosis usually presents with swelling or loss of function often without signs of acute inflammation and toxicity. Radiography reveals lytic lesions often with a sclerotic margin. The spine is affected in over half the cases.

Diagnosis Typically in adults a previously healed Ghon focus or a new infective lesion in the lung breaks down and forms a cavity containing a large number of acid-fast bacilli that are expectorated (so-called post-primary disease). This process is rare before adolescence and in childhood tuberculosis is seldom diagnosed by identifying acid-fast bacilli in a smear of fresh sputum, making diagnosis much more difficult than in adults. Thus greater reliance has to be placed on clinical and X-ray findings together with the results of tuberculin testing; a suggested set of criteria for making the diagnosis in a child is the presence of any two or more of the following:

- A positive tuberculin test.
- Clinical findings compatible with tuberculosis.
- A history of contact.
- A culture of *Mycobacterium tuberculosis* or positive histological findings from a biopsy (can be enough on its own).
- A suggestive chest X-ray.

Tuberculin testing Two forms of the tuberculin test are commonly used in the UK. The *Heaf test* is usually used for screening. This is a multiple puncture test which is easy to perform. The result should be read 3–10 days later and graded on a scale of 0 to IV with a grade II response considered positive (grade III in a child who has had a previous BCG). The *Mantoux test* is performed by giving an intradermal injection of purified protein derivative of tuberculin, either 10 units (0.1 ml of 1:1000), or 1 unit (0.1 ml of 1:10 000); the former concentration should always be used except where there is a likelihood of a very strong hypersensitivity reaction to tuberculin (for example a child with phlyctenular conjunctivitis or erythema nodosum). The test should be performed on the volar aspect of the forearm and has only been properly carried out if a bleb has been raised in the skin. It should be read after 48–72 hours by measuring the transverse diameter of induration in millimetres. Only the diameter of the indurated area that can be palpated and not the area of redness should be recorded. A reaction of 5 mm is considered positive.

Tuberculin tests are less easy to interpret in children who have had a previous BCG. It is thought that a reaction with a transverse diameter of 10 mm or more to a Mantoux test can be suggestive of infection in children who have had a previous BCG, while a reaction of 15 mm is more indicative. However, some children may give a response of over 15 mm due to BCG alone.

Culture and histology Isolating *Mycobacterium tuberculosis* from culture remains the 'gold standard' for the diagnosis of tuberculosis. Unfortunately, as infected children harbour only a small number of organisms, specimens are often negative, and in only about 30% of children is the diagnosis confirmed by culture or histology. Early-morning gastric washings taken on three successive days remain the best way to obtain specimens from which mycobacteria can be cultured. Bronchoalveolar lavage is less effective, probably because only mycobacteria in one bronchial segment at one time will be found, whereas gastric washing specimens contain all the mycobacteria that have been coughed and swallowed overnight. Early-morning urine specimens are less useful but may be positive in disseminated tuberculosis. Induced sputum using nebulized saline can also be useful, but must be undertaken away from other patients to prevent cross-infection. Microscopy is often negative and it takes 6–8 weeks for *M. tuberculosis* to grow on culture. Histological examination of lymph nodes will reveal caseating granulomas and acid-fast bacilli may be demonstrated, but such results must be interpreted in the clinical context as it is not possible to distinguish infection with *Mycobacterium tuberculosis* from atypical mycobacterial infection.

Radiology Tuberculous infection is suggested by the presence of hilar or mediastinal lymphadenopathy particularly when it is unilateral. Pulmonary, cervical or abdominal calcification may be a further clue and in children who have disseminated disease the characteristic expanded lucent lesions may be present in many bones even when there is no clinical evidence of disease at that site.

Other diagnostic techniques There is a great need for quick, reliable and specific diagnostic tests that will detect tuberculosis in children. Detecting mycobacterial DNA by polymerase chain reaction or mycobacterial lipids by gas–liquid chromatography, as well as changes in humoral or cell-mediated responses, may eventually be useful tests, but none is yet available for general clinical use.

MANAGEMENT

As children rarely have cavitatory disease they are not normally infective and so do not pose a direct risk to other patients. However, it may be wise to nurse them in a cubicle while contact tracing is being completed because of the possibility that a visiting relative has pulmonary tuberculosis.

Pulmonary and glandular tuberculosis Medication should be given in collaboration with a physician in paediatric or adult medicine who is experienced in tuberculosis therapy. That said, the present antituberculous regimens have been derived from extensive and carefully conducted studies in adults with cavitating disease and less is known about the best regimens for children. However, it seems that the 6-month 'short course chemotherapy' regimen is both effective and safe. The recommended regimen is:

- Isoniazid for 6 months.
- Rifampicin for 6 months.
- Pyrazinamide for the first 2 months.

When compliance is very poor intermittent supervised regimens where medication is given three times a week have been shown to be as effective. Peripheral neuropathy as a complication of isoniazid therapy can be prevented by pyridoxine, though this is now recommended only for malnourished children. Skin rashes and liver function test abnormalities can complicate treatment with rifampicin, isoniazid and pyrazinamide, the latter also occasionally causing photosensitivity. However, on the whole side-effects are unusual in children. Ethambutol is not recommended for therapy because young children will not be able to report the early signs of ocular toxicity. Streptomycin is too otoxic and nephrotoxic for routine use, but it and other second-line agents—cycloserine, capreomycin, amikacin and ciprofloxacin—may be considered in the unusual (for the UK) occurrence of resistance to front-line agents.

Extrapulmonary tuberculosis including tuberculous meningitis Few studies have been performed to determine the best treatment for extrapulmonary tuberculosis, particularly tuberculous meningitis. Most people use the same drug regimen as for pulmonary disease but a longer course of treatment is recommended for tuberculosis meningitis, usually rifampicin or isoniazid for 12 months with pyrazinamide for at least the first 2 months. Concomitant steroid therapy is recommended for tuberculous meningitis, tuberculous pericarditis or where a hilar lymph node is obstructing a bronchus. Expert advice should be sought and it may be necessary to give steroids for 6–8 weeks.

Infants born to mothers with tuberculosis There is rarely a need to separate mothers with tuberculosis from their infants. However, such infants should be investigated carefully and managed as if they had the disease. Babies born to mothers with infectious pulmonary tuberculosis should receive chemoprophylaxis (usually isoniazid) for 6 months and then be tuberculin tested: if negative, BCG should be given; if strongly positive, further therapy should be considered. Such babies may be breast-fed. Isoniazid-resistant BCG is now not used in such cases.

Congenital tuberculosis due to genital tract tuberculosis in the mother is rare and is a difficult diagnosis to make. Infants present with non-specific features of congenital infection such hepatosplenomegaly, fever, leucopenia and jaundice. A high index of suspicion is vital and these children should be treated as for extrapulmonary tuberculosis.

Multidrug-resistant tuberculosis Resistant strains of *Mycobacterium tuberculosis* are relatively rare in the UK although alarmingly more common in other parts of the world. Patterns of drug resistance in children tend to mirror those found in adults from the same populations. Resistance is most common to streptomycin and isoniazid and is still rare for rifampicin (see the second-line agents listed above).

PREVENTION OF FURTHER CASES

Prompt treatment of infectious cases of tuberculosis and thorough contact tracing are the most important preventive measures. Vaccination with BCG and the screening of entrants to the UK from high-incidence countries* make supplementary contributions to the prevention of tuberculosis in the UK.

BCG vaccination Bacillus Calmette–Guérin (BCG) vaccine was developed in France in the early years of this century and has been used routinely in Britain since the 1950s. It is hardly used at all in North America. Its effectiveness is disputed as studies in different populations have given very varying results. However, there is a consensus that BCG does protect against disseminated disease and tuberculous meningitis in particular. Studies in the UK suggest BCG

***Tuberculosis incidence more than 40 per 10^5 population per annum.**

offers about 75% protection against all forms of disease. It is recommended for all infants born into a household where there is a recent history of tuberculosis or whose families are Asian or African in origin, for immigrants from countries with a high incidence of tuberculosis, tuberculin-negative contacts of open tuberculosis cases, health care workers at risk and all tuberculin-negative schoolchildren (the schools programme). Contraindications to BCG vaccination are:

- An acute febrile illness—defer vaccination until the child is better.
- Tuberculin-positive individuals.
- Children born to HIV-positive mothers and those at risk of severe combined immunodeficiency (i.e. a positive family history of this condition).

The vaccination is given as an intradermal injection of 0.05 ml in children under 3 months old and 0.1 ml in children over 3 months old. Percutaneous injection may also be used for infants and neonates *but the strength of BCG is different for the two methods and must not be confused.* It should be given at the site of the insertion of the left deltoid muscle, though in generalized severe septic skin conditions care should be taken to make the injection away from affected skin. In most individuals a papule forms 2–6 weeks after immunization. This often discharges and needs no treatment, although parents may wish to use a dry non-occlusive dressing (or a waterproof dressing when swimming). More severe reactions including prolonged deep ulceration, lymphadenitis and osteomyelitis are most commonly caused by faulty technique resulting in subcutaneous rather than intradermal injection. Treatment with isoniazid for 6 weeks is often helpful. Specialist advice should be sought in these circumstances.

The school BCG programme BCG is recommended for tuberculin-negative school children between the ages of 10 and 13 years. Initial Heaf testing and BCG are not necessary for children with a definitive BCG scar. Heaf grades 0 and I receive BCG; no action is taken for those with grade II reactions unless there are other signs, symptoms or a suspicious history. Children with grade III and IV reactions should be referred for specialist examination. Even if the children are normal to examination, chemoprophylactic treatment may be given if they have been in contact with tuberculosis or resident in high-prevalence countries in the preceding 2 years. The school programme is under review as with the decline of tuberculosis in the 1980s BCG vaccination was considered barely cost-effective and some districts with very low incidence have stopped the programme prior to a national decision.

Screening of immigrants All immigrants to the UK from Asia, Africa, South and Central America and the Caribbean and other countries where tuberculosis is common should be screened. In addition all refugees should be screened. Initial screening may take place at the port of entry but it is more important that information on new immigrants is passed to the consultant in communicable disease control in the district of intended residence so that comprehensive screening can be arranged. Screening consists of an interview about health status, current symptoms and previous BCG vaccination. Screening by tuberculin testing is not needed in asymptomatic individuals with a definite BCG scar. Individuals with suggestive symptoms or strongly positive Heaf tests (grades II, III and IV in children, III and IV in adults) must be referred for specialist opinion. Heaf-negative (grade 0 and I) children should receive BCG.

Isolation Older children and adults with smear-positive pulmonary disease (sufficient bacilli to be seen on direct examination) should be regarded as infectious and segregated in a single room or managed at home. If the organism is fully sensitive they will become non-infectious after 2 weeks of medication containing rifampicin and isoniazid (see comments above on the need for initial isolation of the hospitalized child with tuberculosis).

Contact tracing Ten per cent of tuberculosis cases are diagnosed by contact tracing. Thorough and effective tracing of all children exposed to tuberculosis is vital as all will be at risk of developing potentially life-threatening disease. Children under the age of 5 years who are close contacts of a smear-positive adult are particularly at risk and should be evaluated promptly following their contact being established. Children should be examined for evidence of disease and a chest X-ray should be performed, as should a Heaf or Mantoux test. Some authorities have as policy that all children under the age of 5 years should be given a 6-month course of isoniazid regardless of the results of the initial screening. Children over the age of 5 years should be re-evaluated after 6 weeks (as screening tests performed during the incubation period may have given a false negative result). Children who have a negative tuberculin test and a normal chest X-ray are then given BCG vaccination. If they are tuberculin-positive (grade II Heaf or 5 mm × 5 mm Mantoux if no previous BCG, and grade III Heaf or 10 mm × 10 mm Mantoux if given BCG) but have a normal chest X-ray and no clinical signs of disease, isoniazid alone is given for 6 months ('chemoprophylaxis'). If there is clinical evidence of disease then the children should be given standard triple therapy. If the source case was smear-positive it is probably wise to review the children after 6 months and a year even if initial screening was negative. Most children are infected by an adult in the same household and it should be remembered that there is likely to be an infectious adult for every case in a child. The contacts of children with tuberculosis should also be screened, not to identify individuals infected by the child (as children are rarely infective) but rather to identify the source case from whom the child was infected.

Protection of staff at risk All health care workers should report symptoms suggestive of tuberculosis and they should also be protected by Heaf testing and BCG vaccination if non-immune (Heaf grade 0 or I). Evidence of infectious tuberculosis should be sought among prospective national health service staff and students, teachers and nursery staff.

FURTHER READING

Joint Tuberculosis Committee of the British Thoracic Society (1994) Control and prevention of tuberculosis in the United Kingdom: Code of Practice 1994. *Thorax* **49**: 1193–1200.

Smith MHD, Starke JR & Marquis JR (1992) Tuberculosis and opportunistic mycobacterial infections. In *Textbook of Paediatric Infectious Disease*, 3rd edn, (eds Feigin RD, Cherry JD) pp. 1321–1362.

TYPHOID AND PARATYPHOID FEVER

Typhoid and paratyphoid are notifiable diseases

ORGANISMS

Typhoid is caused by *Salmonella typhi* and paratyphoid by *S. paratyphi* A, B and C. Salmonellae are Gram-negative bacilli. The main reservoir for *S. typhi* and *S. paratyphi* is in humans, though rarely domestic animals are found to be infected with *S. paratyphi*, and as both organisms can exist for some time outside the body. Sewage, water and food contaminated by sewage can act as environmental reservoirs.

EPIDEMIOLOGY

Typhoid and paratyphoid occur worldwide. Both are endemic in developing countries and most cases reported in industrialized countries such as the UK are imported. In the UK most imported cases of typhoid come from India and Africa. Paratyphoid is indigenous in the UK. In 1994 there were 227 cases of typhoid reported in England and Wales and 2117 cases of paratyphoid.

Transmission of both infections is usually by food or water contaminated by faeces or urine from an infected person. Because heat destroys the bacteria uncooked foods, salads, cold drinks and milk products are the most common vehicles. Typhoid infection can be long-term and symptomless with the organism reproducing in the biliary tree and being excreted with faeces.

Incubation period for both infections is 1–3 weeks depending on the size of the infecting dose. The dose for *S. typhi* can be particularly low (10^2 organisms).

NATURAL HISTORY AND CLINICAL FEATURES

Clinically the presentations of both infections are similar, though paratyphoid fever is rarely as severe as typhoid and if there is fever the onset may be more abrupt and the outcome is rarely fatal. In contrast to *S. typhi*, infection with *S. paratyphi* can cause diarrhoea. Both infections are systemic bacterial diseases which can range from being totally asymptomatic to severe enteric fever with systemic spread and intestinal perforation. Enteric fever is characterized by slow onset of a sustained fever, malaise, headache and constipation though diarrhoea tends to occur in young children. Physical findings can include splenomegaly, bradycardia and rose-coloured spots on the trunk, and the organisms can be isolated from the blood early in the diseases and from faeces and urine after the first week.

Diagnosis is by isolation of organisms from cultures of stool, rectal swabs and blood or bone marrow. Paired serology specimens may confirm a diagnosis but are rarely usefully clinically.

MANAGEMENT

Antibiotics are recommended for invasive diseases. The drugs of first choice are ampicillin, trimethoprim, chloramphenicol and ciprofloxacin, though many organisms acquired in developing countries are resistant to the more common established antibiotics. Ceftriaxone may also be useful. Treatment for enteric fever is for a minimum 14 days. Even so relapses may occur. If there are foci in abscesses or osteomyelitis treatment may need to be parenteral and prolonged for up to 6 weeks, especially in the immunocompromised patient.

PREVENTION OF FURTHER CASES

Cases must be notified by the doctor providing care, and the local consultant in communicable disease control or the director of public health should be informed. For both infections enteric precautions must be applied (Chapters 26 and 27). Family and close contacts need to be screened by stool specimens. Infected food handlers and others at high risk of causing transmission should be excluded from work until their infection is demonstrated to have cleared by six negative stool specimens taken at two week intervals starting two weeks after completing antibiotics. Staff caring for children may return to work 48 hours after their first normal stool, while in children there should be three negative stool specimens at weekly intervals. Long-term carriers may have their infection cleared by a course of ciprofloxacin Occasionally persistent carriers have been cured by cholecystectomy.

Vaccine The current parenteral vaccine against typhoid is not very effective. Although it is widely employed, especially for travellers going to developing countries, many authorities do not recommend its use, preferring to emphasize the importance of general enteric precautions to avoid gastrointestinal infections in general. Two newer vaccines (one live, one killed) seem to be more successful and are to be preferred.

99 TYPHUS

There are two forms of typhus: epidemic (louse-borne) and endemic (flea-borne).

ORGANISM

Rickettsia prowazekiipi is responsible for epidemic, louse-borne typhus fever and *R. prowazeki var mooseri* for endemic, flea-borne typhus fever.

EPIDEMIC TYPHUS

EPIDEMIOLOGY

Infection occurs in all ages, but disease tends to be less severe in children. It occurs worldwide in association with poverty, overcrowding and poor sanitary conditions. Hence it is common among refugees and in war zones and outbreaks occur in the winter.

Transmission is from human to human by the body louse. People are infective during the febrile illness and for 2 days afterwards. The louse infects by first biting an infected person and then excreting *R. prowazeki* in its faeces which are rubbed into a bite on another person through scratching. Rickettsiae remain viable in the dead louse.

Incubation period is 1–2 weeks from the bite in the recipient.

NATURAL HISTORY AND CLINICAL FEATURES

There is an abrupt onset of high fever and malaise with shivering and general body pain in the older patient. A maculopapular rash appears 5–7 days later on the trunk and spreads to the axillae (a useful diagnostic feature) and the limbs. Face, palms and soles are spared. The rash becomes haemorrhagic (petechial or generalized) and then turns brown. Severe complications include myocardial and renal involvement; these are more common in older children and adults and can be fatal.

Diagnosis See below.

MANAGEMENT

Antibiotic treatment with chloramphenicol is given for 10 days. Specific supportive measures must also be given if there are complications. Tetracycline may be used in those age 9 years or more.

PREVENTION OF FURTHER CASES

Patients and close contacts must be deloused. Suitable agents are lindane and permethrin-containing topical treatments. All clothing and bedding must be deloused.

ENDEMIC TYPHUS

EPIDEMIOLOGY

Rats and mice are the natural hosts and transmission only occurs occasionally and sporadically via bites of fleas. Distribution is worldwide, but the disease is uncommon in the UK.

Incubation period is 1–2 weeks from the bite.

NATURAL HISTORY AND CLINICAL FEATURES

The disease process is similar to but milder than epidemic typhus and is rarely complicated or fatal even in adults. Fever occurs, as does a non-haemorrhagic maculopapular rash. Without treatment the disease is self-limiting in 2 weeks.

Diagnosis Both epidemic and endemic typhus are best diagnosed clinically with confirmation coming from rising titres of antibodies or agglutinins in convalescent versus acute serum.

MANAGEMENT

One dose of doxycycline (5 mg/kg, max 200mg) is curative in children and adults.

PREVENTION OF FURTHER CASES

Measures against rats and mice should be taken including use of residual insecticides and good waste disposal.

VIRAL HAEMORRHAGIC FEVERS

100

Notifiable disease

Viral haemorrhagic fevers (VHFs) are severe viral infections, in which haemorrhage is an important clinical feature. Several different VHFs exist and the pathogenesis of the bleeding differs between them. The importance of managing potential VHFs lies in the differential diagnosis from other, more treatable, life-threatening haemorrhagic diseases such as malignant malaria or meningococcal disease.

ORGANISMS

Several groups of viruses are responsible for viral haemorrhagic fevers. Most have an animal reservoir and several are transmitted by an insect vector (Table 100.1).

EPIDEMIOLOGY

Arboviruses The Flaviviridae and Alphaviridae were previously grouped as arboviruses (ARthropod-BOrne). All are able to replicate both in the insect vector and their vertebrate host.

Yellow fever is an important endemic and epidemic disease of tropical and subtropical Africa and South America. Its insect vector is the mosquito (*Aedes aegypti*) which is no longer found in Europe. Jungle or sylvatic yellow fever is transmitted from non-human primates. Urban yellow fever is transmitted from infected humans. Both types occur in all age groups with equal frequency and where further transmission is possible through mosquitoes cases must be isolated (see Chapter 102).

Dengue is present in the tropics and subtropics worldwide. Its insect vector is also *Aedes aegypti* and in epidemics can have a very high attack rate. Dengue haemorrhagic fever is usually confined to children. It occurs when a child is re-infected with a heterologous Dengue serotype (there are four serotypes), and is thought to be due to pre-existing antibody binding to virus and facilitating infection of monocytes or macrophages via Fc receptors. Dengue haemorrhagic fever occurs more frequently in south-east Asia.

Other arboviral haemorrhagic fevers may have a reservoir in chimpanzees or monkeys. They have a similar course to dengue, but without a rash.

ARENAVIRUSES

Lassa fever occurs in West Africa. It persistently infects the multimammate rat (*Mastomys natalensis*) and humans become infected by inhaling or ingesting infected urine. Other haemorrhagic fevers caused by arenaviruses, Machupo, Junin and Sabia, are transmitted from persistently infected *Calomys* species in South America.

Bunyaviruses The nairovirus causing Crimean–Congo haemorrhagic fever (CCHF) is transmitted to humans from many vertebrate species including hares, hedgehogs and domestic animals via the tick (*Hyalomma* spp.). This fever has been described in Russia, Bulgaria, former Yugoslavia, Pakistan, Iraq, Tanzania, Zaire, Uganda, Burkina Faso and South Africa. Infection can spread from person to person by aerosol to hospital staff or to other family members, often with increased severity of disease in the recipient.

Hantaviruses cause haemorrhagic fever with renal syndrome (HFRS). Hantaan, which is found in Korea, Japan, the far east of Russia and China, persistently and silently infects fieldmice (*Apodemus agrarius*). Infection occurs when humans enter the fieldmouse's ecological niche or vice versa, and virus is usually transmitted via inhalation of excreta or saliva. Seoul virus is present throughout the world and persistently infects the Norway rat (*Rattus norvegicus*). For example, in Baltimore in the USA, 50% of rats have been found to be excreting virus. Puumala virus persistently infects the bank vole (*Clethrionomys glareolus*) and is found in Scandinavia and other parts of northern Europe. Hantaviruses have been found in human and animal reservoirs in the UK. In most surveys 5–10% of cases are reported in children. Person-to-person spread (apart from two cases of transplacental spread) has not been described. Hantavirus pulmonary syndrome has not been reported in children.

Filoviruses The filoviruses Marburg and Ebola are transmitted via the respiratory route. Ebola virus epidemics have occurred in Zaire and Sudan with high mortality. Marburg virus occurred initially in monkey handlers in a laboratory in Germany, but subsequent sporadic cases occurred in travellers in Kenya and Uganda. Although monkeys have been found to be infected, it is thought that they are not the definitive host. A search for a small rodent or any other host has so far proved fruitless.

Incubation period varies from 1 day to 6 weeks (Table 100.1).

NATURAL HISTORY AND CLINICAL FEATURES

Arboviruses Dengue may be an undifferentiated febrile illness. Nausea and vomiting occur in 60% of cases, more commonly in children and the elderly. Over 50% of patients will have cough. Older children and adults will display the more classical disease. This begins with a sudden onset of fever (which may be biphasic), severe muscle aches, bone and joint pains, severe headache and altered taste (a metallic taste is described). Lymphadenopathy and rash appear 2–3 days after onset of fever. The rash is preceded by skin flushing and can be maculopapular, petechial or purpuric. There is a spectrum of disease from mild dengue fever (DF) to dengue haemorrhagic fever (DHF) and dengue shock syndrome (DSS), but DHF and DSS should not be diagnosed unless the criteria in Table 100.2 are met. Dengue haemorrhagic fever usually occurs in two stages. The first resembles classical dengue with fever, malaise, headache, anorexia and vomiting. Two to five days later the condition worsens with the onset of shock. There is restlessness, irritability, cold extremities, narrowed pulse pressure and petechiae on the face and extremities. Frank ecchymoses (10% of cases) and bleeding from gums and venepuncture sites can occur, and the tourniquet test will produce petechiae. Children will also have thrombocytopenia and haemoconcentration which helps to differentiate early or low-grade DHF from dengue. If there is circulatory failure (hypotension or narrowed pulse pressure) this is diagnostic of DSS. Approximately 30% of children with DHF progress to DSS. The mortality rate of DHF is 5–10%.

Arenaviruses It is estimated that Lassa fever virus (LFV) affects up to 50 000 persons each year in west Africa. In a study in Sierra Leone it was estimated that 12% of 3849 hospital admissions were for Lassa fever and that LFV was responsible for 30% of the deaths in hospital. Nevertheless, not all cases are severe. Infection begins insidiously with generalized myalgia, chills, sore throat, fever and dry cough. This can progress with manifestations of increased capillary permeability such as pulmonary oedema and subconjunctival oedema. Subsequently haemorrhagic complications such as epistaxis, haemoptysis, haematemesis, petechiae at pressure points and oozing from venepuncture sites develop. This terminates with abrupt shock and death. The overall mortality is 7–10% but rises to 30% in the first trimester of pregnancy. Viraemia is heavier in pregnant women.

Bunyaviruses Crimean–Congo haemorrhagic fever (CCHF) begins abruptly with

Table 100.1 Viruses and haemorrhagic fevers

Virus group	Virology	Reservoir	Vector	Direct person-to-person spread	Incubation period (days)	Geographical distribution
FLAVIVIRIDAE	Enveloped RNA					
Yellow fever		Monkeys, humans	Mosquito (*Aedes aegypti*)	No	3–6	Tropics and subtropics
Dengue		Humans	Mosquito (*Aedes aegypti*)	No	2–7	Tropics and subtropics
Omsk haemorrhagic fever		Musk rats	Ticks (*Dermatocentor*)	No	3–7	Russia, Romania
TOGAVIRIDAE	Enveloped RNA					
Chikungunya*		Humans (?monkeys)	Mosquito (*Aedes aegypti*)	No	1–6	Sub-Saharan Africa India, SE Asia
ARENAVIRIDAE	Unenveloped RNA					
Lassa fever		Multimammate rats	Aerosol (urine)	Yes	10–11	Sub-Saharan Africa
Junin (Argentinian fever)		*Calomys musculinus*	Aerosol (urine)	Yes	10–11	South America
Machupo (Bolivian haemorrhagic fever)		*Calomys callosus*	Aerosol (urine)	Yes	10–11	South America
Sabia (Venezualan haemorrhagic fever)		?	Aerosol (urine)	Yes	10–11	South America

BUNYAVIRIDAE	Enveloped RNA					
Phlebovirus:						
Rift Valley fever		Sheep, cattle, goats	Mosquito, sandfly	No	3–12	Sub-Saharan Africa
Nairovirus:						
Crimean-Congo HF		Many vertebrates	Ticks (*Hyalomma*, etc.)	Yes†	3–12	Russia, sub-Saharan Africa
Hantavirus:						
Hantaan		Fieldmice (*Apodemus*)	Aerosol (excreta)	No	7–42	Far East
Seoul		*Rattus norvegicus*	Aerosol (excreta)	No	7–42	Worldwide
Puumala		Bank voles (*Clethrionomys*)	Aerosol (excreta)	No	7–42	Northern Europe
FILOVIRIDAE	Enveloped RNA					
Ebola		Unknown‡	Contact with secretions	Yes	7–9	West and central Africa
Marburg		Unknown‡	Aerosol	Yes	7–9	West and central Africa

***Usually causes arthritis and fever but in children produces a bleeding diathesis.**
†Nosocomial infection via blood and interfamilial aerosol spread.
‡Isolated from monkeys but these are thought not to be the definitive host.

Table 100.2 Diagnosis and staging of DHF and DSS

Clinical	
Acute high fever	> 2–7 days
Haemorrhage	Tourniquet test positive (> 20 petechiae per inch or per 2.5 cm). Plus one or more of epistaxis, gum bleeding, melaena, haematemesis, ecchymoses
Hepatomegaly	
Shock	Hypotension, narrow pulse pressure, cold clammy skin
Laboratory	
Thrombocytopenia	(< 100,000/μl)
Haemoconcentration	Haematocrit increase by 20% or more
Staging	
Grade I	Fever, non-specific symptoms, positive tourniquet test
Grade II	As above plus spontaneous bleeding
Grade III	Circulatory failure, rapid weak pulse, hypotension narrowing pulse pressure
Grade IV	Profound shock with blood pressure not measurable

Adapted from Belshe RB, ed. (1991) *Textbook of Human Virology* pp. 651–652. Mosby, New York.
DHF, dengue haemorrhagic fever; DSS, Dengue shock syndrome

fever, myalgia, malaise and headache. This lasts 2–3 days when the patient then has full development of haemorrhagic features. Petechiae develop over the chest and abdomen and epistaxis is common. Spreading cutaneous ecchymoses and bleeding from every orifice together with neurological signs indicate very severe disease. Death occurs following circulatory collapse. There may be hepatomegaly and occasionally splenomegaly.

Haemorrhagic fever with renal syndrome (HFRS) varies in severity. That due to hantaan virus (sometimes termed Korean haemorrhagic fever) is the most severe. Classically it evolves through five phases (febrile, hypotensive, oliguric, diuretic and convalescent). Mild haemorrhagic signs occur first in the hypotensive phase which lasts from 2 hours to 3 days. Major haemorrhages and most of the deaths occurs in the oliguria phase (3–7 days). The diuretic phase lasts from days to weeks with polyuria (3–6 litre/day), and convalescence takes weeks to months. A mortality rate of 15% is not uncommon. Balkan HFRS is due to a similar virus, has a similar clinical pattern but is acquired from the yellow-necked fieldmouse (*Apodemus flavicollis*). Nephropathia epidemica (NE) occurs in northern Europe and is due to

Puumala virus. It is far milder than Hantaan virus infection, indeed only 1 in 15–20 cases of infection are symptomatic and the mortality is below 1%. Seoul virus infection occurs worldwide and is intermediate in severity between Hantaan and Puumala. It usually does not show phase progression but patients do show hepatomegaly. There is some evidence that hantavirus infection might predispose to development of chronic renal failure.

Filoviruses Illness due to filovirus usually begins with fever, myalgia and headache. Two to three days later diarrhoea and a morbilliform rash appear. This is followed by widespread haemorrhagic manifestations. Mortality is high (Marburg 50% ; Ebola 80%).

Diagnosis Travel history and history of contact with arthropods and animals will help in reaching a diagnosis. Malaria, meningococcal septicaemia and rickettsioses are part of the differential diagnosis. The specific diagnosis depends upon detection of virus or a serological response to it. Great care must be exercised in handling specimens from patients with VHF. Samples will need to be examined under category 4 containment at specialist centres.*

MANAGEMENT AND PREVENTION

All viral haemorrhagic fevers require specialist care and advice. Infections with arenaviruses, filoviruses and CCHF are transmissible person-to-person and cases (suspected or proven) should be managed in a high-security infectious disease unit. Supportive therapy includes fluid management and administration of fresh frozen plasma and platelets. Ribavirin (intravenous) may be of benefit in arenavirus, bunyavirus and filovirus infections. Immune plasma may also be of benefit in some cases of VHF.

If VHF is considered possible or likely the consultant in communicable disease control must be informed immediately by telephone. The names and addresses of family and health care contacts should be noted in case the VHF is one that is transmissible person-to-person.

A vaccine is available to prevent yellow fever.

WARTS AND VERRUCAE

101

ORGANISM

The human papillomavirus (HPV) belongs to the papovavirus group of DNA viruses. At least 60 types have been recognized as pathogenic in humans.

EPIDEMIOLOGY

Warts occur worldwide and in all ages, but different types have a predilection for different age groups. Plantar warts (verrucae) are most common in school-age children; common and flat warts predominate in young children, and genital warts in the sexually active. The only reservoir for human warts is humans.

***In the UK, contact PHLS Virus Reference Division (telephone 0181-200-4400). Out of working hours contact the on-call doctor for the Communicable Disease Surveillance Centre (telephone 0181-200-6868).**

Transmission Infectivity is low and spread occurs with direct contact. Genital warts in children should always raise the possibility of sexual abuse. Laryngeal papillomas are most probably transmitted from the mother's cervix at birth.

Incubation period is from 1 month to 2 years.

NATURAL HISTORY AND CLINICAL FEATURES

Plantar warts are flat hyperkeratotic lesions on the soles of the feet. They are frequently painful. Laryngeal papillomas occur on the vocal cords and epiglottis in young children. Skin warts may be flat or raised, smooth or rough, varying in size from a pinhead to over a centimetre. Genital warts (condyloma acuminatum) are fleshy growths seen most commonly in moist areas in and around the genitalia and anus.

Diagnosis is clinical. Earlier hopes that typing of genital warts might distinguish those with a sexual mode of spread have not been confirmed.

MANAGEMENT

Most warts are self-limiting though it may take a year or more for some warts to regress. Where treatment is needed, cryotherapy can be used except on those in the genital region. For these podophyllin is more appropriate. Curettage and/or salicylic acid plasters are often used for verrucae. Laryngeal warts are removed by laser therapy or surgery.

102 YELLOW FEVER

See also Chapters 20 and 100.

ORGANISM

Yellow fever is caused by an enveloped RNA virus of the genus *Flavivirus*.

EPIDEMIOLOGY

The reservoir of infection is among monkeys and other vertebrates and the mosquito (*Aedes aegypti*) is the vector. *Aedes aegypti* is no longer found in Europe. Yellow fever occurs in two endemic zones in central Africa and northern South America with a natural reservoir in forest monkeys; however, cases occur in both urban and rural settings with a relatively high mortality. The disease is almost unheard-of in the UK, but British travellers to endemic zones are at risk.

Transmission is by specific mosquitoes, notably *Aedes aegypti*, either from monkeys to humans (jungle or sylvatic yellow fever) or from human to human (urban yellow fever). Blood of patients is infective via mosquitoes from onset of fever for up to 5 days.

Incubation period is 3–6 days following the mosquito bite.

NATURAL HISTORY AND CLINICAL FEATURES

Yellow fever is a disease of varying severity which in severe forms manifests as sudden-onset fever, malaise proceeding to jaundice, haemorrhagic symptoms and death.

Diagnosis is by isolation of the virus or serological testing. If there is haemorrhage or coma important differential diagnoses include malaria, meningococcal disease and the other viral haemorrhagic fevers (see Chapter 100).

MANAGEMENT

Treatment is supportive. Therapy will include fluid management and may involve administration of fresh frozen plasma and platelets.

PREVENTION OF FURTHER CASES

Yellow fever immunization is highly effective. It is strongly recommended for those travelling to endemic countries. It is also required in many countries for those travelling from endemic zones.

YERSINIOSIS 103

ORGANISMS

Yersinia enterocolitica and *Y. pseudotuberculosis* are Gram-negative bacilli.

EPIDEMIOLOGY

The main reservoir of these organisms is in farm animals and rats. Infections occur following ingestion of contaminated food. Infection is more common and more serious in individuals with iron overload such as thalassaemia patients on long-term transfusion programmes. It is commoner in temperate and cool climates.

Transmission is from contaminated food, especially undercooked pork, or directly from farm animals.

Incubation period is 4–6 days, range 1–14 days.

NATURAL HISTORY AND CLINICAL FEATURES

Yersinia enterocolitica causes acute diarrhoea often with blood and mucus in the stools and associated with fever and pain. The pain may be so severe as to mimic appendicitis or other acute surgical problem. Bacteraemia and non-intestinal disease such as osteomyelitis may occur. Erythema nodosum and reactive arthritis may complicate the infection and occur most commonly in adults. *Yersinia pseudotuberculosis* causes fever and abdominal pain usually without diarrhoea. This usually results from an acute ileitis and/or mesenteric adenitis. There is fever and there may be a blotchy red rash.

Diagnosis Both organisms can be identified in the stool and blood early in the illness. Stool isolation requires cold enrichment and prolonged culture under special conditions. Inform the laboratory when this diagnosis is suspected. Serological tests looking for agglutinating antibodies are also available through reference laboratories but false positive results can occur.

MANAGEMENT

Co-trimoxazole, aminoglycosides, cefotaxime and (in those over 9 years old) tetracycline are all useful in systemic (blood culture positive) infection. Their benefits in disease confined to the intestine is unproven but it is reasonable to treat if symptoms are severe or prolonged.

PREVENTION OF FURTHER CASES

Strict food hygiene should be observed. Children visiting farms and handling animals should always be made to wash their hands before eating.

APPENDIX I: MORTALITY AND MORBIDITY FROM INFECTIOUS DISEASE IN THE UK

Numbers and rates of deaths among children in the UK from selected causes during the years (1988–1992) are shown for infants (children under age 1 year) in Table I.1 and for all children (14 years and under) in Table I.2. These show a gradually declining number of deaths from infectious and parasitic disease 'combined infections' and all causes. It should be noted that in 1992 the introduction of *Haemophilus influenzae* type b (Hib) vaccination seemingly reduced deaths from invasive *Haemophilus* disease and there was also a sharp fall in deaths from sudden infant death syndrome and respiratory causes in infants.

Morbidity and immunization data are shown graphically for the vaccine-preventable diseases, selected gastrointestinal infections, vertically acquired human immunodeficiency virus (HIV), meningococcal disease and respiratory syncytial virus using notifications, clinical and laboratory reports variously for England and Wales, England, Wales and Northern Ireland, and the UK as available.

Diphtheria notifications (Figure I.1) show the dramatic effect of immunization which began after 1940. In contrast, laboratory reports of gastrointestinal infections and food poisoning have increased substantially with steady rises in reports of *Salmonella* and *Campylobacter* spp. and a particular rise in shigella dysentery in 1991 and 1992 (Figure I.2). Laboratory reports of *Haemophilus influenzae* type b (Figure I.3) have fallen dramatically since the introduction of Hib vaccine in 1992. Numbers of cases of HIV-1 infections and acquired immune deficiency syndrome (AIDS) cases (Figure I.4) through mother-to-child infection are increasing steadily. In this figure the decline in numbers of births to HIV-1 infected mothers is artefactual, reflecting underidentification of maternal infection and unresolved infection status of children born after 1992. Notifications of Measles from 1940 to 1993 (Figure I.5) show a characteristic two-yearly epidemic subsiding after immunization began in 1968, (Figure I.6) indicates the success of the measles and rubella (MR) vaccination campaign of the autumn of 1994. Meningococcal infections (Figure I.7) have shown slow rises and falls apart from the dramatic epidemic that took place during the Second World War. Pertussis was largely controlled in the 1950s but experienced a resurgence in the late 1970s and early 1980s (Figure I.8) following a controversy over vaccine safety and it took a decade to make up the lost ground. The graph for polio (Figure I.9) demonstrates the large-scale epidemics that took place after the Second World War and the protective effect of the introduction of the Salk and Sabin vaccines. Epidemics of respiratory syncytial virus infections occur every winter (Figure I.10). The decline in tetanus notifications and deaths (Figure I.11) lagged behind the introduction of routine childhood immunization in the mid-1950s because of the large number of unimmunized adults who remained unprotected. Notifications of tuberculosis in children show a recent rise in infections in children over 2 years old (Figure I.12). Vaccine coverage data (Figure I.13) show a steadily improving picture over the period 1988 to 1994 but these national data conceal poor coverage in a number of districts.

Diphtheria

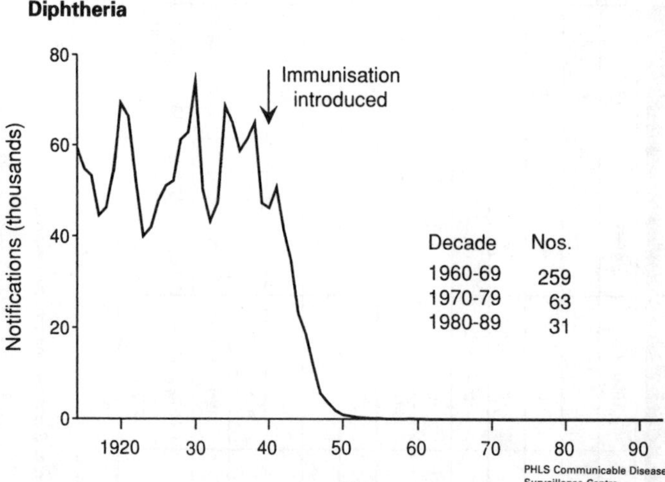

Figure I.1 Diphtheria notifications (all ages), England and Wales 1914–1993.

Gastrointestinal infections

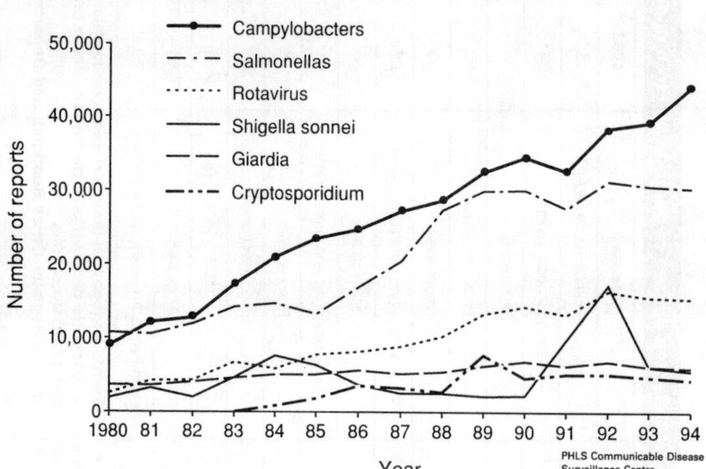

Figure I.2 Laboratory reports of selected gastrointestinal infections (all ages), England and Wales 1980–1994.

Table I.1 Selected causes of death in children under 1 year old in the UK 1988–1992 (rates per thousand births)

ICD code	Disease	1988	1989	1990	1991	1992
001-009	Intestinal infectious disease	15	27	15	16	10
036	Meningococcal infection	34	51	50	48	36
038	Septicaemia	8	24	13	14	19
030–041	Other bacterial disease*	50	78	75	67	59
045–079	Viral disease	23	14	16	11	6
001–139	All infectious and parasitic disease	92 (0.11)	125 (0.16)	114 (0.15)	97 (0.12)	81 (0.10)
320–322	Meningitis	35	34	27	35	27
466	Acute bronchitis and bronchiolitis	61	55	49	48	20
480–486	Pneumonia	145	107	101	88	60
	Combined infections*†	333 (0.43)	321 (0.41)	291 (0.38)	268 (0.33)	188 (0.24)
798	SIDS	1532 (1.97)	1304 (1.69)	1190 (1.53)	975 (1.23)	504 (0.64)
	All causes*	7061 (9.06)	6542 (8.48)	6272 (9.09)	5825 (7.34)	4961 (6.30)
	Denominators (thousands) of live brths	779.6	770.8	775.7	794.1	787.4

***Includes totals for meningococcal infection and septicaemia.**
†All infections and parasitic disease, plus meningitis, acute bronchitis and pneumonia.
SIDS, sudden infant death syndrome.
Source: OPCS, General Register Office Scotland, and Department of Health and Social Services, Northern Ireland.

Table I.2 Selected causes of death in children aged 14 years and under in the UK 1988–1992 (rates per hundred thousand child population)

ICD code	Disease	1988	1989	1990	1991	1992
001-009	Intestinal infectious disease	21	31	21	22	15
036	Meningococcal infection	117	134	121	120	100
038	Septicaemia	16	42	32	28	20
030–041 (excl. 036, 038)	Other bacterial disease*	147	184	169	159	140
045–079	Viral disease	61	46	37	38	20
001–139	All infectious and parasitic disease	235 (2.26)	273 (2.52)	246 (2.27)	228 (2.06)	192 (1.71)
320–322	Meningitis	62	70	65	69	58
466	Acute bronchitis and bronchiolitis	84	84	64	66	35
480–486	Pneumonia	195	159	149	150	92
	Combined infections*†	576 (5.56)	586 (5.41)	524 (4.79)	513 (4.64)	377 (3.37)
798	SIDS	1566	1339	1226	1017	531
All causes	All causes*	9696 (93.59)	9143 (84.42)	8793 (80.45)	8316 (75.19)	7180 (64.16)
	Population denominators (10^5s)	103.6	108.3	109.3	110.6	111.9

***Includes totals for meningococcal infection and septicaemia**
†All infections and parasitic disease, plus meningitis, acute bronchitis and pneumonia.
SIDS, sudden infant death syndrome.
Source: OPCS, General Register Office Scotland, and Department of Health and Social Services, Northern Ireland.

Haemophilus influenzae type b infection

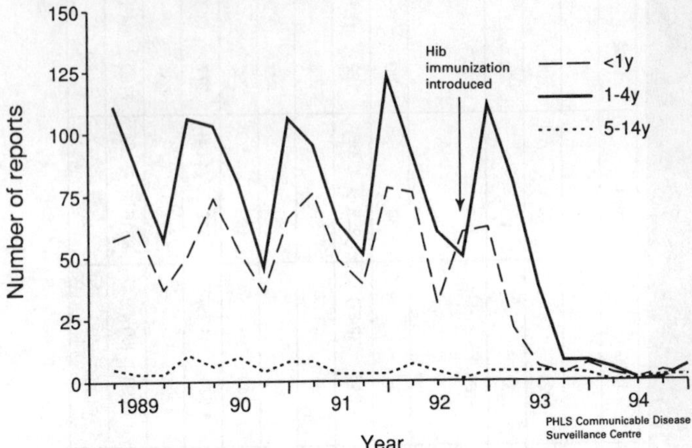

Figure I.3 Laboratory reports of *Haemophilus influenzae* type b (bacteraemia and meningitis), England and Wales 1989–1994.

Human Immunodeficiency virus infection–mother to child transmission

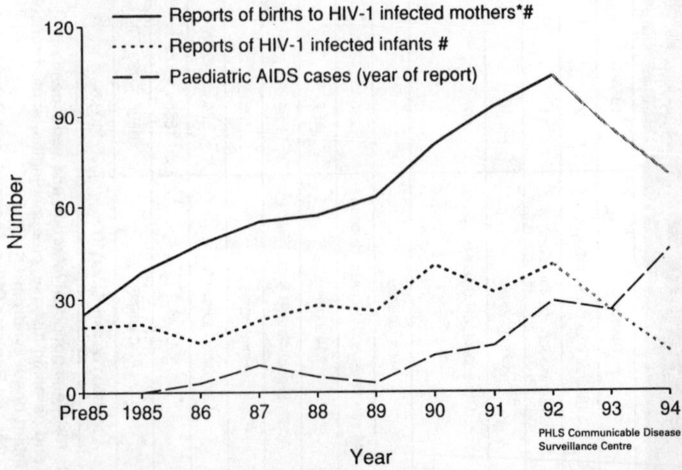

Figure I.4 Human immunodeficiency virus 1 (HIV-1) and acquired immune deficiency syndrome (AIDS) through mother-to-child transmission in the UK 1994.

[Caption continued on facing page]

[Caption I.4 continued]

The decline in the reports of HIV infection in 1993 and 1994 reflects under-identification of HIV-1 infections in mothers, and infection status in exposed infants being unresolved. Sources include voluntary confidential reports by obstetricians, paediatricians and microbiologists. Data collated by the Institute of Child Health, London, in collaboration with the Communicable Disease Surveillance Centre and the Scottish Centre for Infection and Environmental Health.

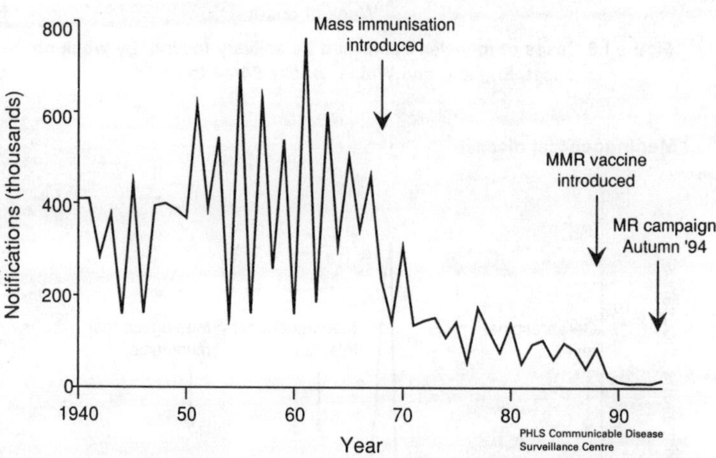

Figure I.5 Measles notifications (all ages), England and Wales 1940–1994.

Measles (1994–1995)

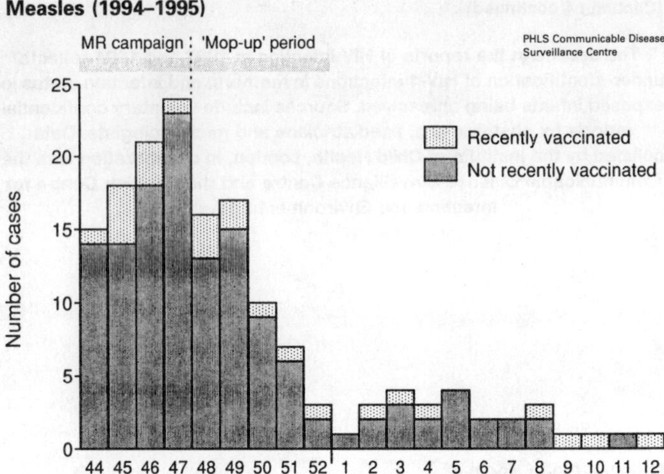

Figure I.6 Cases of measles confirmed by salivary testing, by week on onset, England and Wales, weeks 94/44 to 95/04.

Meningococcal disease

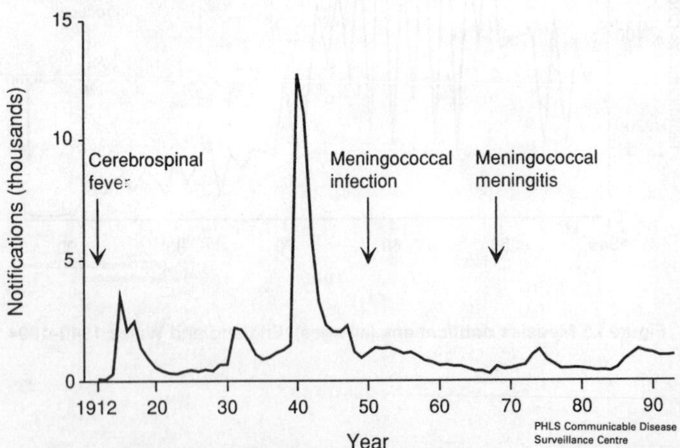

Figure I.7 Meningococcal infection and meningococcal meningitis notifications (all ages), England and Wales 1912–1993 (1993 data provisional).

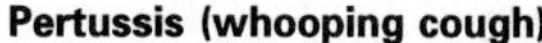

Pertussis (whooping cough)

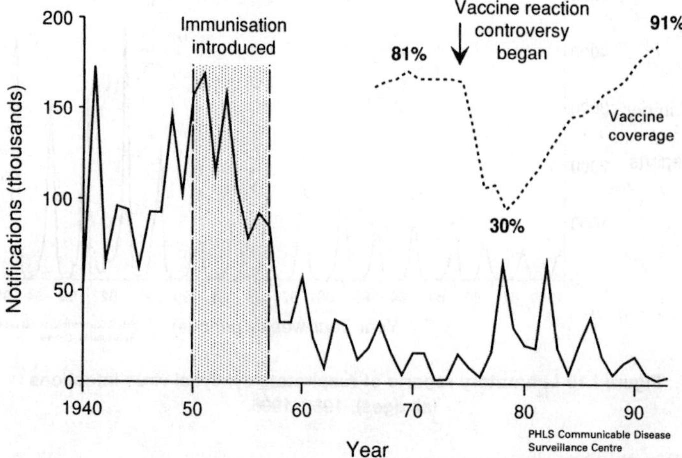

Figure I.8 Whooping cough notifications (all ages) and vaccine uptake rate, England and Wales, 1940–1993.

Poliomyelitis

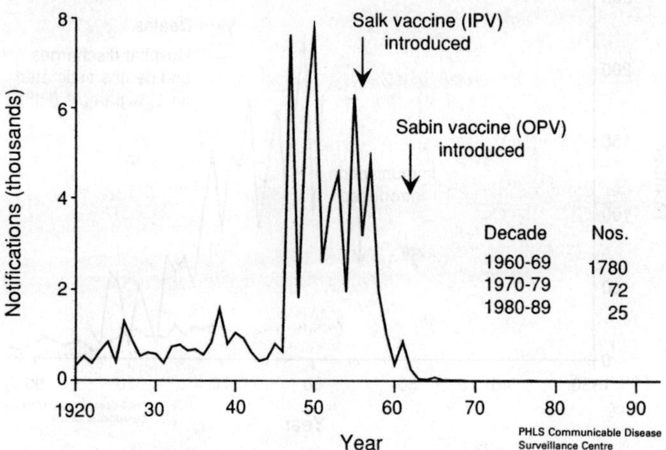

Figure I.9 Poliomyelitis notifications (all ages), England and Wales 1920–1993. Actual numbers are: 1960–1969, 1780; 1970–1979, 72; 1980–1989, 25.

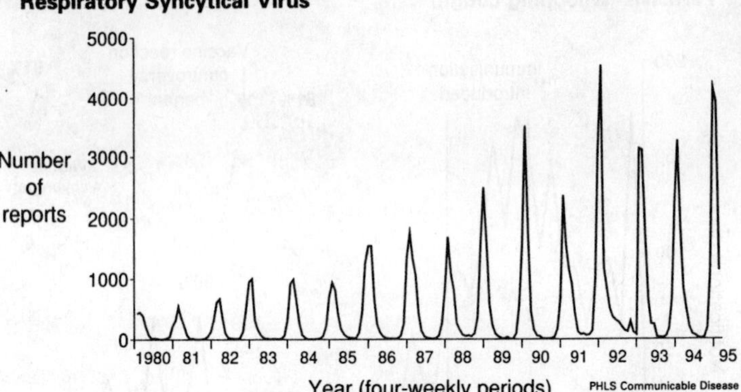

Figure I.10 Laboratory reports of respiratory syncytial virus infections (all ages), 1980–1995.

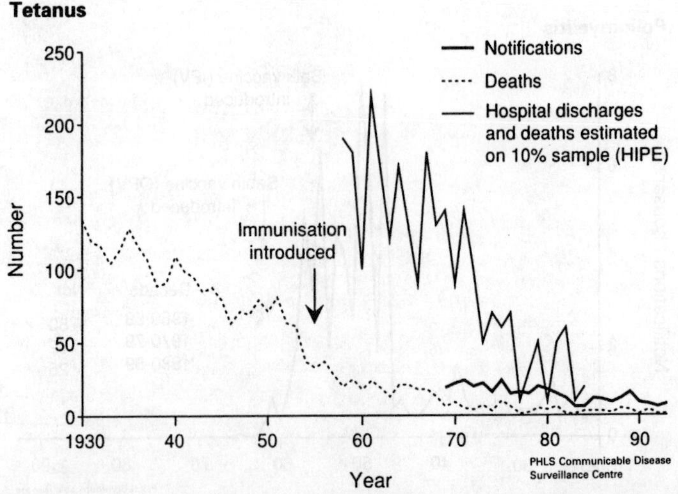

Figure I.11 Tetanus notifications, deaths and hospital discharges and deaths (all ages), England and Wales 1930–1993.

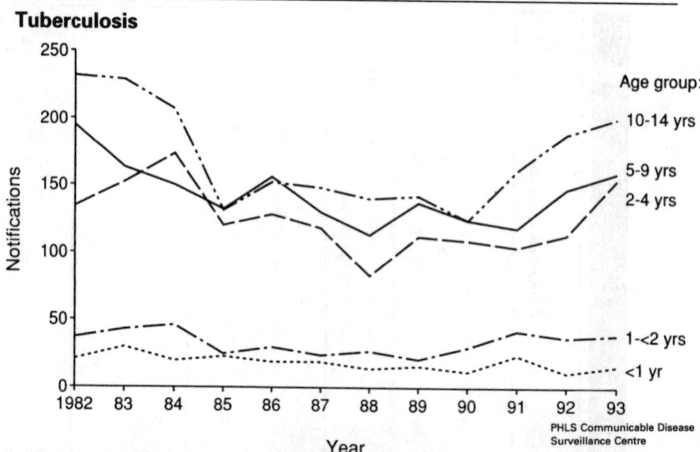

Figure I.12 Notifications of tuberculosis (all forms) in children, England and Wales, 1982–1993.

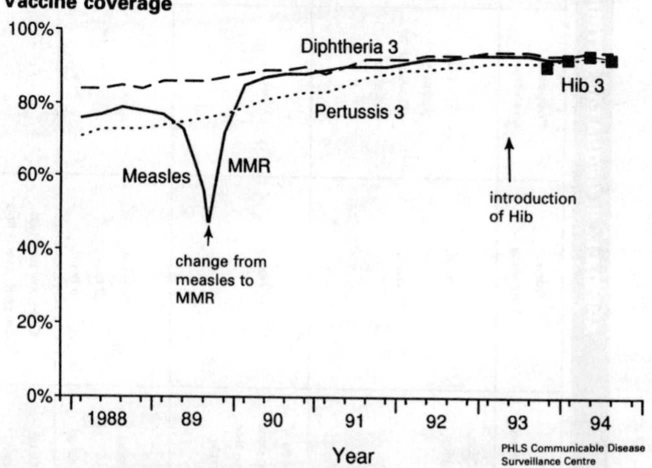

Figure I.13 Vaccine coverage February 1988 to August 1994 for England, Wales and N. Ireland. Percentage coverage of third dose diphtheria and pertussis, single antigen measles, measles, mumps and rubella (MMR) and *Haemophilus influenzae* type b (Hib) vaccines (all reporting districts). From 1991 onwards, coverage of immunization was based on uptake at 12 months of age; previously it was based on uptake at 18 months. Uptake of measles/MMR is at 24 months of age. Sources: COVER (Cover of Vaccination Evaluated Rapidly); Public Health Laboratory Service Communicable Disease Surveillance Centre

APPENDIX II: NEONATAL ANTIBIOTIC DOSAGES

Antibiotic	Single dose	Dose frequency	Post-natal age (days)	Weight	Administration and notes
Acyclovir	*IV infusion* 10 mg/kg	12 hourly	< 33 weeks gestation	Any	Administer over 1 hour in a max concentration of 25 mg in 1 ml
		18 hourly	> 33 weeks gestation	Any	*Reduce dose frequency in renal failure* Serum creatinine: 70–100 μmol/l, give every 12 hours; 110–130 μmol/l, give every 24 hours > 130 μmol/l or urine output < 1 ml/kg per hour, give 5 mg/kg every 24 hours
Amikacin 100 mg/2 ml ampoules	*IV or IM* Loading dose 10 mg/kg then 7.5 mg/kg	12 hourly	Any	Any	Slow IV bolus or infusion over 30 min Levels at third dose: peak 20–30 mg/l (1 hour after dose) trough < 10 mg/l (before dose)
Amoxycillin 125 mg/5 ml oral suspension	*Oral* 30 mg/kg	12 hourly	< 7	Any	
		8 hourly	> 7	Any	
	50 mg/kg	8 hourly	Any	Any	
Amphotericin	*IV infusion* 25 μg/kg	Once only as a test Dose given over 1 hour			

	THEN 200 μg/kg increasing to 1mg/kg	24 hourly	Any	Any	Increase by 200 μg/kg daily *to a* maximum 1 mg/kg daily Maximum total dose 15 mg kg Infuse over 4–6 hours (a) Administer only in pH tested glucose 5% (b) Avoid other nephrotoxic drugs (c) Protect from light (d) Do not filter (e) Monitor renal function and treat hypokalaemia early with potassium supplement and/or amiloride
Amphotericin liposomal	*IV infusion* 1 mg/kg increasing to 3 mg/kg	24 hourly	Any	Any	For use in infants with moderate or severe renal impairment or if conventional amphotericin not tolerated
Ampicillin 250 mg vial	*IV or IM* 50 mg/kg 50 mg/kg	 12 hourly 8 hourly	 0–7 > 7	Any	
Azlocillin 500 mg vial	*IV or IM* 50 mg/kg 100 mg/kg 100 mg/kg	 12 hourly 12 hourly 8 hourly	 0–7 0–7 > 7	 < 2 kg > 2 kg Any	
Aztreonam	*IV* 30 mg/kg	 12 hourly 8 hourly 8 hourly 6 hourly	 < 7 < 7 > 7 > 7	 < 2 kg > 2 kg < 2 kg > 2 kg	IV infusion over 20–60 min at concentration not exceeding 20 mg in 1 ml Reduce dose by 50% in severe renal impairment

Antibiotic	Single dose	Dose frequency	Post-natal age (days)	Weight	Administration and notes
Benzylpenicillin 600 mg vial (=1 million units)	*IV or IM* 60 mg/kg	12 hourly 8 hourly 8 hourly 6 hourly	< 7 < 7 > 7 > 7	< 2 kg > 2 kg < 2 kg > 2 kg	Reduce dose by 50% in severe renal impairment as may cause convulsions
Cefotaxime 500 mg vial	*IV* 50 mg/kg	12 hourly 12 hourly 8 hourly	< 7 > 7 > 7	Any < 2 kg > 2 kg	In severe infections up to 200 mg/kg per day. Reduce dose by 50% in severe renal impairment
Ceftazidime 250 mg vial	*IV* 30 mg/kg	12 hourly 8 hourly 8 hourly	< 7 > 7 > 7	Any < 2 kg > 2 kg	Increase dose interval to 24 hourly in severe renal impairment
Cefuroxime 250 mg vial 750 mg vial	*IV* 30 mg/kg	12 hourly 8 hourly	< 7 > 7	Any Any	Reduce dose in severe renal impairment. In severe infections can use up to 50 mg/kg per dose
Chloramphenicol 300 mg vial	*IV only* 25 mg/kg	24 hourly 24 hourly 12 hourly	< 7 > 7 > 7	Any < 2 kg > 2 kg	Avoid if possible Monitor blood levels and adjust dose. Levels at fifth dose: peak 10–20 μg/ml 30 min after dose trough < 10 μg/ml levels decreased by phenobarbitone and phenytoin Beware 'grey baby' syndrome

Ciprofloxacin 100 mg/200 ml vial	*IV* 5 mg/kg	12 hourly	Any	Any	Infuse over 30–60 minutes. Only use when benefit outweighs risk as may cause arthropathy
Powders	*Oral* 7.5 mg/kg	12 hourly	Any	Any	Prescribed on a named patient basis.
Erythromycin 500 g vial 125 mg/5 ml oral suspension	*IV infusion or oral* 10 mg/kg 15 mg/kg	12 hourly 8 hourly 8 hourly	< 7 > 7 > 7	Any < 2 kg > 2 kg	Infuse over 30–60 min. Caution in jaundice as displaces bilirubin. May increase serum levels of digoxin, theophylline and carbamazepine
Flucloxacillin 250 mg vial 125 mg/5 ml oral suspension	*IV or oral* 30 mg/kg	12 hourly 8 hourly	< 7 > 7	Any Any	Increase dose interval in severe renal impairment
Fluconazole	*IV or Oral* 1–2 mg/kg 3–6 mg/kg	24 hourly 24 hourly	Any Any	Any Any	Superficial candidiasis Invasive candidiasis Reduce dosage in renal impairment
Flucytosine 2.5 g in 250 ml infusion	*IV or oral* 25 mg/kg	6 hourly	< 28	Any	Infuse over 30 min. Monitor blood levels. Trough level 30–50 mg/l. Peak level < 80 mg/l Increase dose interval in renal impairment. Monitor blood count
25 mg/ml suspension	50 mg/kg	6 hourly	> 28	Any	Usually combined with amphotericin B

Appendix II continued

Antibiotic	Single dose	Dose frequency	Post-natal age (days)	Weight	Administration and notes
Fusidic acid	See sodium fusidate				
Gentamicin 20 mg in 2 ml ampoules	*IV or IM* 4 mg/kg	36 hourly	< 7	Gestation < 28 weeks	At all gestational ages: Predose (trough) and 1 hour post-dose (peak) levels around fourth dose. Levels: predose < 2 mg/l; post-dose 6–10 mg/l
	4 mg/kg, then 24 hours later 2.5 mg/kg	Loading dose, 24 hourly	> 7	< 28 weeks	
	3 mg/kg	24 hourly	< 7	28–32 weeks	
	4 mg/kg, then 18 hours later 2.5 mg/kg	Loading dose, 18 hourly	> 7	28–32 weeks	
	2.5 mg/kg	18 hourly	< 7	32–38 weeks	
	2.5 mg/kg	12 hourly	> 7	32–38 weeks	
	2.5 mg/kg	12 hourly	< 7	> 38 weeks	
	2.5 mg/kg	8 hourly	> 7	> 38 weeks	
Imipenem with cilastatin 250 mg vial	*IV* 20 mg/kg	8 hourly	< 7	Any	Infuse over 60 min. Increase dose interval to 12 hourly in severe renal impairment. Convulsions may occur—stop drug
		8 hourly	> 7	< 2 kg	
		6 hourly	> 7	> 2 kg	

(may be superceded by meropenem, which less neurotoxic.)

Metronidazole 100 mg/20 ml ampoules 200 mg/5 ml suspension	*IV or oral* 7.5 mg/kg	8 hourly	Any	Any	Infuse over 30 min. Increase dose interval to 12 hourly in severe renal impairment. Injection solution may be given rectally
Neomycin eye-drops		6 hourly			
Netilmicin	*IV* 3 mg/kg 2.5 mg/kg	18 hourly 12 hourly 12 hourly 8 hourly	< 7 < 7 > 7 > 7	< 2 kg > 2 kg < 2 kg > 2 kg	Give as slow IV bolus 3–5 min or as an IV infusion 30 min. Monitor blood levels around *third* dose Peak 5–12 mg/l (1 hour after start of infusion or IV bolus), trough < 3 mg/l.
Piperacillin	*IV* 75 mg/kg 100 mg/kg	12 hourly 8 hourly 8 hourly 6 hourly	< 7 < 7 > 7 > 7	< 2 kg > 2 kg < 2 kg > 2 kg	Give as an infusion over 30 min or bolus over 3–5 mins. Increase dose interval in severe renal impairment Hypokalaemia may occur
Sodium fusidate 500 mg sodium fusidate in each vial	*IV* 5 mg/kg	8 hourly	Any	Any	Infuse over 6 hours though possible over 3 hours if via central line. Do not use alone —combine with flucloxacillin
175 mg/5 ml	*Oral* 10–15 mg/kg (0.3 ml/kg of suspension)	8 hourly	Any	Any	*Note—all doses calculated as sodium fusidate*

Appendix II continued

Antibiotic	Single dose	Dose frequency	Post-natal age (days)	Weight	Administration and notes
Teicoplanin	*IV infusion*				
	16 mg/kg loading dose, then 8 mg/kg	24 hourly	Any	Any	Infuse over 30 min Dosage reduced in renal impairment
Trimethoprim	*IV*				
100 mg/5 ml ampoules	3 mg/kg	12 hourly	Any	Any	Reduce dose in severe renal failure. Give as a slow bolus or infusion
Suspension	*Oral*				
10 mg/ml	2 mg/kg	12 hourly	Any	Any	
	1–2 mg/kg	at night	Any	Any	Prophylaxis
Vancomycin	*IV infusion*			*Gestation*	Monitor levels: aim for predose < 10 mg/l; post-dose 25–40 mg/l
500 mg ampoules	20 mg/kg	24 hourly	< 7	< 28 weeks	Predose (trough) and 1 hour after infusion completed (peak) levels *around third dose*
	15 mg/kg	24 hourly	> 7	< 28 weeks	
	20 mg/kg	24 hourly	< 7	28–32 weeks	
	20 mg/kg	18 hourly	> 7	28–32 weeks	
	20 mg/kg	18 hourly	< 7	32–38 weeks	
	15 mg/kg	12 hourly	> 7	32–38 weeks	

	15 mg/kg 10 mg/kg	12 hourly 8 hourly	< 7 > 7	> 38 weeks > 38 weeks	
	15 mg/kg	Once	Any	Any	Prophylaxis prior to central venous line or ventriculoperitoneal/ ventriculoatrial shunt insertion
Parenteral preparation given orally	*Oral* 10 mg/kg	6 hourly	Any	Any	To treat *Clostridium difficile* pseudomembraneous colitis or staphylococcal enterocolitis

APPENDIX III: ANTIMICROBIALS FOR THE INFANT AND CHILD (excluding neonates)

Drug	Route	Times daily	Single dosage at age			Comments
			1 year	7 years	14 years	
Acyclovir	IV	3	250–500 mg/m^2	250–500 mg/m^2	250–500 mg/m^2	Used for neonatal HSV infection, herpes encephalitis, eczema herpeticum and varicella in immunocompromised
	O	5			800 mg	Higher doses in herpes encephalitis and immunocompromised
	O	4	20 mg/kg	20 mg/kg		
	O	3–4	100 mg	200 mg	200 mg	Prophylaxis cf. H. Simplex
Amikacin	IV	2	7.5 mg/kg	7.5 mg/kg	7.5 mg/kg	Aminoglycoside sometimes used for severe Gram-negative infections (e.g. in cystic fibrosis) atypical mycobacterial infection Check renal function prior to use Trough should be < 8 mg/l, peak 20–30 mg/l In prolonged use: check drug levels weekly and check hearing regularly even when drug levels normal
Amoxycillin	O, IV	3	62.5 mg	125 mg	250 mg	Treatment of otitis media, pneumonia, etc.; standard course 5 days

Amphotericin B	IV (infuse over 6 hours)	1	250 μg starting dose increasing to maximum of 1000 μg/kg	250 μg starting dose increasing to maximum of 1000 μg/kg	250 μg starting dose increasing to maximum of 1000 μg/kg	Fungal (especially candidal) septicaemia, usually in an immunocompromised child Increase dose gradually over several days to 1 mg/kg Several weeks' therapy may be required. Watch renal function and plasma K^+ levels
Amphotericin B (liposomal)	IV	1	1 mg/kg starting dose increasing to 3 mg/kg	1 mg/kg starting dose increasing to 3 mg/kg	1 mg/kg starting dose increasing to 3 mg/kg	Better tolerated than conventional amphotericin Use in renal failure or failure to tolerate conventional amphotericin
Ampicillin	O IV	4 4	125 mg 50–100 mg/kg	250 mg 50–100 mg/kg	500 mg 50–100 mg/kg	Otitis media, pneumonia and meningitis
Azithromycin	O	1	10 mg/kg	10 mg/kg	500 mg	Macrolide persists in tissues 3-day course equivalent to full course of other antibiotics Good *Haemophilus* cover
Azlocillin	IV	3	100 mg/kg	100 mg/kg to maximum of 5 g	100 mg/kg to maximum of 5 g	Treatment of *Pseudomonas* infection in immunocompromised child and in cystic fibrosis. Combine with an aminoglycoside
Aztreonam	IV	3–4	30–50 mg/kg	30–50 mg/kg to maximum of 2 g	30–50 mg/kg to maximum of 2 g	A monocyclic beta-lactam Active against Gram-negative bacteria including *Pseudomonas aeruginosa, Haemophilus influenzae* Low risk of hypersensitivity in children with penicillin allergy

Appendix III continued

Drug	Route	Times daily	Single dosage at age			Comments
			1 year	7 years	14 years	
Benzylpenicillin		See penicillin G				
Cefotaxime	IV	3–4	25–50 mg/kg	25–50 mg/kg	25–50 mg/kg	Treatment of septicaemia, meningitis and life-threatening infections Reduce dose in renal failure Maximum doses in meningitis
Ceftazidime	IV	3	25–50 mg/kg	25–50 mg/kg	25–50 mg/kg	Broad spectrum Particularly effective in *Pseudomonas aeruginosa* infections Use high dose in children with cystic fibrosis, meningitis, and the immunocompromised
Ceftriaxone	IV, IM	1	50–80 mg/kg	50–80 mg/kg	50–80 mg/kg	Once-daily treatment for serious bacterial infections including meningitis–use maximum dose. Reduce dosage in combined renal and hepatic impairment

Cefuroxime	IV	3	25–80 mg/kg	25–80 mg/kg	25–80 mg/kg	Serious bacterial infections esp. *H. influenzae* infections Reduce dose in renal impairment
Cephradine	O	4	25–50 mg/kg 125 mg	250 mg	500 mg	Treatment of urine infections if resistant organisms Reduce dose in renal impairment
Chloramphenicol	O, IV	4	25 mg/kg for 48 hours then 12.5 mg/kg	25 mg/kg for 48 hours then 12.5 mg/kg	25 mg/kg for 48 hours then 12.5 mg/kg	Only used for treatment of meningitis, Cerebral absess, epiglottitis and some cases of typhoid Monitor levels Well absorbed orally
Chloroquine	O		Initially 10 mg/kg (max: 600 mg) 6 hours later 5 mg/kg per day (max: 300 mg) daily dose for 2 days	Initially 10 mg/kg (max: 600 mg) 6 hours later 5 mg/kg per day (max: 300 mg) daily dose for 2 days	Initially 10 mg/kg (max: 600 mg) 6 hours later 5 mg/kg per day (max: 300 mg) daily dose for 2 days	Treatment of simple malaria when chloroquine resistance is not a problem For prophylaxis see Chapter 68
Ciprofloxacin	O IV	2 2	3.75–7.5 mg/kg 5 mg/kg	3.75–7.5 mg/kg 5 mg/kg	3.75–7.5 mg/kg 5 mg/kg	*Pseudomonas* infection in cystic fibrosis; invasive salmonellosis and typhoid Theoretical risk of arthropathy
Clarithromycin	O	2	7.5 mg/kg	7.5 mg/kg	7.5 mg/kg	Macrolide Pyogenic bacterial infections, atypical mycobacterial infection

Appendix III continued

Drug	Route	Times daily	Single dosage at age			Comments
			1 year	7 years	14 years	
Clindamycin	O	4	3–6 mg/kg	3–6 mg/kg	3–6 mg/kg	Staphylococcal bone and joint infection
	IV	3–4	5–10 mg/kg	5–10 mg/kg	5–10 mg/kg	Watch for pseudomembranous colitis
Clotrimazole	Use topically	3				Fungal infection—tinea pedis (athlete's foot)
Co-amoxiclav	O	3	62.5 mg	125 mg	250 mg	Dose expressed is for amyoxycillin component Clavulanic acid is beta-lactamase inhibitor; broadens spectrum of amoxycillin to include most *Staphylococcus aureus* and
	IV	3–4	25 mg/kg	25 mg/kg	25 mg/kg	other penicillinase-producing strains
Co-trimoxazole	O	2	240 mg	480 mg	960 mg	Chest infections, typhoid, invasive salmonellosis
	IV	4	30 mg/kg for *Pneumocystis carinii* pneumonia	30 mg/kg for *Pneumocystis carinii* pneumonia	30 mg/kg for *Pneumocystis carinii* pneumonia	Drug is mixture of 5 parts sulpha-methoxazole and 1 part trimethoprim (dose = sum of each in mg)
	O	2 (3 days/ week)	450 mg/m^2 max 480 mg	450 mg/m^2 max 480 mg	450 mg/m^2 max 480 mg	Prophylaxis against *Pneumocystis carinii* (PCP)
	O	2 (daily)	12 mg/kg	12 mg/kg	12 mg/kg	Prophylaxis against bacterial and PCP infection in immunodeficient states

Diethyl-carbamazine	O	2	0.5–3 mg/kg	0.5–3 mg/kg	0.5–3 mg/kg	Filariasis Dose increased from min to max over 3 days
Erythromycin	O IV	4 4	125 mg 12.5 mg/kg	250 mg 12.5 mg/kg	500 mg 12.5 mg/kg	Use when definite history of penicillin allergy For otitis, tonsillitis, pneumonia Treatment of *Chlamydia trachomatis, C. psittaci, Legionella* and *Mycoplasma pneumoniae* infection
Ethambutol	O	1	15–25 mg/kg	15-25 mg/kg	15-25 mg/kg	Treatment of tuberculosis, used in conjunction with isoniazid and rifampicin Avoid in renal impairment Visual problems can result and it should not be given to children < 6 years old Test colour vision before and during treatment Reduce dose after 60 days to 15 mg/kg if still required
Flucloxacillin	O IV	4 4	125 mg 25–50 mg/kg	250 mg 25–50 mg/kg (max 2g)	500 mg 25–50 mg/kg (max 2g)	Staphylococcal infections including septicaemia and osteomyelitis May be combined with another antibiotic Drain any abscess surgically
Fluconazole	O IV	1 1	1–2 mg/kg 3–6 mg/kg	1–2 mg/kg 3–6 mg/kg	1–2 mg/kg 3–6 mg/kg	Superficial candida infection Limited experience of use in children For systemic candidiasis, cryptococcal infection and persistent superficial candidiasis Reduce dose in renal impairment

Appendix III continued

Drug	Route	Times daily	Single dosage at age			Comments
			1 year	7 years	14 years	
Flucytosine	O, IV	4	25–50 mg/kg	25–50 mg/kg	25–50 mg/kg	For systemic candidiasis and cryptococcosis Monitor blood count and levels (Trough 30–50 mg/l peak < 80 mg/l)
Fusidic acid	O IV	3 3	250 mg 6 mg/kg	500 mg 6 mg/kg	750 mg 6 mg/kg	*Staphylococcus aureus* infection including osteomyelitis and suppurative arthritis Should be combined with flucloxacillin or erythromycin
Gentamicin	IV	3	2.5 mg/kg	2.5 mg/kg (maximum of 120 mg)	2.5 mg/kg (maximum of 120 mg)	Gram-negative infections, especially cystic fibrosis and immunocompromised states Reduce dose in renal impairment Always monitor trough and peak levels Aim for peak 6–10 mg/l and trough < 2 mg/l
Griseofulvin	O	2	5 mg/kg	5 mg/kg	5 mg/kg	For ringworm of scalp (6 weeks); nails (6 months) May cause photosensitivity

Imipenem with cilastatin (may be superceded by meropenem which is less neurotoxic)	IV	4	15 mg/kg (max. 2 g/day)	15 mg/kg (max. 2 g/day)	15 mg/kg (max. 2 g/day)	A thienamycin beta-lactam antibiotic For aerobic and anaerobic Gram-positive and negative bacteria May cause convulsions
Isoniazid	O, IV	1	10 mg/kg	10 mg/kg (max. 300 mg)	300 mg	Treatment of tuberculosis Combined with other drugs unless for prophylaxis For TB meningitis use 10–20 mg/kg Give pyridoxine to prevent peripheral neuritis
Mebendazole	O	1 (single dose)	Avoid	100 mg	100 mg	For hookworm, threadworm, roundworm and whipworm infections Not recommended in children under 2 years old 2nd dose may be needed after 2 weeks
Mefloquine	O	1 (single dose)	20 mg/kg	20 mg/kg	20 mg/kg	Resistant falciparum malaria needed after 2 weeks Single dose or divided into two, 6 hours apart
Metronidazole	O O O, rectal, IV	1 3 3	500 mg 200 mg 7.5 mg/kg	1 g 400 mg 7.5 mg/kg	2 g 800 mg 7.5 mg/kg	Giardiasis (3 days treatment) Amoebiasis (treat for 5 days) Anaerobic infection

Appendix III continued

Drug	Route	Times daily	Single dosage at age: 1 year	7 years	14 years	Comments
Miconazole	O	4	62.5 mg	125 mg	125–250 mg	Fungal infections especially *Candida*. Oral preparation for oral thrush
	IV	3	12–15 mg/kg	12–15 mg/kg	12–15 mg/kg	IV for systemic infection—need specialist advice
Netilmicin	IV, IM	3	2.5 mg/kg	2.5 mg/kg	2.5 mg/kg	Gram-negative infections, especially in cystic fibrosis and immunocompromised states Always monitor levels (Trough < 3 mg/l, peak 5–12 mg/l)
Nitrofurantoin	O	4	0.75 mg/kg	0.75 mg/kg	0.75 mg/kg	For lower urinary tract infections with multiple organism resistance. May cause nausea and vomiting. Not suitable for pyelonephritis
	O	1 (at night)	1 mg/kg	1 mg/kg	1 mg/kg	Prophylaxis of urinary tract infection
Nystatin	O, topical	4–6	100 000 U	100 000 U	100 000 U	Given for oral thrush or candidal napkin dermatitis Prophylactic usage for immunocompromised children on broad spectrum antibiotics

Penicillin G (benzylpenicillin)	IM IV	4 4–6	150 mg 30–60 mg/kg	300 mg 30–60 mg/kg	600 mg 30–60 mg/kg	1 megaunit = 600 mg Tonsilitis, lobar pneumonia, erysipelas, endocarditis, meningococcal and pneumococcal meningitis Higher dose 4-hourly in meningitis and endocarditis
Penicillin G—domiciliary use in emergency treatment of meningococcal infection	IM, IV	Single dose	600 mg	1200 mg	1200 mg	
Penicillin G as procaine penicillin	IM	1	60 mg/kg	60 mg/kg to maximum of 2.4 g	60 mg/kg to maximum of 2.4 g	For treatment of gonococcal infection and syphilis in childhood Therapeutic level maintained better with probenecid given 30 min before injection
Penicillin V (phenoxymethyl-penicillin) Prophylaxis	O O	4 2	125 mg 62.5 mg	250 mg 125 mg	500 mg 250 mg	Tonsilitis and minor infections, prophylaxis of rheumatic fever and septicaemia after splenectomy and in sickle-cell anaemia
Piperacillin	IV	3–4	50–75 mg/kg	50–75 mg/kg	50–75 mg/kg	For treatment of *Pseudomonas aeruginosa* infection in children with cystic fibrosis and immunocompromised status Combine with aminoglycoside Empirical treatment of febrile neutropenia

Appendix III continued

Drug	Route	Times daily	Single dosage at age			Comments
			1 year	7 years	14 years	
Piperazine	O	Two doses given 14 days apart	$\frac{2}{3}$ sachet	1 sachet	1 sachet	For treatment of threadworms Combined with senna
Pivampicillin	O	3	Avoid	175 mg	250 mg	175 mg in 5 ml Similar antibacterial spectrum to ampicillin wth better absorption Contains sorbitol
Pyrazinamide	O	3	7–12 mg/kg	7–12 mg/kg	7–12 mg/kg	Used in tuberculosis including TB meningitis Monitor liver function
Pyrimethamine	O (give folinic acid supplement)	1	1 mg/kg	1 mg/kg	1 mg/kg	In combination with sulphadiazine for congenital toxoplasmosis in 3-week courses alternating with spiramycin
Pyrimethamine and sulfadoxine	O	(Single dose)	$\frac{1}{2}$ tablet	$1\frac{1}{2}$ tablets	2–3 tablets	Single dose for completing treatment of falciparum malaria 1 tablet contains 25 mg pyrimethamine and 500 mg sulfadoxine

Quinine	O IV (over 4 h)	3 3	125 mg 10 mg/kg	300 mg 10 mg/kg (max. 600 mg)	600 mg 10 mg/kg (max. 600 mg)	Doses given as base. Quinine base, 100 mg = quinine bisulphate; 169 mg = quinine dihydrochloride/hydrochloride or quinine sulphate 122 mg Treatment of malaria, esp. if chloroquine resistance, or cerebral malaria With resistant strains an IV loading dose of 20 mg/kg is required; Always seek specialist advice Treatment usually given for 7 days IV therapy contraindicated below 3 months of age Complete treatment with single dose of pyrimethamine/ sulfadoxine as above
Rifampicin	O, IV	1	20 mg/kg (maximum dosage 600 mg)	600 mg (maximum dosage 600 mg)	600 mg (maximum dosage 600 mg)	Treatment of tuberculosis
Rifampicin	O, IV	2	150 mg	300 mg	600 mg	Severe staphylococcal infection, Brucellosis
Rifampicin as prophylaxis	O O	2 (for 2 days) 1 (for 4 days)	10 mg/kg 20 mg/kg (max. 600 mg)	10 mg/kg 20 mg/kg (max. 600 mg)	600 mg/kg 20 mg/kg (max. 600 mg)	Prophylaxis of *Neisseria meningitidis* infection Prophylaxis of *Haemophilus influenzae* type B infection Drug interaction with oral contraceptive Warn about orange secretions

Appendix III continued

Drug	Route	Times daily	Single dosage at age: 1 year	7 years	14 years	Comments
Spiramycin	O	2	1 g	1–2 g	2 g	For treatment of cryptosporidiosis in the immunosuppressed
	O	2	50 mg/kg	50 mg/kg	50 mg/kg	For congenital toxoplasmosis—alternating with pyrimethamine and sulphadiazine in 3-weekly cycles
Streptomycin	IM	1	15–20 mg/kg	15–20 mg/kg	750 mg–1 g	Treatment of tuberculosis for up to 12 weeks Other antituberculous drugs always given simultaneously
Sulphadiazine	O	2	50 mg/kg	50 mg/kg	50 mg/kg	Congenital toxoplasmosis in combination with pyrimethamine alternated with spiramycin in 3-weekly cycles
Teicoplanin	IV	1	10 mg/kg 12-hourly × 3 doses then 6–10 mg/kg daily	10 mg/kg 12-hourly × 3 doses then 6–10 mg/kg daily	10 mg/kg 12-hourly × 3 doses then 6–10 mg/kg daily	Gram-positive infections especially those due to coagulase-negative staphylococci

Thiabendazole	O	2	25 mg/kg	25 mg/kg	25 mg/kg	Treatment of refractory hookworm, threadworm, whipworm, roundworm, visceral larva migrans, *Strongyloides stercoralis* Treatment given for 3–7 days. Take specalist advice
Tobramycin	IV	3	2.5 mg/kg	2.5 mg/kg	2.5 mg/kg	Treatment of Gram-negative infection in the immunosuppressed Monitor levels; ototoxic Reduce dosage in renal impaiment (Trough level < 2 mg/l peak < 10 mg/l)
Trimethoprim	O	2	50 mg	100 mg	200 mg	For urinary tract infections, invasive salmonellosis including typhoid
	IV	2	3–4.5 mg/kg	3–4.5 mg/kg	3–4.5 mg/kg	Single evening dose as prophylaxis 1–2 mg/kg
Vancomycin	IV	3	15 mg/kg	15 mg/kg	15 mg/kg	Use in multiple-resistant staphylococcal infections Given by slow infusion Ototoxic, nephrotoxic—check levels Reduce dose in renal impairment (Trough < 10 mg/l, peak 20–30 mg/l)
	O	4	10 mg/kg	10 mg/kg	10 mg/kg	For pseudomembranous colitis use IV preparation orally

APPENDIX IV: NOTIFIABLE DISEASES 1995

	England and Wales	Northern Ireland	Scotland
Acute encephalitis	+	+*	0
Acute poliomyelitis	+	+	+
Anthrax	+	+	+
Chickenpox	0	+	+
Cholera	+	+	+
Diphtheria	+	+	+
Dysentery (amoebic or bacillary)	+	+	Bacillary dysentery
Erysipelas	0	0	+
Food poisoning (all sources)	+	+	+
Gastroenteritis (under 2 years of age)	0	+	0
Legionella/legionnaires' disease	0	+	+
Leprosy	+†	0	0
Leptospirosis	+	+	Leptospiral jaundice
Lyme disease	0	0	+
Malaria	+	+	+
Measles	+	+	+
Membranous croup	0	0	+
Meningitis	+	+*	0
Meningococcal septicaemia (without meningitis)	+	+	Meningococcal infection
Mumps	+	+	+
Ophthalmia neonatorum (includes *Neisseria gonorrhoeae* and *Chlamydia trachomatis* infection)	+	0	0

Paratyphoid fever	+	+	+
Plague	+	+	+
Puerperal fever	0	0	+
Rabies	+	+	+
Relapsing fever (*Borrelia* infection)	+	+	+
Rubella	+	+	+
Scarlet fever	+	+	+
Smallpox	+	+	+
Tetanus	+	+	+
Toxoplasmosis	0	0	+
Tuberculosis (all forms)	+	+	+
Typhoid fever	+	+	+
Typhus	+	+	+
Viral haemorrhagic fever	+	+	+
Acute viral hepatitis	+‡	+‡	+‡
Whooping cough	+	+	+
Yellow fever	+	+	0

Notify:
England and Wales—consultant in communicable disease control (or officer performing this function)
N. Ireland—director of public health of the appropriate health and social services board
Scotland—director of public health or consultant in public health in the appropriate health board
Adult Acquired immune deficiency syndrome cases are reported on a special AIDS clinical report form in strict medical confidence to the Director, PHLS CDSC, 61 Colindale Avenue, London NW9 5EQ. (See Chapter 19 for reporting of paediatric cases)
***As acute encephalitis/meningitis (bacterial) or acute encephalitis/meningitis (viral).**
†Reported directly to the Chief Medical Officer, Department of Health.
‡Reported as hepatitis A, B, non-A, non-B or unspecified (likely to include hepatitis C as separate category in the future).

APPENDIX V: EXCLUSION PERIODS

This appendix attempts to set out the incubation period, period of communicability, main sources of infection and suggested period of exclusion from school, nursery or day care for most of the diseases covered in this book (Table V.1). These are only guidelines and should be modified for each individual circumstance. A child who is feeling significantly unwell should not return to school, even if no longer infectious. Where there is an immunocompromised child within a class, periods of exclusion may need to be adhered to strictly, whereas when all the other children are essentially well, the periods can be shortened. In a nursery where the standards of personal hygiene may not be as good as in a secondary school it is important to keep to the exclusion periods for enteric illness because spread within the nursery environment is much more likely.

Whenever there is any doubt, it is important to consult with the school health service and the consultant in communicable disease control (CCDC). Each district should have its own guidelines, which will include details of the circumstances in which the CCDC should be informed of any episodes of infection.

Table V.1 Exclusion periods

Disease	Usual incubation period (range)	Period of communicability	Minimum period of exclusion	Mode of spread
AIDS/HIV	Variable—may be years	Indefinite	None	Blood or sexual contact. Congenital/perinatal
Amoebic dysentery	2–4 weeks (few days to years)	Prolonged (may be years if untreated)	Until 3 stool specimens negative	Food/water, faecal
Arbovirus	1–15 days	Requires arthropod vector from animal host		
Ascaris	4–8 weeks	Not spread directly from person to person		From faeces in soil or contaminated food
Aspergillosis	Unknown	Organism is ubiquitous in the environment. Person-to-person spread is not important		
Botulism	12–36 hours (up to several days) (Infant botulism 3 days to 2 weeks)	Person-to-person spread does not occur		Food-borne
Brucellosis	1–2 months (1 week to several months)	Person-to-person spread is rare. Infection is from infected animals and tissues (including placenta) through cuts/abrasions of the skin, aerosol, oral ingestion or contact with conjunctival mucosa		
Campylobacter enteritis	3–5 days (1–10 days)	Up to 7 weeks but usually 2–3 weeks unless antibiotic given	Until child no longer has diarrhoea	Faecal and contaminated food or milk
Candidiasis	2–5 days	While organism present	None	Person-to-person and environmental

Table V.1 continued

Disease	Usual incubation period (range)	Period of communicability	Minimum period of exclusion	Mode of spread
Cat-scratch disease	3–10 days to appearance of primary lesion, further 2–6 weeks to appearance of lymphadenopathy	Requires bite, scratch or other close contact from an animal vector (cat, dog or monkey)		
Chickenpox	14-17 days (10–21 days)	From 2 days before until 5 days after rash appears	Until vesicles have crusted	Direct contact wth lesions, rarely air-borne
Chlamydia		See main text		
Cholera	1–3 days (range few hours to 5 days)	May be several months until stools are negative, unless treated	Until stools are negative	Contaminated food and water
Conjunctivitis		See main text		Person-to-person
Cryptosporidiosis	2–14 days	Variable, usually while diarrhoea present	Usually while diarrhoea lasts	Faecal, pets, farm animals and water
Cytomegalovirus	?	While virus being excreted	None	Saliva and sexual contact Congenital
Dermatophytoses		See Tinea		
Diphtheria	2–5 days (2–7 days)	2–3 weeks unless treated, in which case 24 hours after treatment started	Until throat swab negative	Contact with discharge from nose, throat, eye and skin lesions of infected person

Enteroviruses (non-polio and non-HFM)	2 hours-6 days	Variable	While symptomatic	Faecal and respiratory
Escherichia coli diarrhoea	See main entry in text			
Fifth disease (parovirus)	4–14 days (4–20 days)	For 7 days before appearance of rash	None	Infectious droplets
Gastroenteritis Adenovirus gastroenteritis Astrovirus gastroenteritis Calcivirus gastroenteritis Norwalk gastroenteritis Rotavirus gastroenteritis	 8–10 days 1–2 days 1–3 days 12–48 hours 1–3 days	 while symptomatic while symptomatic while symptomatic while symptomatic while symptomatic	 while symptomatic while symptomatic while symptomatic while symptomatic while symptomatic	 Faeces Faeces, waterborne Faeces, water or food borne Faeces, water or food borne Faeces
Giardiasis	7–10 days (5–25 days)	Prolonged if untreated	None	Faecal, and food and water
Gonococcal infections	See main entries in text			
Haemolytic uraemic syndrome	about 3–4 days to onset of diarrhoea	See main entry in text		Some food,unpasteurized milk and contaminated water
Haemophilus influenzae infection	Unknown	As long as organism present in resiratory tract	None	Direct contact or respiratory droplet. Not very infectious
Haemorhagic fevers	See main entry in text			
Hand, foot and mouth disease	3–5 days	2–3 days before to weeks after onset	None. Presence of rash does not imply infectivity	Resiratory droplet, faecal and direct contact with rash

Table V.1 continued

Disease	Usual incubation period (range)	Period of communicability	Minimum period of exclusion	Mode of spread
Heliobacter infection	Unknown	Unknown	None	Unknown
Hepatitis A	25–30 days (15–45 days)	From 7 days before to 7 days after onset of symptoms	7 days from onset of symptoms	Faeces, food, water and blood
Hepatitis B	60–90 days (45–160 days)	Prolonged in carriers	None	Blood and body fluids Congenital/perinatal
Hepatitis C	6–8 weeks (2–29 weeks)	Infectious while organism present	None	Blood and sexual transmission Congenital/perinatal
Herpes simplex	2–14 days 2–28 days (perinatal infection) (childhood infection)	Variable	None	Direct contact with lesion
Infectious mononucleosis	30–50 days	Indefinate	None	Spread requires close ('kissing') contact
Impetigo: streptococcal staphylococcal	 7–10 days 1–10 days	While lesions draining	Until lesions healed or 24 hours after antibiotics started	Direct contact with lesion
Influenza	1–3 days	3–7 days from onset of symptoms	Until well	Direct contact, droplets or recently contamined articles

Invasive helminths	For *Toxocara* see later entry, for others see main entry in text			
Kawasaki disease		Evidence in relation to aetiology of disease insufficient		
Legionellosis	2-10 days (pneumonia) 1–2 days (Pontiac fever). Figures are for adults—not clear in children	Person-to-person spread not recorded		Aerosolized contaminated water
Leishmaniasis visceral cutaneous	Few weeks to 6 months A few weeks	Person-to-person spread not recorded		Sandfly bite
Listeriosis		See main entry in text		
Lyme disease	7–10 days (3-32 days)	Person-to-person spread not recorded		Tick bite
Malaria	See main entry in text			
Measles	8-12 days (7–18 days)	From 3–5 days before to 4 days after onset of rash	From appearance of symptoms to 4 days from onset of rash	Infectious droplets
Meningococcal disease	< 4 days (2–10 days)	While organism in throat	Until organism cleared	Infectious droplets—usually close contact
Molluscum contagiosum	2–7 weeks (7 days to 6 months)	While lesions persist	None	Direct contact

Table V.1 continued

Disease	Usual incubation period (range)	Period of communicability	Minimum period of exclusion	Mode of spread
Mumps	16–18 days (12–25 days)	6 days before to 7 days after appearance of swelling	Until 7 days after swelling appears	Infectious droplets
Mycobacterium infection (atypical)	weeks to months		Person-to-person spread does not occur	
Nits (pediculosis capitis)	6–10 days	While nits or lice survive	None	Direct contact or via combs, brushes and hats
Pertussis	7–10 days (6-20 days)	From 7 days after exposure to 21 days after onset of paroxysmal cough	Until 21 days after appearance of paroxysmal cough If treated with appropriate antibiotic—after 7 days treatment	Infectious droplets
Plague				
bubonic	2–6 days	Person-to-person spread only from content of bubo, otherwise spread by flea bite		
pneumonic	2–4 days	While ill	For 3 days after start of treatment	Respiratory droplets
Pneumocystis	Unknown	Unknown		Unknown
Poliomyelitis	7–21 days (3-35 days)	While virus present in stool—usually a few days before onset to several weeks after	On advice of CCDC	Faecal and rarely by food or water
Prion Disease		See main entry in text		

Rabies	2 months (5 days to > 1 year) injuries closer to the brain have shorter incubation periods	No proven case of person-to-person transmission, but found in saliva. Isolation indicated		From bite of infected animal or licking of mucosa or broken skin
Resiratory syncytial virus infection	4–6 days (2–8 days)	Virus shedding may continue for 3–4 weeks	While symptomatic	Infectious droplets or contaminated fomites
Roseola infantum (HHV-6)	8–10 days	Unknown	None	Infectious droplets
Rubella	16-18 days (14–21 days)	7 days before to 4 days after appearance of rash	Until 4 days after onset of rash	Infectious droplets
Salmonellosis	12–36 hours (6 hours–3 days)	While organism present in stool	While organism present in stool	Food or water-borne Faeces Contact with infected animals (including turtles and terrapins), medication and medical instruments
Scabies	4–6 weeks (1–4 days reinfection)	While mite present	Until mites killed	Close personal contact
Shigellosis (bacillary dysentery)	1–3 days (1–7 days)	While organism present in stool	Until 3 stools negative	Faeces
Spongiform encephalopathies (Prion disease)	See main entry in text			

Table V.1 continued

Disease	Usual incubation period (range)	Period of communicability	Minimum period of exclusion	Mode of spread
Staphylococcal infection	See main entry in text			
Streptococcal infection	See main entry in text			
Syphilis (acquired)	3 weeks (10–90 days)	Variable	None	Sexual contact
Tetanus	4 days–3 weeks (1 day to several months)	Not spread from person-to-person		Contaminated wound—may be minor
Threadworms	Unknown	While infected	None	Faecal
Tinea capitis (scalp ringworm)	10–14 days	Unclear	Cover lesion	Direct contact or contaminated combs, sheets, and animals.
Tinea corporis (body ringworm)	? 4–10 days	Unclear	Cover lesion	Direct contact or formites (animal and human)
Tinea pedis (athlete's foot)	Unknown	Unclear	None	Ubiquitous
Tinea unguium	Unknown	Not very contagious	None	Direct contact with skin and nails
Toxic shock syndrome	2 days	See main entry in text	None	See main entry in text

Toxocariasis	Some weeks to several months. Up to 10 years for ocular symptoms	Not spread from person-to-person		Ingestion of faeces from infected dog or, less commonly, cat
Toxoplasmosis	7 days (4–21 days)	Not spread from person-to-person		Ingestion of poorly cooked infected meat or of faeces from infected cat
Tuberculosis	Variable but usually 4–12 weeks	While organism present in sputum	Until live organisms eradicated from sputum	Infectious droplets
Typhoid and paratyphoid fevers	1–3 weeks (3–60 days)	While organism present in stool. Can be prolonged	Until 3 or 6 stools negative on advice of CCDC	Faeces
Typhus endemic	1–2 weeks	Not spread from person-to-person		Transmitted by a bite from a rat flea
Typhus epidemic	1–2 weeks	Spread from person-to-person by body louse		
Warts and verrucae	See main entry in text—except for genital warts, they are not very infectious			
Yellow fever	3–6 days	Not spread from person-to-person		Bite from infected mosquito
Yersiniosis	4–16 days (1–14 days)	For 6 weeks after development of symptoms	While symptomatic	Contaminated food and water Contact with animals ? Faecal

APPENDIX VI: CONTRAINDICATIONS TO IMMUNIZATION

No child should be denied immunization without serious thought to the consequences, both for the individual child and for the community. Where there is any doubt advice should be sought from a consultant paediatrician, consultant in public health medicine or the District or Health Board immunization co-ordinator. The vaccines used in the UK are listed in Table VI.1.

A large number of conditions are *not* contraindications to immunization:

- Family history of any adverse reactions following immunization.
- Family history of convulsions.
- Previous history of pertussis, measles, rubella, mumps, *Haemophilus*, polio, tetanus or other specific infections.
- Prematurity—immunization should not be postponed.
- Stable neurological conditions such as cerebral palsy, spina bifida and Down's syndrome.
- Hay fever or other atopic condition.
- Treatment with antibiotics or locally acting steroids.
- Pregnancy in the child's mother.
- Child being breast-fed.
- History of jaundice after birth.
- Being under a certain weight.
- Over the age recommended in the immunization schedule.
- Recent or imminent surgery.

Table VI.1 Antigens in vaccines licensed for use in the UK

Live vaccines†	Inactivated vaccines†
BCG	Anthrax‡
Measles	cholera
Mumps	Diphtheria (toxoid)
Polio (oral—OPV)	*Haemophilus influenzae* b
Rubella	Hepatitis A
Typhoid (oral)	Hepatitis B
Yellow Fever	Influenza
	N. meningitidis A, C, Y, W135
	Pneumococcal
	Pertussis
	Polio (injected IPV)
	Tetanus (toxoid)
	Typhoid

† A number of the vaccines are available in combinations (e.g. DTP–diphtheria, tetanus pertussis)
‡ Not used in children

TRUE CONTRAINDICATIONS TO IMMUNIZATION

Some contraindications apply to all vaccines, others are related only to live vaccines and a few are relevant only to specific vaccines.

Contraindications to all vaccines

Acute illness If a child is suffering from any acute illness, immunization should be postponed until the child has recovered. However, minor infections without fever or systemic upset, snuffles, etc. are not reasons to postpone immunization.

Previous severe reactions Immunization with the same antigen should not be carried out in individuals who have a history of severe local or general reaction to a preceding antigen. Severe reactions are defined as follows:

- Local—swelling that becomes indurated and involves most of the anterolateral surface of the thigh or a major part of the circumference of the upper arm.
- General—fever equal to or more than 39.5 °C within 48 hours of vaccination; or any of the following within 72 hours:
  - anaphylaxis
  - bronchospasm
  - laryngeal oedema
  - generalized collapse
  - prolonged unresponsiveness
  - prolonged inconsolable or high-pitched screaming for more than 4 hours
  - convulsions or encephalopathy.

The commonest source of reaction is whole cell pertussis vaccines. When these reactions have occurred with DTP vaccine immunization should be completed with DT.

Contraindications to live vaccines

Pregnancy Live vaccines should not be offered to pregnant women. However, the risk would seem to be theoretical rather than real as there is no evidence of specific abnormalities resulting from accidental immunization of pregnant women. Inadvertant immunization of pregnant women with a live vaccine is not in itself a reason for offering a termination of pregnancy. If a pregnant woman is likely to be at particular risk of infection, for example, travelling to countries where yellow fever or polio are highly endemic, then she should be encouraged to accept immunization.

Immunosuppressed individuals (see also Appendix VII) Live vaccines may be ineffective and cause severe adverse effects in certain groups of patients:

- All patients currently being treated for malignant disease with chemotherapy or generalized radiotherapy or within 6 months of terminating such treatment.
- Patients who have received an organ transplant and are on immunosuppressive treatment.
- Children who within the previous 12 months have received a bone marrow transplant.
- Children who receive prednisolone at a daily dose (or its equivalent) of 2 mg/kg for at least a week or 1 mg/kg daily for 1 month.* Corticosteroids administered

---

***For adults an equivalent dose is harder to define but immunosuppression should be considered in those who receive 40 mg a day or more for more than a week.**

through other routes (aerosols, topically or intra-articularly) are not immunosuppressive. Administration of live vaccines should be postponed for at least 3 months after immunosuppressive treatment has stopped or reached levels not associated with immunosuppression. Lower doses of steroids given in combination with cytotoxic drugs and other immunosuppressants should be considered to cause immunosuppression and the advice of the responsible doctor sought.

- Patients with evidence of cell-mediated immunity, for example symptomatic human immunodeficiency virus (HIV) infection, severe combined immunodeficiency and other syndromes. (see Chapter 16)

Patients with minor deficiencies of antibodies are not at risk and those with major antibody deficiencies will be receiving antibodies in their immunoglobulin treatment and hence will not be at particular risk from live vaccines.

Occasionally there may be children on lower doses of steroids or other immunosuppressants for a prolonged period, or who because of their underlying disease may be immunosuppressed and at increased risk of infection. The clinician should discuss their management with a consultant in paediatric infectious disease or other relevant specialist. Individuals who fulfil the above criteria should be given the appropriate immunoglobulin preparation as soon as possible following exposure to measles (HNIG) and chickenpox (VZIG) (see Chapters 37 and 69). However if there has been exposure to varicella it is worthwhile checking the exposed patient for the presence of specific antibody to zoster (anti-VZV). If it is present the rise in circulating anti-VZV gained from administering varicella zoster immunoglobulin (VZIG) will be minimal.

Giving of live vaccines after immunoglobulin Some of the live vaccines may be less efficacious if given within 3 months after injection of normal immunoglobulin. If convenient, live vaccine should be deferred. However, if the risk of exposure is great, then vaccination should still proceed, consideration being given to a later booster. This does not apply to yellow fever vaccine, as normal immunoglobulin in the UK is unlikely to contain antibodies to yellow fever.

Live vaccine and normal immunoglobulin given simultaneously These may be given at the same time with every likelihood that the live vaccination will be successful. However, they should be given in separate syringes and in different sites.

Contraindications to specific vaccines

BCG vaccination Except in infants under 3 months old, BCG (bacillus Calmette–Guérin) should be given only to those individuals who have had a negative tuberculin test.

Pertussis vaccination Where a child has an evolving neurological illness, pertussis immunization should be delayed until the clinical picture is clear. Children who have had a severe reaction (as defined above) to a previous dose of whole cell vaccine should receive no further doses. Consideration may be given to using acellular vaccine (on a named patient basis) for subsequent doses.

Polio vaccination As the live vaccine virus is transmissible, it should not be given to babies in a household where there is an immunosuppressed individual.

Inactivated polio vaccine should be used instead. Steps should be taken to ensure all members of the household have received polio vaccination. Cases of paralytic polio have been recorded in inadequately immunized individuals in close contact with a baby recently given oral polio vaccine.

APPENDIX VII: IMMUNIZATION OF THE CHILD WITH A POTENTIALLY IMPAIRED IMMUNE RESPONSE

When the use of vaccines is considered in the child with impaired immune responses,* the reflex is often to avoid them altogether. This takes its origin in the very real fear of potential damage that live vaccines can do to children with some severe immunodeficiencies, for example live poliovirus vaccine in X-linked agammaglobulinaemia. There is an additional common perception that killed vaccines, which pose no such risk, are 'not worth using' because the child's immune response will be inadequate. Such children are at particularly high risk of serious infections and therefore they are amongst those most in need of protection by immunization, where it can be done safely. Thus there is a great need for specific vaccines to be tested in different groups of 'high-risk' children to assess their safety, immunogenicity and efficacy. Although there is a renewed consciousness of these issues in the context of the small but growing population of children with human immunodeficiency virus (HIV) infection, work has also been going on for some time in children with malignancies and in particular leukaemia. There is good evidence regarding the effectiveness or othewise, of a limited number of vaccines in these groups, but there are also large gaps in our knowledge, so that in many instances recommendations have to be made on the basis of extrapolation from what may be known about other vaccines and conditions, rather than direct evidence.

THE VACCINES

The live vaccines currently licensed in the UK are bacillus Calmette–Guérin (BCG), trivalent oral polio vaccine (OPV), measles, mumps and rubella (MMR), yellow fever and oral typhoid (Table VI.1). A live varicella vaccine is available, though unlicensed in the UK but is rarely used. All other licensed vaccines are not live they include an enhanced inactivated injected polio vaccine (IPV) which is highly immunogenic.

CHILDREN WITH MALIGNANCY, INCLUDING LEUKAEMIA

Although policies vary between centres, families of children diagnosed as having malignant disease and treated with cytotoxic drugs are usually told that the child should avoid all live vaccinations and wait 6 months after the cessation of chemotherapy before resuming the normal programme of immunization.

Chickenpox is usually mild and self-limiting in normal children but can be devastating in children with malignancies, especially leukaemia. Even the child who has previously had chickenpox and has anti-varicella antibody may be at increased risk because of defective cell-mediated immunity. Susceptible patients (i.e. negative for varicella zoster antibody) with a history of exposure to varicella should be passively immunized with varicella zoster immune globulin (VZIG) within 72 hours of exposure although administration of VZ1G up to 10 days after exposure may attenuate disease. Those who develop the disease are treated with high-dose intravenous acyclovir and supportive measures.

An attenuated live varicella vaccine (Merieux, UK) is available in the UK on a 'named patient' basis and has been used in several trials in children with

---

***See also Appendix VI.**

malignancies in the USA and Japan. Skin rashes and fevers occur in 30–40% of leukaemia patients given the vaccine, but severe illness is very rare and no vaccine-associated deaths have been reported. More than 90% given two doses seroconvert. It has been suggested that the vaccine should be given to leukaemic children under the following circumstances:

- The child must have been in remission for at least 1 year.
- The total peripheral lymphocyte count should be at least 0.7×10^9/l on the day of vaccination.
- Immunosuppressive chemotherapy should be withheld for 1 week before vaccination and 1 week afterwards. Steroids should not be given for 2 weeks after vaccination. It is not necessary to withhold chemotherapy at the time of the second dose of vaccine.

Perhaps the vaccine has not been generally accepted because of concern about the use of a live virus which has the capacity to remain latent even in the immunocompetent person. With further experience this may change.

Measles can cause encephalitis, pneumonitis and death in children with malignancy even if passive protection is attempted with gammaglobulin. The incidence of measles has declined in Britain with universal immunization, but vaccinated children may lose their immunity while on cytotoxic therapy. At present herd immunity is relied on to protect the at risk population. It is particularly important to ensure that the immuno compromised patient's siblings and other frequent contacts have been immunized. Gammaglobulin is given to those at risk with a history of exposure, but it does not provide reliable or complete protection. Live measles vaccine (as MMR) is not used in children receiving chemotherapy for malignancy but is usually given 3–6 months after cessation of therapy, whatever the premalignant immunization status. This cautious approach stems from a study carried out in 1962 in the USA. Of 12 children with acute lymphoblastic leukaemia, one died of atypical measles. However, several more recent studies demonstrate that the current live vaccine induces seroconversion without severe adverse effects in children with leukaemia who are in remission but still receiving treatment. Current guidelines state that children with malignancies can receive MMR 6 months after cessation of chemotherapy.

Other vaccines Children who have completed a primary course of immunization before the development of their malignancy are generally considered to be adequately protected against diphtheria, tetanus, pertussis and polio, although measles antibody titres decline in some children. It would however be prudent to check antibody levels against those antigens (not pertussis). Pneumococeal and *Haemophilus influenzae* type b (Hib) antibody titres may also decline. If the child is part-way through the immunization programme when malignancy is diagnosed, diphtheria, pertussis and tetanus (DPT), inactivated polio vaccine (IPV) and Hib vaccines can be continued once the child's condition is stable on treatment. Additional boosters of these vaccines should be given when the child is in remission and again when off treatment for 1 year. Pertussis vaccine should be included in this regimen if the child is under 7 years old. Children with tetanus-prone wounds should receive any boosters in accordance with the guidelines for normal children (Chapter 93). Rubella reimmunization is given as MMR after completion of treatment. In the UK, malignancy in a child is not an indication for giving influenza, pneumococcal or hepatitis B immunization.

CHILDREN WHO HAVE HAD A BONE MARROW TRANSPLANT

Children who have had a bone marrow transplant (BMT) are at much higher and prolonged risk of serious infection than those receiving cytotoxic therapy alone. Reconstitution of the ability to produce good antibody responses particularly against polysaccharide antigens may take up to 2 years. In theory, the recipient of an allogenic BMT should be immunologically naïve. However, this is not always the case, but even though the ability to make secondary antibody can persist, it may decline slowly over 12–24 months. Children who have had a BMT should have antibody levels to diphtheria, tetanus, pertussis, Hib, measles, mumps and rubella checked 6 months after transplantation and immunization given as necessary. Influenza vaccination should be given yearly in the autumn.

CHILDREN WITH HIV INFECTION

The small, but growing, population of children with HIV have predominantly been infected vertically (Chapter 19). Consideration should always be given to the possible need for both passive and active immunization, in a few cases extensive infection with BCG has followed immunization of infected individuals. As tuberculosis incidence is low in the UK and most children born to HIV-infected mothers are followed closely, BCG is not usually given. If the child is found to be not HIV infected, then BCG is given.* For similar reasons many physicians prefer to give IPV rather than OPV, though extensive disease with OPV is extremely rare. The MMR vaccine seems to be safe and efficacious in HIV-infected children (see Chapter 19). Immunization with Hib and pneumococcal vaccines is important. As poor responses occur in advanced disease antibody responses should be measured. In the case of pneumococcal polysaccharide vaccine there is a dilemma between wanting to immunize early (before immune function declines) and knowing that even in normal children responses are poor below 2 years of age. If vaccination is attempted below this age it is therefore particularly important to check for a response and reimmunize if necessary. The arrival of conjugate vaccines (which should be immunogenic at a younger age) may help with this problem.

CHILDREN WITH PRIMARY IMMUNODEFICIENCIES

The seroresponse to specific vaccine antigens is used increasingly in the investigation of children with suspected immunodeficiency (see Chapter 16). However, immunization is also an important part of their management and, as with children with malignancies, efforts should be made to provide these children with as much protection as possible, bearing in mind that in some cases they may be unable to respond to vaccines. Patients with minor deficiencies of antibodies should receive all the usual vaccines. Those with major antibody deficiencies will be receiving antibodies against some infections in their immunoglobulin treatment. Children with evidence of severe deficiences in cell-mediated immunity should not receive live vaccines. Unfortunately, the routine use of BCG and polio vaccine

***If, however, the child is shortly returning to a country where tuberculosis is prevalent and will not be closely followed, he or she should receive BCG at birth; this is the World Health Organization policy for developing countries.**

occasionally reveals the unsuspected underlying diagnosis of severe immunodeficiency. This is one of the factors that has prompted some to call for the routine use of killed polio vaccine, as in Scandinavia and France. It is important to remember that children with defects of non-specific immunity such as low numbers or deficient function of neutrophils or complement—are at no increased risk from live vaccines and should receive them in the normal way.

CHILDREN WITH SICKLE-CELL DISEASE AND OTHER CAUSES OF HYPOSPLENISM

Individuals with absent spleens or reduced splenic function, including those with sickle-cell disease, are not at any increased risk from viral infections nor from live vaccines. These can be given according to the standard programme. Annual influenza vaccine is advised as it reduces the possibility of serious bacterial respiratory superinfection. Overwhelming pneumococcal infection is a significant hazard. The current vaccine (23 valent unconjugated polysaccharide) has a lower efficacy in children under 2 years old, but should be given to older children. When splenectomy is a planned procedure, the vaccine should be given as far in advance as possible. Reimmunization may be required and vaccination against pneumococcal antigen does not replace the need for prophylactic penicillin as not all serotypes are included.. Invasive Hib infection sometimes occurs in hyposplenic individuals well beyond the age of 5 years, and meningococcal infection can also be a problem. Vaccines should also be given. Hib conjugate vaccine should be given to asplenic/hyposplenic children of all ages. A single dose is efficacious over age 2 years (Chapter 52). Currently licensed meningococcal vaccine only protects against A, C, Y and W135 strains and gives 3 to 5 years protection from a single dose (Chapter 70). Clear recommendations regarding reimmunization cannot be made, although antibody titres may be helpful.

CHILDREN WITH MALNUTRITION AND CHRONIC DISEASE

Chronic malnutrition may influence the immune responses to both infections and vaccines in developing countries and in highly deprived children in the industrialized world. However this is not of major importance in the UK. Children with chronic diseases in whom adequate nutrition can be a problem—such as those with cystic fibrosis—should receive all the routine immunizations and be offered additional protection with pneumococcal, meningococcal and influenza vaccine, and Hib vaccine if they have not already had it.

CHILDREN WITH NEPHROTIC SYNDROME

Children with nephrotic syndrome are at increased risk of pneumococcal infection and should be immunized with pneumococcal vaccine. They suffer from loss of immunoglobulin G and should be offered antibacterial vaccines as above. They also require passive immunization after exposure to measles and varicella.

CHILDREN BORN PREMATURELY

While children born prematurely respond appropriately to most immunizations, there is some evidence that after Hib and hepatitis B vaccination, a small number of premature babies may not be adequately protected. However it remains a firm recommendation that all immunizations should be scheduled on the basis of the child's actual date of delivery and no allowance should be made for prematurity.

CHILDREN TREATED WITH SYSTEMIC CORTICOSTEROIDS

Children being treated with replacement doses of steroids should receive all the usual immunizations. A number of conditions require pharmacological doses of steroids. The dose and period of systemic steroid treatment that results in significant immunosuppression is usually given as prednisolone 2 mg/kg per day for more than a week or 1 mg/kg per day for more than a month (see Appendix VI for full criteria). The general rules concerning use of immunization apply: avoid live vaccines, but give non-live vaccines normally. Any child on pharmacological doses of steroids (even if less than 2 mg/kg per day) should receive ZIG if exposed to chickenpox, unless they are known to have had chickenpox previously. The situation becomes increasingly unclear with lower doses or alternate day regimens for longer periods, and individual discretion is called for. The current recommendation is that a child on 2 mg/kg per day or more of prednisolone should receive normal immunoglobulin if in contact with measles, unless known to be immune. Live vaccines can be given once the child has been off steroids for 3 months. Corticosteroids administered topically are rarely immunosuppressive.

FUTURE DEVELOPMENTS

Better, more immunogenic vaccines against the pneumococcus, and perhaps other common bacterial and viral pathogens may become available soon. These will be of particular importance to children potentially at risk of such infections because of immunodeficiency or other chronic disease. In the meantime there is an urgent need for further specific studies of the safety and efficacy of existing vaccines in well-defined high-risk groups so that clearer recommendations can be made.

FURTHER READING

Plotkin SA & Mortimer EA, eds (1994) *Vaccines*. WB Saunders, Philadelphia.

APPENDIX VIII: FURTHER READING

Clinical paediatrics

Feigin RD & Cherry JD, eds. (1992) *Textbook of Paediatric Infectious Disease*, 3rd edn. WB Saunders, Philadelphia. *Recognized as the main reference work in its field*.

Report of the Committee on Infections Diseases (1994) "*Red Book*". American Academy of Paediatrics. 23rd edition.

Remington JS & Klein JO (1995) *Infectious Disease of the Fetus and Newborn Infant*, 4th edn, WB Saunders, Philadelphia. *The authoritative work on neonatal infection*.

General Infectious Disease

Mandell GL, Bennett JE, Dolin R. (1995) *Principles and practise of Infectious Disease*. Churchill Livingstone, New York. Fourth edition. A good comprehensive all age textbook.

Public health and immunization practice

Beneson AS, ed. (1990) *Control of Communicable Disease in Man*, 15th edn. American Public Health Association. *Comprehensive guide to public health management of infectious disease.*

Department of Health *Immunisation Against Infectious Disease*. HMSO,London. *The authoritative guide to immunization practice in the UK*. (A new edition is due to be published in 1996.)

Microbiology

Belshe , ed. (1990) *A Textbook of Human Virology*. Mosby/Year Book, St Louis.

Shanson DC, (1989) *Microbiology in Clinical Practice*. Wright, London.

Immunology

Janeway CA & Travers P (1994) *Immunobiology: The Human System in Health and Disease*. Blackwell, Oxford.

Steihm ER (1989) *Immunological Disorders in Infants and Children*, 3rd edn. W B Saunders, Philadelphia.

Travel and Immunization

Department of Health, Welsh Office, Scottish Home and Health Department, DHSS (Northern Ireland) with the Public Health Laboratory Service Communicable Disease Surveillance Centre, (1995) *Health Information for Overseas Travel*, HMSO, London.

INDEX

Note: Subjects dealt with in detail are paginated in **bold** type; data in Tables and Figures are paginated in *italic* type. Further drug and immunization data are given in the appendices.

Individual Drug Dosages are to be found in Appendix II (Neonates) p 340 and III (Infants and Older Children) p 348

Acute encephalitis, **60–62**
  causative organisms, *60*
Acute pericarditis, 56
  see also under Cardiac *and also* Heart *aspects*
Acute phase proteins, 135
Adenovirus, 290–291
Adopted children, 122–123
Age, and mortality, 330–339
AIDS, **104–108**
  see also HIV
Aminoglycosides, 158–159
Amoebiasis, **176**
Amphotericin, *see under* Antifungal drugs, 95–99
Animal bites, 111, 285–286
Animal-transmitted diseases, *see* Zoonoses, 124–134
Antenatal HIV testing, 108
Antibiotic-associated diarrhoea, 39
Antibiotic combinations, *8*
Antibiotics, **152–161**
  clinical use of, 160–161
  dosages, 340–361
    neonates, 340–347
    older children, 348–361
  and HIV, *see under* HIV
  in the immunocompromised child, 89–94
  in immunodeficiency, 87–88
  for late-onset sepsis, 11–12
  in meningococcal disease, 260–264
  mode of action, *153–154*
  and sepsis-causing organisms, *9*
  therapeutic use of, 160–161
    in prophylaxis, 160–161
  in vesicoureteric reflex, 45–46
  see also Neonatal infection; *see also under specific drug names and also specific bacterial diseases*
Antibody deficiency, 90–91
Antibody or antigen detection, 137, 288
  agglutination (LPA), 137
  counter current immunoelectrophoresis (CIE), 137
  enzyme-linked immunosorbent assay (ELISA), 137
  latex agglutination, 137
  radioimmunoassay, 137
Antimalarial chemoprophylaxis, 253
Antimicrobials, for infants/children (excl. neonates), **348–361**
  see also under Antibiotics
Antimicrobials for neonates **340–347**
Antiretroviral therapy, 106
Arboviruses, 177, 322
Arenaviruses, 323–324
Ascaris (roundworm), **177–178**
Aspergillosis, 100, **178–179**
Astroviruses, 291
Ataxia-telangiectasia *84*
Athlete's foot (Tinea Pedis), 198–199
Azidothymine (AZT), *see* Zidovudine, 106
Azithromycin, 159–160
AZT, *see* Zidovudine, 106
Aztreonam, 155–156

Bacillus Calmette-Guérin (BCG), 316–318
  at school, programme for, 317
  contraindications to the use of, 374
  at school, programme for, 317
Bacitracin, 154
Bacteria, laboratory detection of, 138
  see also under specific bacterial infections
Bacterial meningitis, **57–59**
  causative organisms, *57*
Bacterial sepsis in neonates, 7
Bacterial tracheitis, 25
  see also under Croup, 24
Balkan haemorrhagic fever with renal syndrome (HFRS), 322
Bartonella henselae (Cat scratch disease), 185
BCG vaccination, 316–318
  contraindications to the use of, 374
Bejel, 304
Benzylpenicillin, 155
Beta-lactams, 155–156
Bilharzia, 237–241
Bismuth, 218
Bites, *see specific type of, e.g.* Animal bites, Dog bites
  Rabies, 284–286

Individual Drug Dosages are to be found in Appendix II (Neonates) p 340 and III (Infants and Older Children) p 348

Blood-borne infection control, 169
Bone-marrow transplantation, 88
  and immunization, 380
Bone infections, **34–35**
Bordetella parapertussis, 273–276
Bordetella pertussis, 273–276
Borrelia burgdorferi, 247–248
  see also under Acute encephalitis *and also* Lyme disease
Botulism, **179–182**
  see also under Food poisoning
British Paediatric Association Surveillance Unit (Reportable Infectious Diseases), viii
Brucellosis, 117, **182**
Bubonic plague, 276–277
Bunyaviruses, 322–324, *325*

Caliciviruses, 291–292
Campylobacter infection, **183**
Campylobacteriosis, *125*
Cancer, immunization in, 378–379
  chickenpox and, 378–379
  measles and, 379
Candida spp., 99–100
  see also under Fungal infections
Candidiasis, 17, 99–100, **184**
  see also under Fungal infections
Capnocytophagea canimorsus, 129
Cardiac infections, **51–56**
  laboratory diagnosis of, *150*
Cat-scratch disease, *129*, **185**
Cell-mediated immune deficit, 91–93
Cell-membrane disruption, and antibiotics, 156
  nitroimidazoles, 156
  nystatin, 156
  polymyxins, 156
Cell-wall replication, antibiotics and, 152–156
  bacitracin, 152
  beta-lactams, 155–156
  glycopeptides, 155
Cephaloridine, 155
Chickenpox, 18–20, **185–188**
  maternal, 18–19, **185–188**
  neonatal, 19–20, **185–188**
  use of immunoglobulin in prevention, 18–20
  vaccination for, in cancer, 378–379
  see also Herpes zoster *and also* Varicella zoster
Chlamydia pneumoniae infection, **188**
Chlamydia psittaci infection, **189**
Chlamydia spp., *129*, **188–191**
Chlamydia trachomatis infection, **190–191**
Chronic granulomatous (CGD) disease, 87
Clarithromycin, 159–160
Chloramphenicol, 159
Cholera, 112, **191–192**
Chronic persistent diarrhoea, 42
  see also under other forms of Diarrhoea *and also* Food poisoning
Clindamycin, 159–160
Clostridium difficile, see Pseudomembranous colitis
Clostridium tetani, **306–307**
CMV, *see* Cytomegalovirus infection, 20, **195–196**
Common cold (acute coryza), 22
Community-acquired pneumonia, *28–29*
Community, infection control in the, 168–172
  blood-borne infections, 169
  faecal–oral infection, 168–172
  objectives of, 170–172
  urgent conditions, *171*
Complement tests, 87
Congenital infections, **3–6**
  cytomegalovirus, 195–196
  heart disease (CHD), 51–54
  HBV, 221–227
  HIV, 107–108
  rubella, 292–293
  summary of, 4–6
  syphilis, 301–303
  toxoplasmosis, 307–308
  tuberculosis, 315
Conjunctivitis, 17–18, **193–194**
Contraindications, to immunization, **374–377**
Corticosteroids, and immunization, 382
Corynebacterium diphtheriae, 199–201
Co-trimoxazole, 158
Cowpox, *127–128*, 282
C-reactive protein, 135
Creutzfeldt–Jakob disease, **283–284**
Crimean–Congo haemorrhagic fever, 322–324, *327*
Cross-infections, 32, 162–172
Croup, **24**, 255
Cryptococcosis, 100
Cryptosporidiosis, *125*, **194–195**
Cutaneous leishmaniasis, 243–244
Cysticercosis, 237–241
Cytokines, 88, 135
Cytomegalovirus, 20, **195–196**

DDC, *see* Dideoxycytidine, 106
DDI, *see* Didanosine, 106
Dehydration, 39–40
  clinical assessment of, *40*
  fluid requirements in, *41*

Individual Drug Dosages are to be found in Appendix II (Neonates) p 340 and III (Infants and Older Children) p 348

Delta hepatitis, *see* Hepatitis D, 228
Dengue haemorrhagic fever (DHF), 322–327
Dengue shock syndrome (DSS), 322
2′-Deoxy-3-thiacytidine, *see* 3TC, 107
Dermatophytoses, *127*, **197–199**
Diarrhoea, **36–42**, 204–206, 212
  antibiotic-associated, 39
  bloody diarrhoea, *210–213*
  chronic persistent, 42
  with pus (dysentery), 298–299
  travellers', 115–116
  and vomiting, **36–42**
  see also Food poisoning
Didanosine (001), 106
Dideoxycytidine (DDC, zalcitabine), 106
Diphtheria, 111–112, 117, **199–201**, 330–331
  biotypes, of *Cornynebacterium diphtheriae*, 199–201
  immunization, 202
Disseminated intravascular coagulation (DIC), 66
DNA replication, antibiotics and, 156–158
  co-trimoxazole, 158
  flucytosine, 156–157
  griseofulvin, 157
  metronidazole, 157
  nitrofurantoin, 157
  quinolones, 157
  sulphonamides, 157–158
  trimethoprim, 158
Dogs, toxocariasis and, 308–309
  rabies and, **284–287**
Drug-resistant tuberculosis, 316
Duncan's syndrome, 234
Duodenal ulcers, *see under Helicobacter pylori* infection, **217–219**
Dysentery (diarrhoea with pus), 299

Ear infections, 23
Ear swabs, 10
Early-onset neonatal sepsis, 7–11
Ebola virus, 323
Echinococcisis, *see* Hydatid disease, *129*, **237–241**
ELISA or EIA test, 137
Enanthems, diagnosis, *143–144*
Encephalitis, 60–62, 255
Encephalopathy, HIV, 102
Endocarditis, 51–54
  prevention, *53–54*
Endotoxin, 135
Entamoeba histolytica, 117
Enterovirus infection, **202–203**
Enteroviruses, 20–21, **202–203**
Epididymo-orchitis, 267
Epiglottitis, 24–25
Epstein–Barr virus, 234–235
Erythema infectiosum, **272–273**
Erythromycin, 159
Escherichia coli, 204–206
  Enterobius vermicularis, 304–305
  Enteroaggregative *E. coli*, 204–206
  Enterocolitis, *see* Necrotizing enterocolitis
  Enterohaemorrhagic *E. coli*, 204–206
  Enteroinvasive *E. coli*, 204–206
  Enteropathogenic *E. coli*, 204–206
  Enterotoxigenic *E. coli*, 204–206
  types of, *204*
  VTEC, *see under* Haemolytic uraemic syndrome, 210–212
Escherichia coli diarrhoea, 204–206
  see also other forms of Diarrhoea
Exanthem subitum, **288**
Exanthems, diagnosis of, *143*
Exclusion periods, for infections, **364–373**
Eye infections,
  conjunctivitis, 17
  gonococcal, 208–209
  ophthalmia neonatorum, *see* Conjunctivitis
  toxocariasis, 308

Faecal-oral transmission, 168–169
Falciparum malaria, 248
Fasciola hepatica, 237–240
Fever of unknown origin, *see* Pyrexia of unknown origin, 74–80
Fifth disease, 272–273
Filoviruses, 323, *325*
Flucytosine, 156–157
  see also Antifungal drugs, 95–99
Fluid requirements, daily, *41*
Food-borne botulism, 178–182
Food-borne infections, 109–110
  see also under Food poisoning
Food poisoning, *38*,
  outbreaks, 172
  salmonellosis, 296–297
Foreign travel, 37–42, **109–114**, 115–133, 221, 265
  infections contracted abroad, 115–121
  preparation for, 109–114
  rabies and, 284
  refugees, 122–134
  and tuberculosis, 317
Fungal infections, 95–100
  see also Antifungal drugs, 95–99
  laboratory detection of, 138

Individual Drug Dosages are to be found in Appendix II (Neonates) p 340 and III (Infants and Older Children) p 348

Fungal sepsis, 13–14
Fusidic acid, 160

Gammaglobulin, 88
Gastroenteritis, 15, **36–42**
  agents causing, in the UK, *37*
  endemic, 37
  food/water-borne, 37
  see also under Food poisoning
Gastrointestinal infections, *125–127*, *331*
  laboratory diagnosis, *140*
  see also Food poisoning
Genetic counselling, 88
Genital mycoplasmas, 270
Genitourinary tract infections, laboratory diagnosis, *145*
Genome detection, 137, 290
Geography, and travel diseases, 118–121
  see also under Foreign travel, 109–114
Gerstmann–Straussler syndrome, 283
Giardiasis, *125*, **207–208**
Glandular fever (Infectious mononucleosis), **234–235**
Glasgow Meningococcal Septicaemia Prognostic Score, 261
'Glue ear', 23
Glycopeptides (antibiotics), 155
Gnathostoma spingerum, 237–240
Gnathostomiasis, 237–240
Gonococcal infections, **209–210**
Granulomatous disease, 87
Griseofulvin, 157
Growth factors, 88
Guillain–Barré syndrome, 235, 280

Haemolytic complement test, 87
Haemolytic uraemic syndrome, *126*, **210–212**
Haemophilus influenzae infection, **213–216**
  immunization, 215–216
  type b, *334*
Haemorrhagic fever, 321–327
  with renal syndrome (HFRS), 322
Haemolytic uraemic syndrome (HUS), *126*, **210–213**
Hand, foot and mouth disease, **216–217**
Hantaviruses, 322–323
Head lice, **271–272**
Health care workers, 318
  and chicken pox/varicella, 19
  and hepatitis B, 226
  and rubella, 296
  and tuberculosis, 318
Heart, infections, 51–56
  laboratory diagnosis, *150*
  and septic shock, 65
Helicobacter pylori infection, **217–219**
  urea test for, breath, 218
  urease test, 218
Helminthiasis, 237–241
Hepatitis A, 112, **219–222**
  and foreign travel, 222
Hepatitis B, **222–228**
  Immunization, 226
  serological markers for, *225*
Hepatitis C, **229–230**
Hepatitis D (Delta agent), 228
Hepatitis E, **230–231**
Herpes infections, **231–234**
Herpes simplex virus, 18
Herpes zoster, 185–188
  see also Chickenpox
HIV, **101–108**, *334*
  antenatal testing for, 108
  bacterial infections, 104
  community care, 107
  encephalopathy, 104
  and immunization, 376
  manifestations of, *103*
  and opportunistic infections, 102
  polymerase chain reaction, 105
  psychological aspects of, 107
  social aspects of, 107
  vertical transmission, 102, 107–108
    reduction of, 107–108
    risks, 102
  see also under Immunodeficiency
Hospital cross-infection, 32–33, 163–164
Hospital staff, *see under* Health care workers
Hospitals, and infection control, **162–167**
  control teams, 165
  host factors, 164
  pathogens in, 163
  patients involved, 162
  problems encountered, 162
  site of, 162–163
  spread of, 164
  techniques in, 165–167
    example of, *166*
Human herpesvirus, 288
  see also Herpes infection, **231–234**
Hydatid disease, *129*, **237–243**
Hygiene, 169
  and travelling, 109–110
Hymenolepiasis, *126*
Hyper IgE (Job's) syndromes, *85*

Imipenem, 156

Individual Drug Dosages are to be found in Appendix II (Neonates) p 340 and III (Infants and Older Children) p 348

Immigrants, 316
see also Refugees, **122–123**
Immunization –
contraindications, 374–377
BCG, 376
live, 375
pertussis, 376
polio, 376
diphtheria, 202
Haemophilus influenzae, 215–216
hepatitis B, 226
and HIV, 105–106
of the immunocompromised child, **378–382**
bone-marrow transplantation, 380
cancer, 378
corticosteroids and, 382
HIV and, 380
malnutrition, 381
nephrotic syndrome, 381
premature birth, 381
primary immunodeficiency, 380
sickle-cell disease, 381
influenza, 237
Japanese B encephalitis, 117
measles, 256
after exposure, 256
routine, 256
MMR, 267
pertussis, 275
polio, 280–281
and previous severe reaction, 375
rabies, 285
post-exposure, 285
pre-exposure, 285
status, *123*, 170
and steroids, 384
tetanus, 306
tick borne encephalitis, 113
for travel abroad, **111–114**
advice centres, **113–114**
typhoid, 320
and unknown status, *123*, 170
vaccines available, in the UK, *374*
varicella zoster, 187–188
yellow fever, 329
Immunocompromised child, with infection, **89–94**
antibody deficiency in, 90–91
cell-mediated immune deficit, 92–93
neutropenia, 89–90
neutrophil dysfunction, 90
pathogens associated with, *92*
prophylaxis in, *93*
vaccination in, **378–382**
see also HIV
Immunodeficiency, 81–86
antibiotic use in, 87–88
blood counts in, 81
bone-marrow transplantation, 88
cytokines and, 88
gammaglobulin in, 88
genetic counselling, 88
growth factors and, 88
primary disorders, *83–85*
tests in, 81, 85–87
antibody, 85
complement, 87
Immunoglobulin tests, 86
lymphocyte, 81, 86
Immunosuppression, and live vaccines, 375–376
Incubation periods, 364–373
see also under specific diseases
Infant botulism, 178–182
Infants, and sepsis risks, 8
Infection control in the community, **168–172**
Infection control in hospitals, **162–167**
see also under specific types of infection
Infectious monocleosis (Glandular fever), 234–235
Infective endocarditis, 51–54
Influenza, **235–236**
Immunization, 237
Insect bites, 110–111
Interleukins, *see* Cytokines, 88, 135
International travel, 109–133
Itraconazole, *see under* Antifungal drugs, 95–99
Intravenous rehydration therapy, 41–42
see also Dehydration

Japanese B encephalitis, 117
Joint infections, 34–35
laboratory diagnosis of, *148–149*
Juvenile chronic arthritis, 241

Kala-azar, *see* Visceral leishmaniasis
Katayama syndrome, 117
Kawasaki disease, 5, 55, 67, **241–243**
Ketoconazole, *see under* Antifungal drugs, 95–99
Korean haemorrhagic fever, 322
Kuru, 283

Individual Drug Dosages are to be found in Appendix II (Neonates) p 340 and III (Infants and Older Children) p 348

Laboratory diagnosis, of infection, **135–151**
  antibody detection, 137
  antigen detection, 137
  bacteria, 138
  bone infection, *148–149*
  cardiac infection, 150
  CNS, 139
  enanthems, *143–144*
  exanthems, *143–144*
  fungi, 138
  gastrointestinal infection, *140*
  genome detection, 137
  genitourinary tract infection, *145*
  joint infections, *148–149*
  muscle infections, 148, *149*
  non-specific tests, 135
  normal flora, *138*
  parasitic infections, 151
  respiratory tract infections, *141–142*
  skin infections, *146*
  specific tests, 135–151
  types of, *136*
  viruses, 138
Laryngotracheobronchitis, *see* Croup, **24**, 253
Lassa fever, 117, 324
Late onset neonatal sepsis, 9–13
Legionnaires' disease, **243–244**
Leishmaniasis, *130*, **244–245**
Leptospirosis, *130*
Leucocyte adhesion, 87
Leucocyte function antigen (LFA-1), 87
Lice, *see* Head lice, 271–272 and Typhus, 322
Light microscopy, 135–137
Lincomycin, 159–160
Listeriosis, *131*, **245–247**
Lower respiratory tract infections, **26–33**
  clinical features of, *30*
  risk factors for, *26*
Lumbar puncture, 10
  contraindications in meningitis, 14
Lung infections, 26–33
Lyme disease, 117, *131*, **247–248**
Lymphocyte tests, 82, 87
Lymphocytic interstitial pneumonitis, 104

Macrolides, 159
Malaria, 113, **248–253**
  drug regimen for, *252*
    prophylaxis, *251*
Marburg virus, 323
Measles, 111–112, 253–257, *335–336*
  immunization, in cancer, 378
  mumps and rubella (MMR), 267
Meningitis, 14–15, 57–59, 212, 314
Meningococcal disease, **257–265**, *336*
Meningococcal meningitis, 257–265
Meningoencephalitis, 235
Metronidazole, 157
Miconazole, *see under* Antifungal drugs
Migrants, 295
  see also under Refugees
Molluscum contagiosum, 281–283
Moniliasis,
  Candidiasis, 184–185
Monospot test, 235
Morbidity statistics, in the UK, **330–339**
Mortality, from infectious diseases, in the UK, **330–339**
Mosquito bite avoidance, 253
Mucocutaneous lymph node syndrome, *see* Kawasaki disease
Mumps, **266–268**
  CNS and, 266
Mycobacteriosis, *127*
Mycobacterium infection (atypical), **268–269**
Mycobacterium tuberculosis, 311–318
Mycoplasma infections, 269–270
Mycoplasma pneumoniae, 269–270
Mycoplasma hominis, 269–270
Myocarditis, 55
  see also Cardiac infections, 51–56

Nail ringworm, 198–199
Necrotizing enterocolitis, 16
Neonatal antibiotic dosages, **340–347**
Neonatal infections, **7–21**
  late inset sepsis, 9–13
Nephropathica epidemica, 326
Nephrotic syndrome, and immunization, 381
Neutrophil disorders, 89–90
Neutrophil function disorders, 90
Nitroblue tetrazolium test (NBT), 87
Nitrofurantoin, 157
Nitroimidazoles, 156
Nits, **271–272**
Non-venereal treponematoses, 303–305
Norwalk virus, 292–293
Nosocomial infection, 163–164
Notifiable diseases, in the UK 1995, **362–363**
Nystatin, 156

Ocular larva migrans, 308
Ophthalmia neonatorum, 192–193, 209
Oral vaccine (polio), 281
Oral rehydration therapy, 39, 41
Orf, *128*

Individual Drug Dosages are to be found in Appendix II (Neonates) p 340 and III (Infants and Older Children) p 348

Ornithosis, *129*
Osteomyelitis, 16–17, 34–35
Otitis media, 23, 255

Parasites, 151
  see also under individual organisms
Paratyphoid fever, 319–320
Paronychia, 17
Parvovirus infection, **272–273**
Pasteurellosis, *128*
Paul–Bunnell test, 235
Pediculus humanus capitis, 271–272
Pericarditis, 55–56
  see also Cardiac infection, 51–56
Peritonsillar abscess (quinsy), 23
Pertussis (whooping cough), **273–276**, *337*, 381
  vaccine contraindications, 376
Pharyngitis, 22–23
Pinta, 306
Pinworm, 307–308
Plague, **276–277**
Plantar warts, 328
Plasmodium, see under Malaria
Pneumocystis carinii pneumonia (PCP), 104, **277–279**
Pneumonia, 15, 253, 277–279
  community acquired, *28–29*
Pneumonic plague, 275–276
Pneumonitis, lymphocytic interstitial, 104
Poliomyelitis, 111, **279–281, 337**
  vaccine, 280–281
  vaccine contraindications, 376
Polymerase chain reaction, and HIV, 105
Polymyxins, 156
Poxvirus infection, **281–283**
  see also Molluscum contagiosum
Pregnancy, 187–188, 271, 293–295, 308
  congenital infections, *4–6*
  cytomeglovirus, 195–196
  rubella and, 295
  varicella (chicken pox) and, 187–188
Prion disease (spongiform encephalopathy), **283–284**
Psittacosis, *129*
Pseudomembranous colitis, 39
Pulmonary tuberculosis, 315
Pyrexia of unknown origin (PUO), **74–80**
  age and, *76*
  causes of, *75–76*
  diagnostics of, *77–79*

Q fever, 117, 128
Quinolones, 157
Quinsy, *see* Peritonsillar abscess, 23

Rabies, *131*, **284–286**
  see also Zoonoses
Rash, **68–73**
  types of, 69–73
  see also Skin
Refugees, **122–123**
  immunization of, *123*
Rehydration, fluid requirements, *41*
  see also Dehydration
Reiter's syndrome, 117
Renal imaging, UTIs, *46*
Renal scarring, 45, 46
Respiratory syncytial virus infection, **287**, *338*
Respiratory tract infections, 22, 26–33, *142*
  lower, 26–33
  upper, 22–25
Respiratory viruses, 18
Retropharyngeal abscess, 23
Rheumatic fever, 51
Rifampicin, 159–160
Ringworm, *127*
  body, 197
  nail, 198–199
Roseola infantum, **288**
Rotavirus, **288–293**
Roundworm, 30
Rubella, **293–296**
  vaccine, 381

Salmonella spp., 15
  see also Food poisoning
Salmonella typhi (Typhoid), 319–320
Salmonellosis, *126*, **296–297**
Sarcoptes scabei, 298
Scabies, 298
Scalp ringworm, 196–197
Schistosomiasis, 117, 237–249
Sepsis, neonatal, 7–14
  see also specific forms
Septicaemia, 257–265
Septic shock, **63–66**, 259
  cardiovascular support in, 65
  corticosteroids for, 66
  definition of, 63
  DIC in, 66
  fluid balance in, 66
  immediate therapy, 64
  intensive care and, 65
  nitric oxide synthetase inhibitors in, 66
  plasmapheresis in, 66
Septic spots, 17

Individual Drug Dosages are to be found in Appendix II (Neonates) p 340 and III (Infants and Older Children) p 348

Severe combined immunodeficiency (SCID), *see under* Immunodeficiency, *83–85*
Sexual abuse, 47–50
Sexually transmitted disease, **47–50**
  infections (summary), *48*
  see also HIV, Chlamydia trochomatis; Gonorrhoea; Hepatitis B; Syphilis
Shigellosis, **298–300**
Shock, *see under* Septic shock
Sickle cell disease, 268
  and vaccination, 381
Sinusitis, 23–24
Sixth disease, **288**
Skin, *146*
  in leishmaniasis, 244
  in Lyme disease, 247–248
  scalded, 67
  see also Rash
Slapped cheek syndrome, 272–273
Spiramycin, 160
Spongiform encephalopathies, 283–284
Staphylococcal infections, **300–302**
Staphylococcal scalded skin syndrome, 67
Staphylococcus aureus, in osteomyelitis, 16–17
Steroids, and immunization, 382
Stevens–Johnson syndrome, 242, 270
Still's disease, 55
Streptococcal infections, **302–303**
Strongyloides stercoralis, 237–241
Strongyloidiasis, 237–241
Subacute sclerosing panencephalitis, 254
Sulphonamides, 157–158
Suspected immunodeficiency, **81–88**
Syphilis, **303–304**

Taenia solium, 237–241
Tapeworm infection, *126*
3TC (2-deoxy-3-thiacytidine), 107
Teicoplanin, 155
Tetanus, 112, **306–307**, *338*
Tetracyclines, 159
Threadworms, **307–308**
Thrush, *see* Candidiasis
Tinea capitis, 196–197
Tinea corporis, 197
Tinea pedis, 198
Tonsillitis, 22–23
Tourists, *see* Foreign travel
  see also Refugees
Toxic shock syndrome, **67**
Toxocara canis, 308–309
Toxocariasis, *132*, **308–309**
Toxoplasmosis, *132*, **309–311**
Transcription, DNA, and antibiotics –
  fusidic acid, 160
  rifampicin, 159–160
Translation, DNA, and antibiotics, 158–159
  aminoglycosides, 158–159
  chloramphenicol, 159
  macrolides, 159
  tetracyclines, 159
Transverse myelitis, 235
Travel, *see* Foreign travel
Travellers' diarrhoea, 115–121
  see also other forms of Diarrhoea; *see also* Food poisoning
Treponema pallidum, 303–305
Trichinella spiralis, 237–241
Trichinosis, 237–240
Trimethoprim, 158
Tuberculin testing, 314
Tuberculosis, 112, **311–319**, *339*
  in nursing mothers, 317
Tuberculous meningitis, 314
Tumour necrosis factor, *see* Cytokines
Typhoid, 112, 117, **308–310**
Typhus, **320–321**

Umbilical sepsis, 17
Upper respiratory tract infection, 22–25
Urea breath test, 217
Ureaplasma urealyticum, 269–270
Urease test, 217
Urinary tract infections, 15, **43–46**
Urine sampling, 43–44

Vaccination, *see* Immunization
Vaccines, Live and Inactivated, in use in the UK, *374*
Vancomycin, 155
Varicella zoster, 18–19, 185–188
  see also Chickenpox
Verotoxins, *see under* Haemolytic uraemic syndrome, 210–212
Verrucae, 327–328
Vesicoureteric reflux, 45, 46
Vibrio cholerae, 191–192
Viral capsid antigen, 234
Viral haemorrhagic fever, **321–327**
Viruses, laboratory detection of, 138
  see also specific viruses by name
Visceral larva migrans (VLM), 309
Visceral leishmaniasis, 244–245
Vomiting, 36–42
VTEC, Verotoxin producing *E. Coli. see* Haemolytic uraemic syndrome, 210–212

Individual Drug Dosages are to be found in Appendix II (Neonates) p 340 and III (Infants and Older Children) p 348

Warts, **327–328**
Water-borne infections, 109–110
  typhoid, 319
Water quality, *see under* Foreign travel
Weil's disease, *130*
White cell counts, 135
Wiskott–Aldriche Syndrome, *84*
Whooping cough, *see* Pertussis, 273–276
Wound botulism, 179–180

X-linked lymphoproliferative disorder, 234
X-linked severe combined immunodeficiency (SCID)
X-linked gammaglobulins (Bruton's) Syndrome, 83

Yaws, 304
Yellow fever, 112–113, 319–321, 328–329
Yersinia enterocolitica, 329
Yersinia pestis, 276–277
Yersinia pseudotuberculosis, 329
Yersinosis, 117, *127*, 329

Zalcitabine, *see* Dideoxycytidine
Zidovudine (azidothymidine, AZT), 106
Zoonoses, **124–134**, 170
  hantaviruses, 322
  see also Animal bites *and also* Rabies

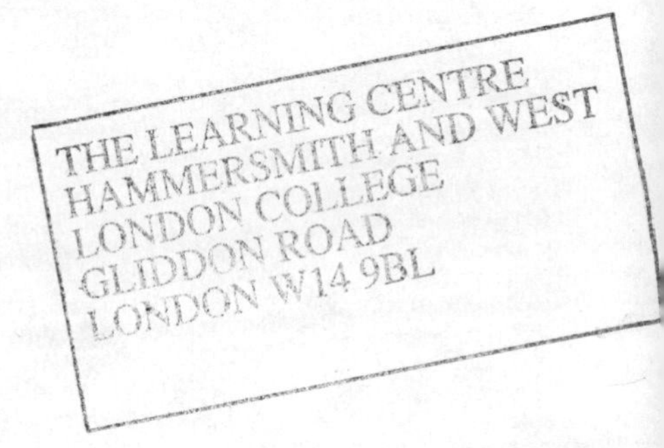